Atlas of Angioaccess Surgery

Atlas of Angioaccess Surgery

Pedro A. Rubio, M.D., Ph.D.
Chief, Department of Surgery
Medical Center Del Oro Hospital;
Clinical Faculty of Surgery
University of Texas
Health Science Center at Houston
Houston, Texas

Edward M. Farrell, M.D.
Cardiovascular Surgical Center
Houston, Texas

Foreword by
Denton A. Cooley, M.D.

YEAR BOOK MEDICAL PUBLISHERS, INC.
Chicago • London

Library of Congress Cataloging in Publication Data

Rubio, Pedro A.
Atlas of angioaccess surgery.

Includes bibliographical references and index.
1. Arteriovenous shunts, Surgical. 2. Arteriovenous shunts, Surgical—Complications and sequelae. 3. Fistula, Arteriovenous—Surgery—Complications and sequelae. 4. Arterial catheterization. I. Farrell, Edward M. II. Title. [DNLM: 1. Arteriovenous shunt, Surgical—Atlases. 2. Catheters, Indwelling—Atlases. WG 17 R896a]
RD598.5.R83 1983 617′.413 82-17643
ISBN 0-8151-7451-9

Seldom does one have the opportunity to express gratitude to those who have made indelible marks in one's life and have shared the responsibility for one's accomplishments.

To Esther and Isaac, my parents, who gave me life and unselfishly taught me responsibility, dignity, and decency by their example, and always gave me loving support.

To Sandy and Eddie, my children, who have suffered from my compulsive search for success and fulfillment in my surgical career.

To Connie, my lady, who has given me love and understanding during my ups and downs and endless working days and nights.

To the memory of Mirna Linda, my late sister, and Moises, my late uncle, who despite their untimely tragic transition will always live within me.

To Denton A. Cooley, my main source of educational and inspirational influence, whose moral and academic support has been invaluable during my career. His friendship above all will always be treasured deep in my heart. I hope that I prove worthy of such trust.

To Edward M. Farrell, for his loyalty and friendship. His endless energy and dedication have made this atlas a reality.

It is with humility that this book is dedicated to them.

PEDRO A. RUBIO

To my family, for the inspiration and support they have given me over the years.

To the memory of H. Wynne Pearce, who by his example instilled in me the desire to become a physician.

To Joseph M. Croley, whose dedication and perseverance in the face of adversity have been inspirational to me.

To Fred and Ruth Leppard, who gave me my most treasured possession, my wife Ruth.

To my friend and mentor, Pedro A. Rubio, a master surgeon who has invested countless hours in training my mind and whose support and guidance have been invaluable in my growth as a surgeon.

It is with affection and gratitude that I dedicate this book to them.

EDWARD M. FARRELL

Contents

Foreword

MEDICINE as practiced today has taken the physician beyond the standard methods of one or two decades ago. New therapeutic techniques such as hemodialysis, plasmapheresis, chronic cancer chemotherapy, intravenous alimentation, chronic antibiotic infusion, and developments still on the horizon have charged the surgeon with creating new portals of access to the circulatory system. Since the early years of the twentieth century and Carrel's monumental experiments on vessel anastomoses, but especially during the past 30 years, advances in vascular surgery have prepared the way for the emergence of a new surgical specialty, which demands immediate results from the surgeon. The properly trained vascular surgeon in the present era should therefore be capable of connecting arteries and veins to each other or to a variety of synthetic fabrics and tubes, homologous or heterologous tissue substitutes, etc. The modern surgeon can thus draw upon the accumulated experience of recent generations of vascular surgeons to solve problems and fulfill the particular needs of the specialist and patient involved in modern therapeutic methods.

The surgical consultant must collaborate closely with both therapist and patient in selecting the most appropriate implantation site. As therapy continues over a prolonged period, almost inevitably complications seem to arise. Indeed, in some patients, it may appear that another angioaccess site is not available. That is when the innovative and creative surgeon may rescue the patient from death. Management of complications such as thrombosis, embolism, infection, and hemorrhage often requires emergency measures that place constant demand upon the surgeon's time. That is when instant communication among physician, surgeon, and patient is most essential.

In this new endeavor one should not overlook the patient's role as a human being struggling for health and life in a situation which only a few years ago was ultimately hopeless. Prolongation of life with comfort and quality should be the objective of the surgeon. He must adopt an attitude of concern and understanding for his patient. Admittedly, dealing with the chronically ill patient whose life often depends upon so many others, whose economic means are overtaxed, and whose emotional stability may have been exhausted, places the surgeon in a difficult role. He must act with equanimity and stability because the patient's life and welfare depend upon him.

This atlas is one of the first of its kind, and I predict it will be widely used and accepted. My admiration goes out to the authors for their contribution to a new surgical technology. Dr. Rubio, one of my most aggressive and able students, has paid me a high compliment by requesting that I write this foreword. In actuality; I am only indirectly familiar with the techniques described herein. But my surgical colleagues who perform these tedious and sometimes frustrating procedures will benefit from this manual. My admiration is also extended to the talented medical illustrator, Patrick McDonnell, whose drawings are indeed superb. This atlas should be available to physicians, surgeons, and even patients undergoing treatment to expand their knowledge of this new subspecialty in medicine.

"Necessity, who is the mother of invention," was attributed to Plato more than 2,000 years ago. During the nineteenth century Howard Spencer said, "Progress, therefore, is not an accident, but a necessity. . . . It is a part of nature." The rapidity of progress during the present era, which has become known as the "Space Age," almost overwhelms us; but the challenge to keep abreast will inspire dedicated people to respond.

Denton A. Cooley, M.D.
Surgeon-in-Chief
Texas Heart Institute
Clinical Professor of Surgery
University of Texas
Health Science Center at Houston

Preface

THIS BOOK is intended as a guide to creating and maintaining adequate angioaccess in patients requiring it. The importance of adequate circulatory access cannot be overstated. The application of these techniques will continue to be the main factor in granting patients an improved quality of life as well as extended lifetimes.

Advancements in hemodialysis have served as the impetus for perfecting angioaccess techniques. However, in recent years a number of other diagnostic and therapeutic modalities have been introduced that depend on the availability of circulatory access. Cancer chemotherapy and plasmapheresis are two such modalities. Consequently, angioaccess is no longer the exclusive realm of a relatively small number of surgeons. We hope the techniques detailed in this book will be of use to surgical generalists who have recourse to angioaccess procedures. And since much of the value of the book is in the illustrations, we are grateful to Patrick McDonnell, a talented medical illustrator at Baylor College of Medicine, who created the artwork.

PEDRO A. RUBIO

EDWARD M. FARRELL

Arteriovenous Shunts

1

AN ARTERIOVENOUS SHUNT is an external device that allows an admixture of the arterial and venous circulations and is constructed with indwelling cannulas. By contrast, in an arteriovenous fistula the connection between the circulations is internal. Since its introduction in 1960, the Quinton-Scribner shunt has been the mainstay for acute angioaccess. Use of a Quinton-Scribner shunt requires adequate peripheral vessels, the distal flow of which can be sacrificed without adverse results. Consequently, patency of the ulnar artery must be assured before a radiocephalic shunt is inserted in the wrist. Also, the relatively low pressure system of a peripheral artery precludes dislodgment of the Teflon vessel tips. If peripheral vessels are not available, the Allen-Brown and Thomas shunts should be considered. The Dacron graft portions of these shunts permit an end-to-side configuration that allows normal distal arterial flow.

Recent developments in the field of percutaneous catheters have significantly reduced the need for shunts requiring operative insertion.

Quinton-Scribner Shunt in the Wrist

A Following confirmation of radial and ulnar artery patency with an Allen test, a longitudinal incision approximately 5 cm long should be made midway between the radial artery and the cephalic vein and proximal to the carpal ligament.

B The vessels are identified and mobilized, and the cephalic vein is ligated with 3-0 silk suture distal to the site of the intended venotomy. While the ligature is used for retraction, a stab wound is made with a no. 11 blade and expanded into a T-shaped incision. Dilators of increasing size are then inserted until the vein is of sufficient caliber to accommodate the vessel tips. Care should be taken not to overdilate the vein and injure the intima.

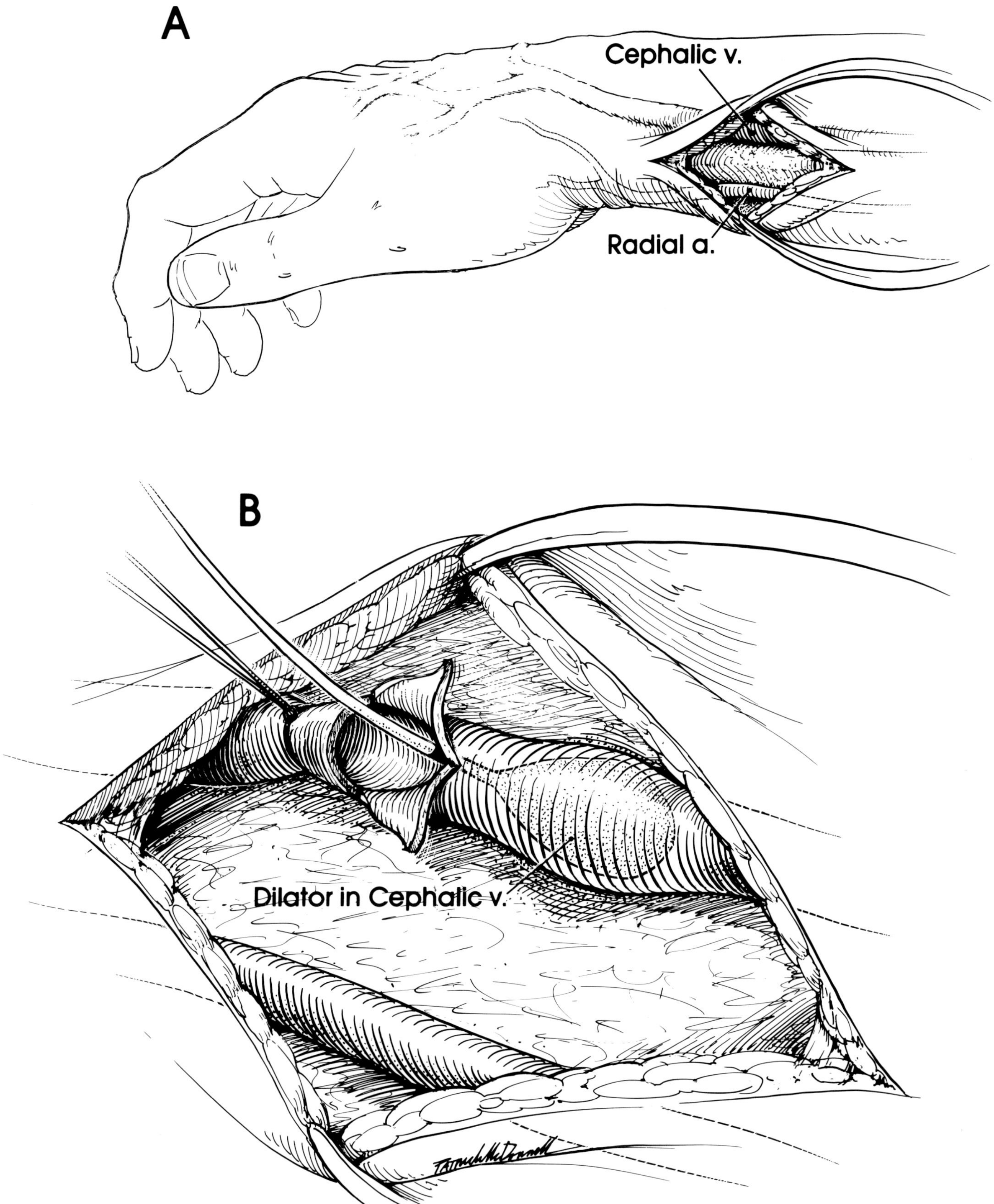
A
Cephalic v.
Radial a.
B
Dilator in Cephalic v.

C A vessel tip slightly smaller than the diameter of the dilator is selected and connected to the standard deviation cannula. Both the vessel tip and cannula should have been submerged in heparinized saline prior to use. While the venotomy flaps are used for retraction, the vessel tip is gently inserted into the venous lumen, with care to avoid dissecting the intima. This ligature is tied and the distal venous tie is used to further secure the cannula in place.

D A pocket in the subcutaneous tissue is created for the curved portion of the standard deviation cannula. Adequate dissection is necessary to avoid crimping of the cannula and shunt failure, and the flap should be thick enough to avoid skin necrosis.

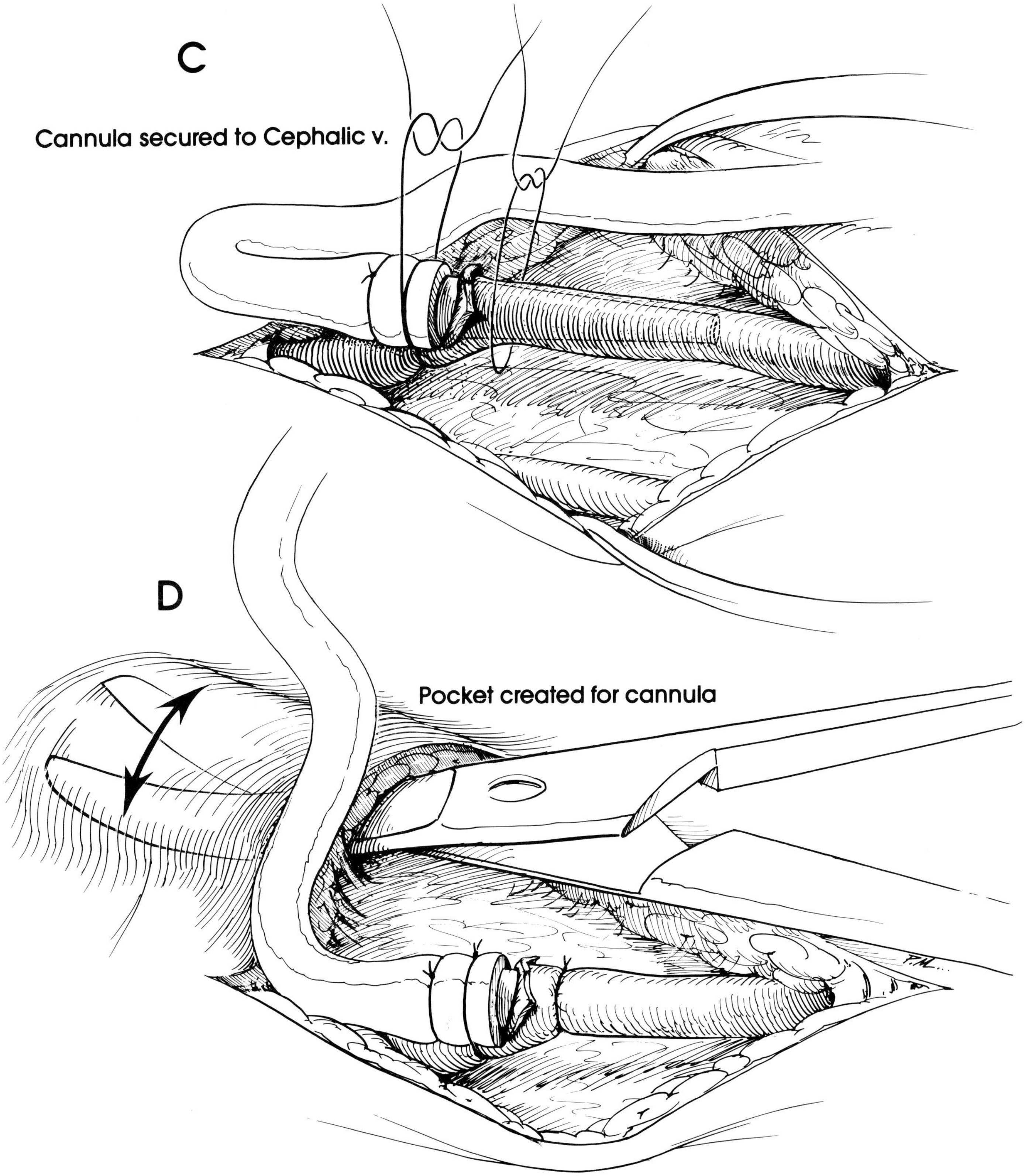
C
Cannula secured to Cephalic v.
D
Pocket created for cannula

E A stab wound is made immediately adjacent to the skin incision to serve as an exit site for the stepped-up portion of the cannula. Heparinized saline is injected through the venous limb of the shunt, and, if there is no evidence of restriction to flow, the cannula is clamped. A Ramirez winged cannula may be used in lieu of a curved cannula. The straight configuration of the Ramirez cannula facilitates thrombectomy, should that become necessary. However, the straight catheter does cross the wrist joint and is therefore more cumbersome for the patient.

F Once the distal vein is ligated, the radial artery is clamped proximally with a microvascular bulldog clamp, and a transverse arteriotomy is performed. The incision is extended into a T configuration, and the artery is sized with venous dilators. To avoid intimal fracture, the artery is not dilated.

E

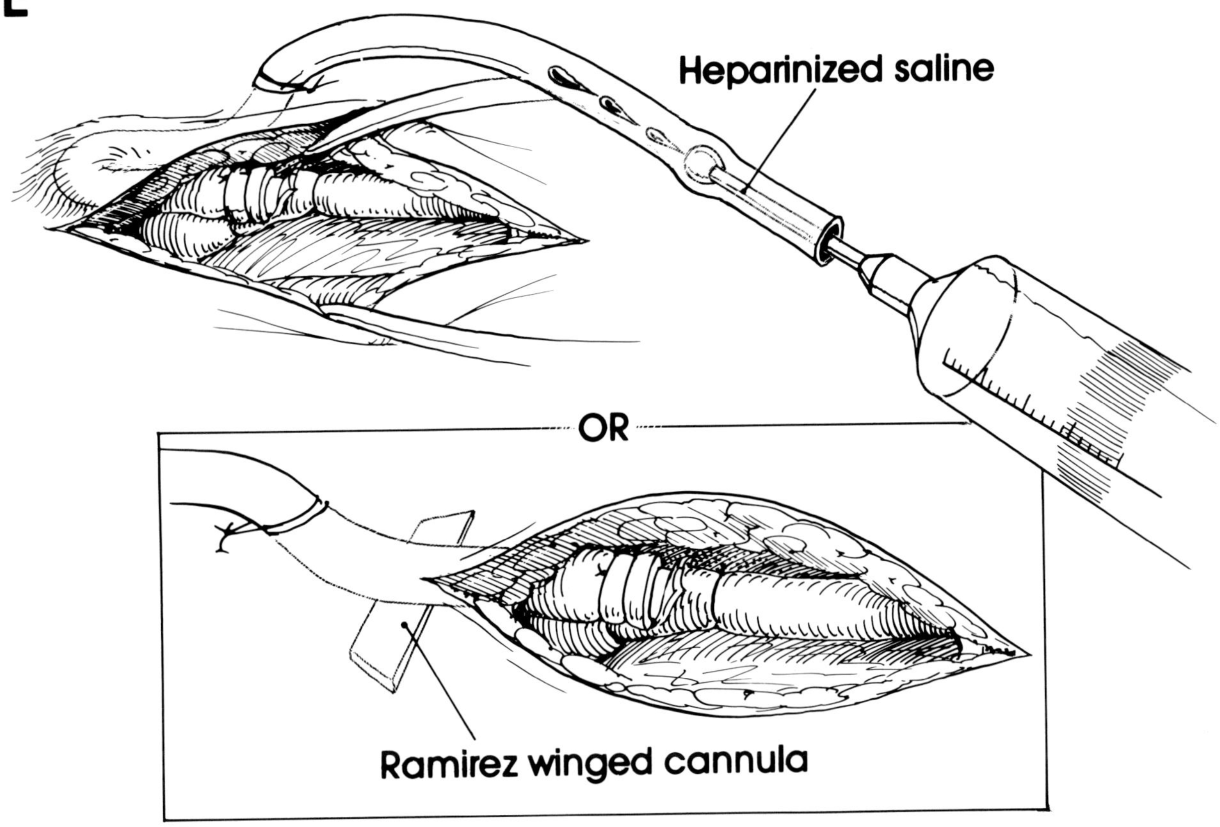

F

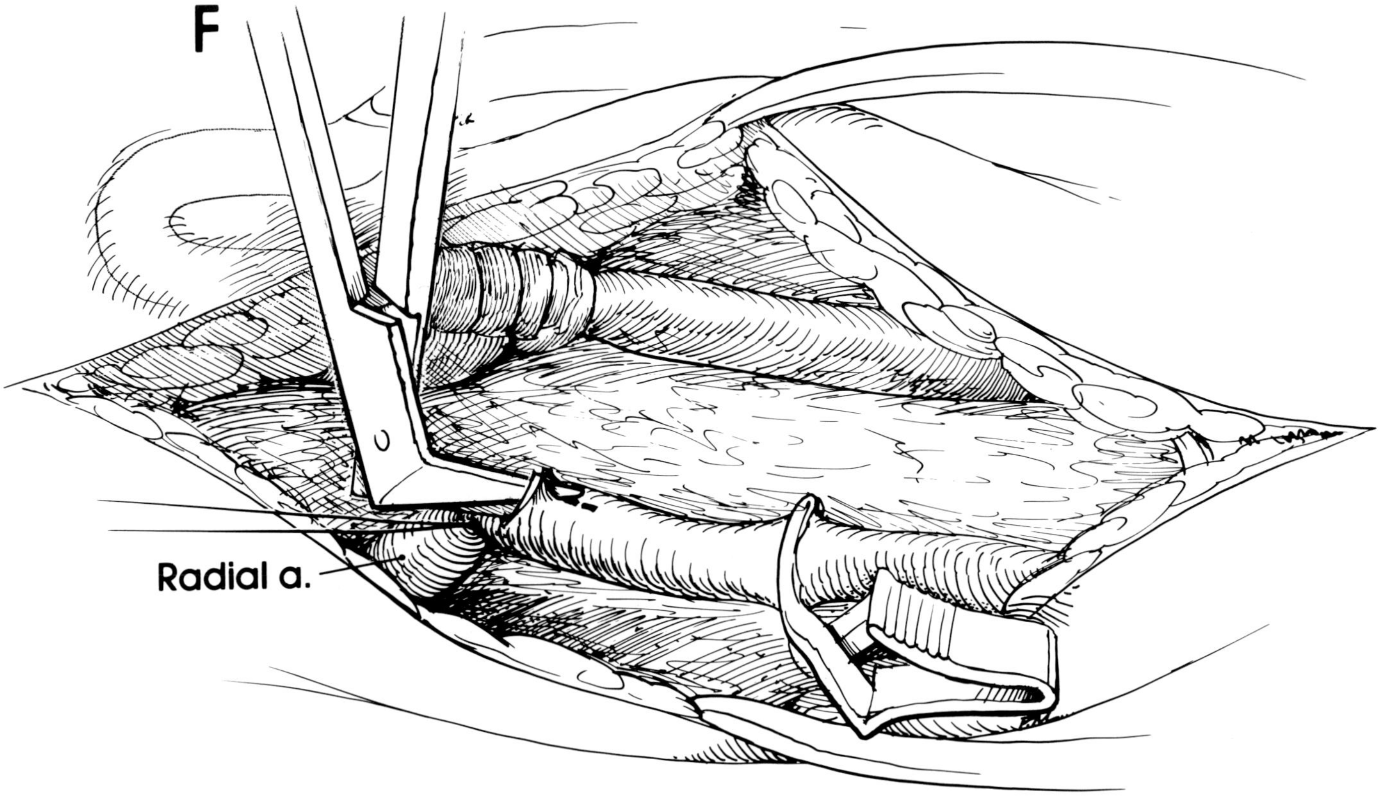

G The appropriate vessel tip is connected to the arterial cannula and secured with 3-0 silk suture. The flaps of the arteriotomy are used for retraction, and the vessel tip is introduced into the arterial lumen. At this point the bulldog clamp is removed, and the insertion completed. Care must be taken to avoid intimal dissection. A 3-0 silk suture is passed beneath the segment of the artery containing the vessel tip and, along with the proximal ligature, is used to secure the cannula in place.

H The cannula is positioned in the subcutaneous tissue and brought out through a stab wound. The arterial limb is tested for any impedance to flow and heparinized. A heparin reservoir is connected to the clamped arterial cannula and filled with heparinized saline. The reservoir is inserted into the venous cannula, which completes the shunt.

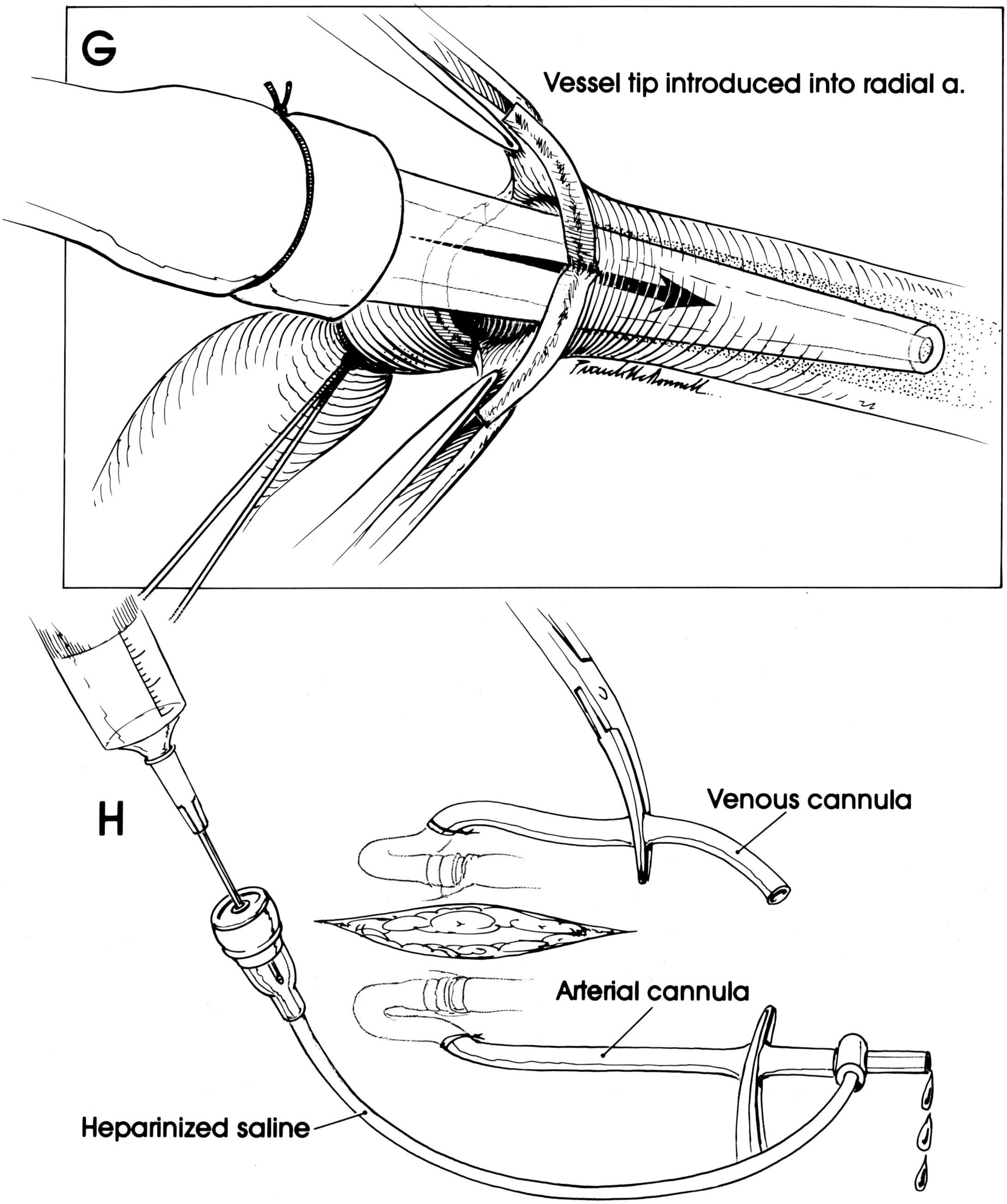
G
Vessel tip introduced into radial a.
H
Venous cannula
Arterial cannula
Heparinized saline

I, J The ascending limb of the reservoir should be positioned perpendicular to the skin to maintain a low blood level in the heparin lock. Irrigation of the shunt is accomplished by flushing first the arterial and then the venous limbs with heparinized saline. This technique should be used during operation and for maintenance irrigation as well. Failure to occlude the venous limb to allow retrograde flow of the antegrade flow of the heparinized saline will result in shunt failure due to critical accumulation of clot in the arterial vessel tip.

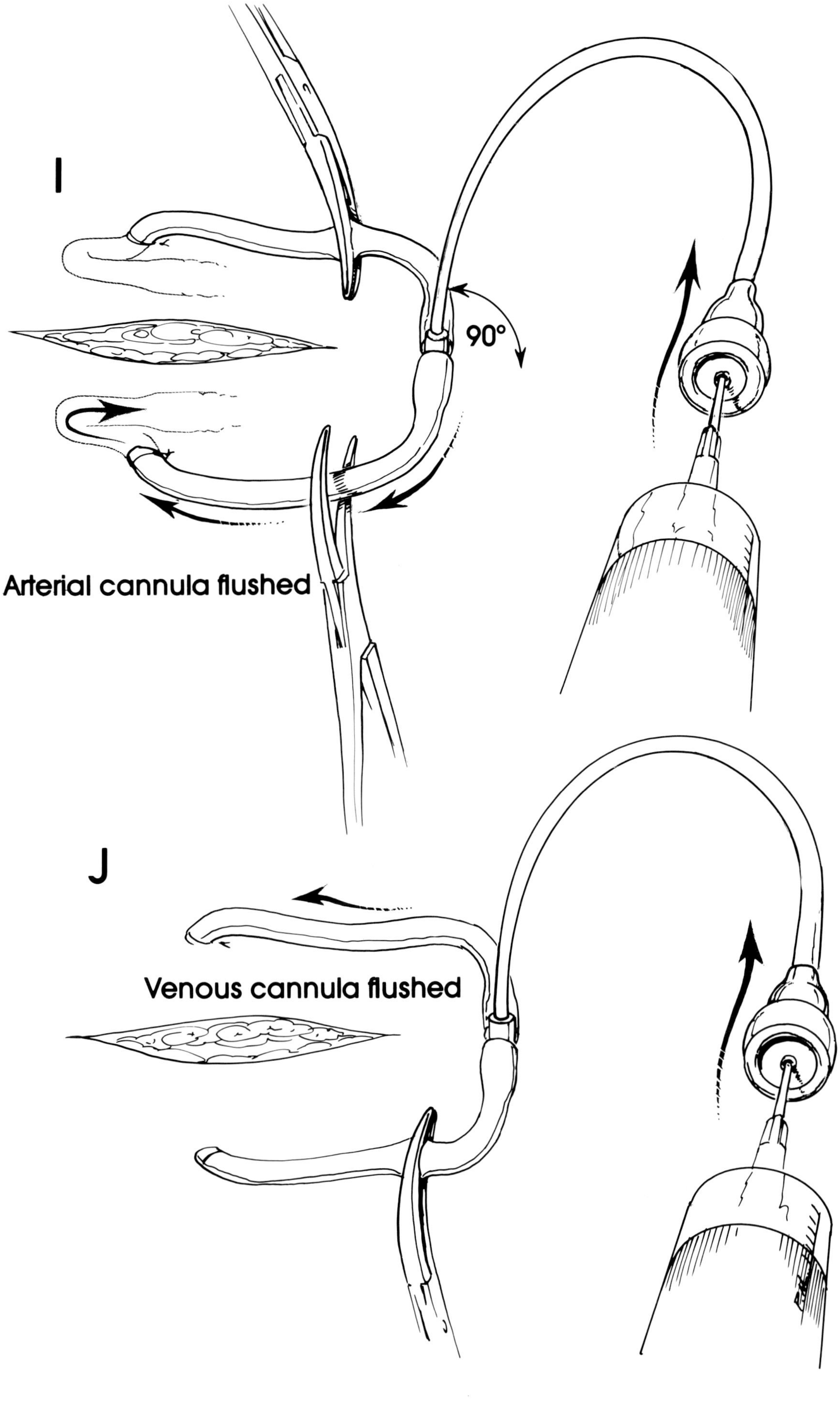
I
90°
Arterial cannula flushed
J
Venous cannula flushed

K The needle in the reservoir cap is removed while positive pressure is maintained on the syringe, thereby priming the heparin lock.

L The cannulas are anchored at the skin with 3-0 nylon suture. The incision is closed with a single layer of absorbable sutures for the subcutaneous tissue and with staples for reapproximation of the skin. The shunt is wrapped lightly with gauze to prevent snagging and accidental dislodgment. Maintenance heparinization is performed every 3 to 4 hours, using approximately 20 cc of a solution of 5% dextrose in water containing 5,000 units of beef-lung heparin per liter. Sutures are removed on the tenth postoperative day to avoid possible skin necrosis and infection.

Ramirez winged cannulas may be used in lieu of the standard deviation cannulas, and a straight connector may be used in place of the T-shaped heparin reservoir, thereby obviating maintenance heparinization. However, the straight connector does not permit visual confirmation of function.

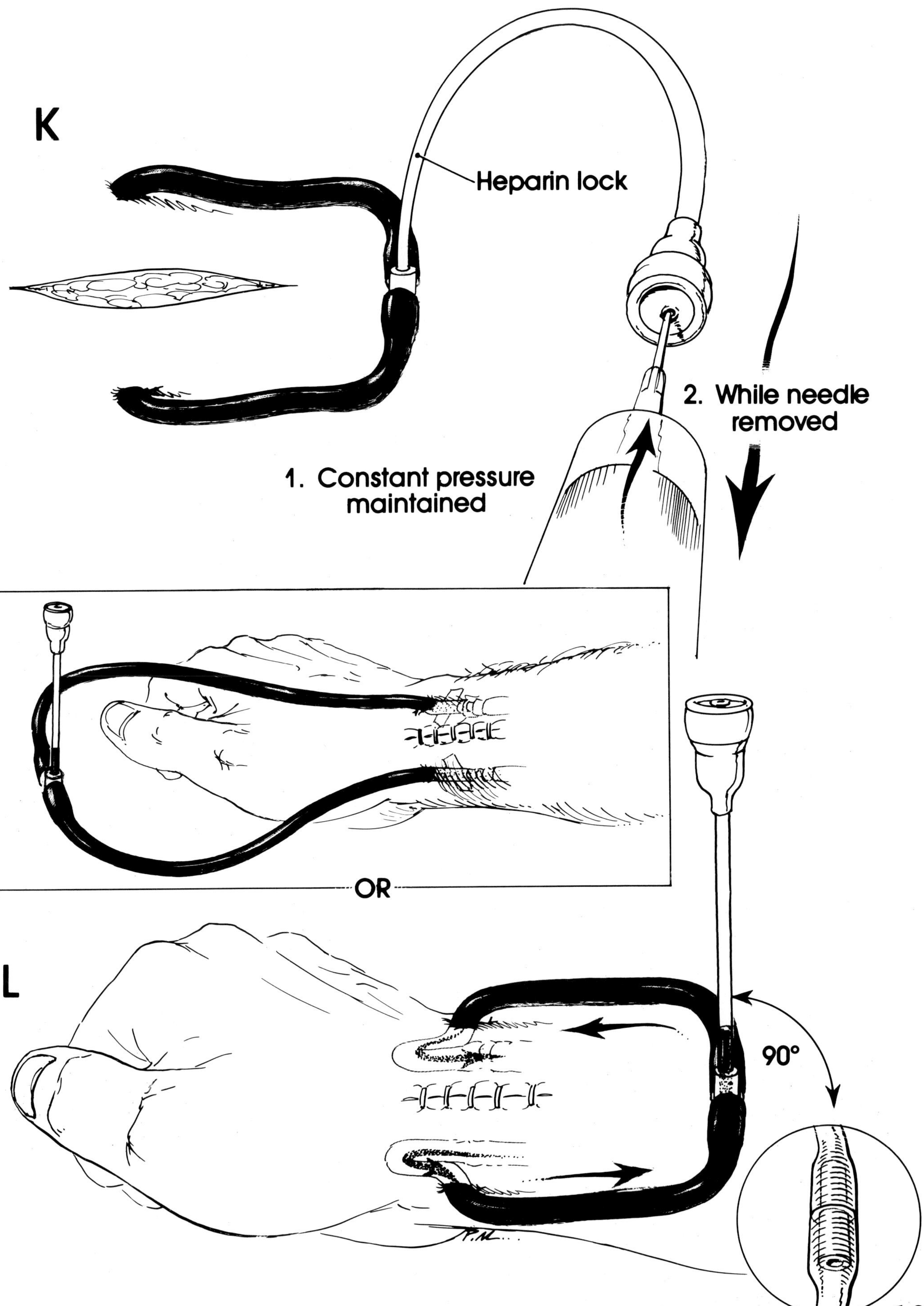
K
Heparin lock
2. While needle removed
1. Constant pressure maintained
OR
L
90°

Quinton-Scribner Shunt in the Ankle

A Shunt insertion may also be performed in the ankle, using the saphenous vein and posterior tibial artery. The technique is identical to that for wrist shunts. In ankle shunts as well as wrist shunts, standard deviation curved cannulas (**B**), Ramirez winged cannulas (**C**), and straight connectors are all options to consider.

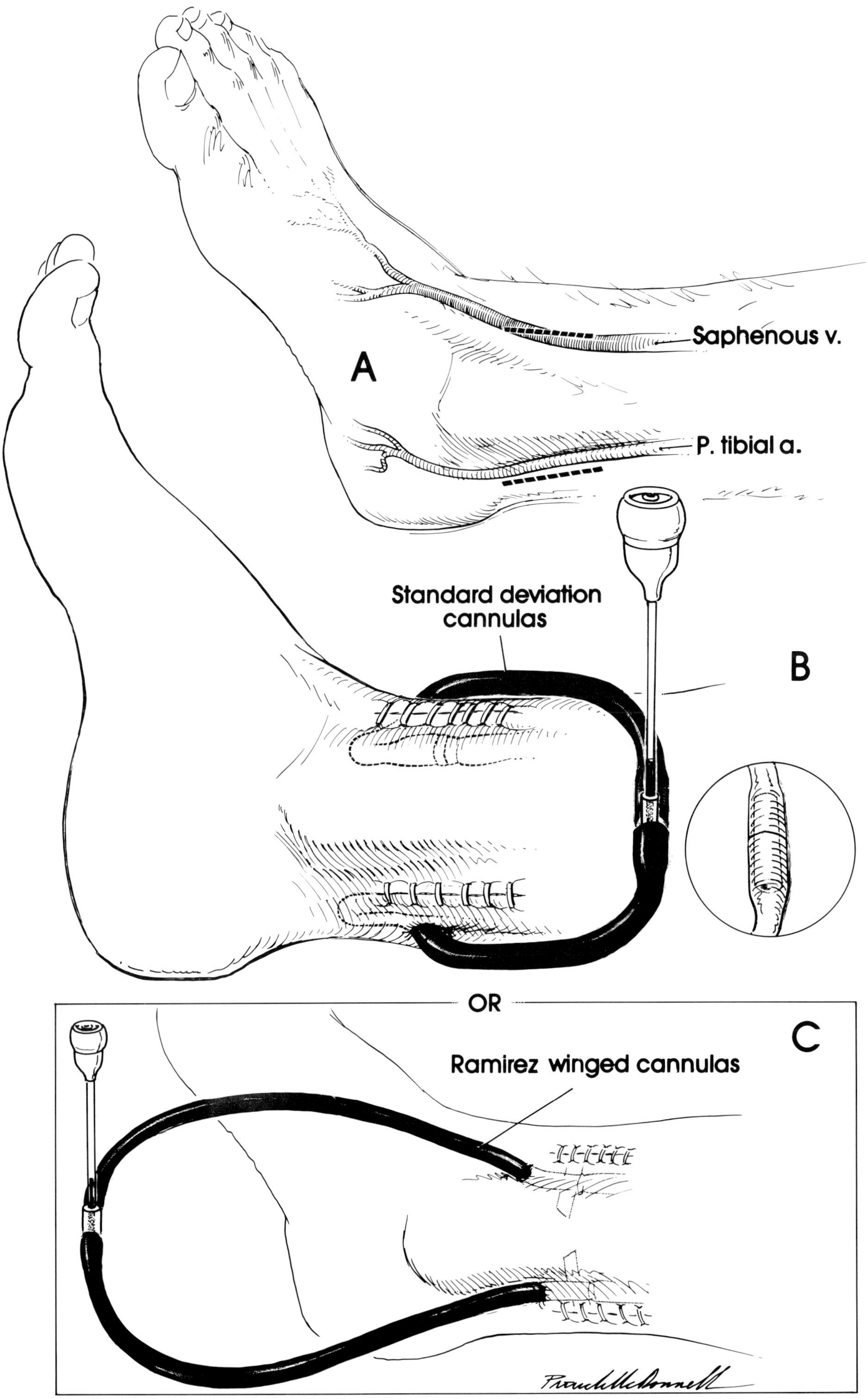
Saphenous v.
A
P. tibial a.
Standard deviation cannulas
B
OR
C
Ramirez winged cannulas

Allen-Brown Shunt
Thomas Applique Shunt

A–C A longitudinal incision approximately 8 cm long is made below the inguinal ligament and just medial to the femoral pulse. The greater saphenous vein and common femoral artery are identified and mobilized, and a retraction loop is placed around the artery. A ligature is placed on the saphenous vein, and a transverse venotomy is done. With Potts scissors, the venotomy is extended into a T-shaped incision. The ligature is used for retraction as dilators of increasing diameter are inserted into the vein. The appropriate Teflon vessel tip is selected, connected to a straight Silastic cannula, and secured with a 3-0 silk tie. With the venotomy flaps used for retraction, the vessel tip is inserted into the vein. A 3-0 silk suture is passed below the vein and tied, holding the vessel tip in place. The cannula is further secured by tying the retraction suture. The cannula is then irrigated and any resistance noted. A stab wound is then made below the incision and the cannula is drawn through the skin, heparinized, and clamped. The cannula should pass smoothly and gradually through the subcutaneous tissue and skin. Too large an angle of exit will cause crimping of the cannula.

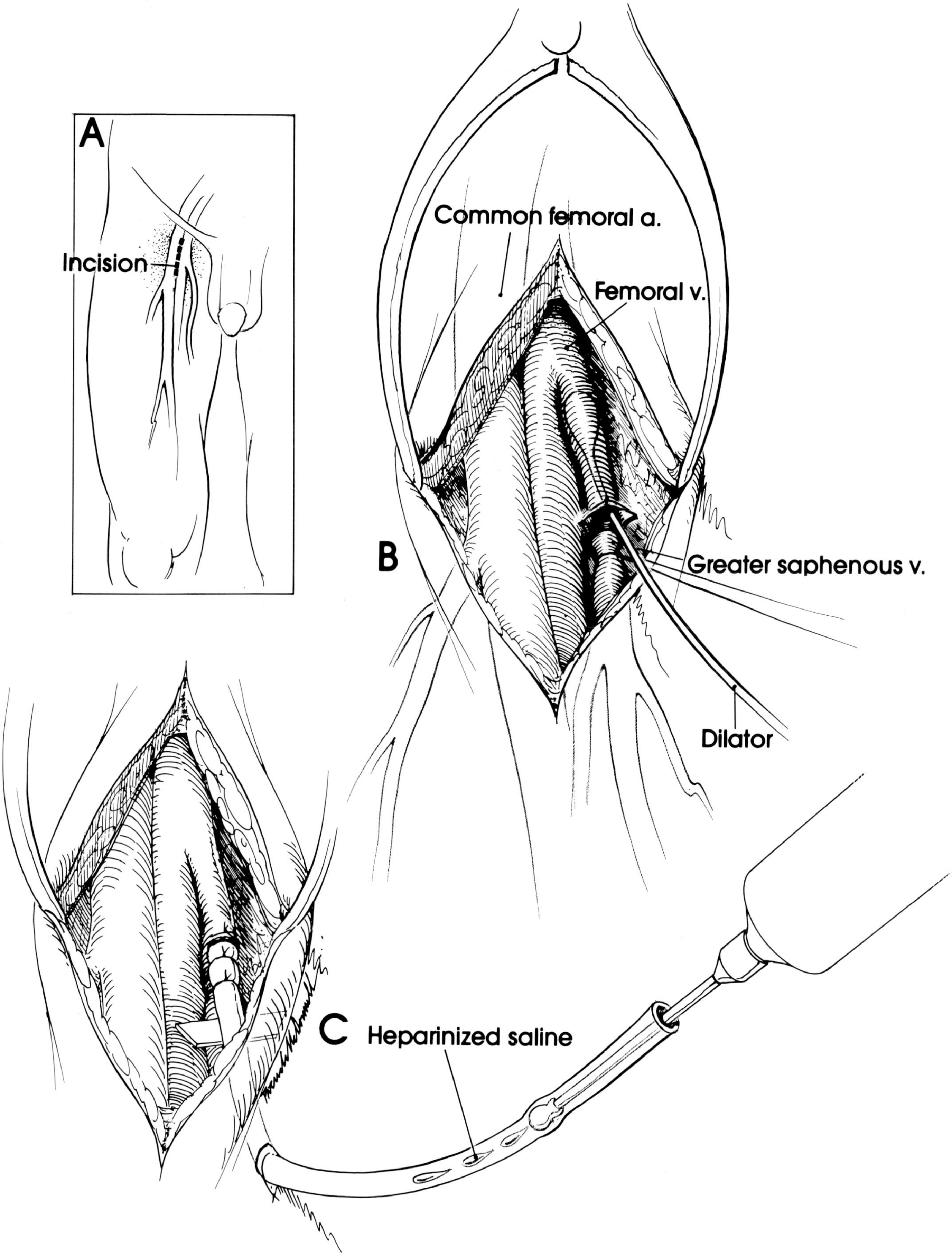
A
Incision
B
Common femoral a.
Femoral v.
Greater saphenous v.
Dilator
C
Heparinized saline

D–E A vascular clamp is placed proximally, and a longitudinal arteriotomy is made in the common femoral artery. The clamp is removed and heparinization is carried out, the vessel loop being used for control. The clamp is replaced, the retraction loop is removed, and distal heparinization is done. A distal clamp is then placed, and the arteriotomy is extended to accommodate the Dacron tube graft of the Allen-Brown cannula. The tube graft is tapered appropriately and incorporated into the arteriotomy with running 5-0 vascular silicone-treated Dacron suture. The Dacron graft should be tapered sufficiently to fit an arteriotomy length of at least one and one-half times the diameter of the graft.

The Thomas applique cannula with its Dacron patch graft is an alternative to the Allen-Brown arterial cannula.

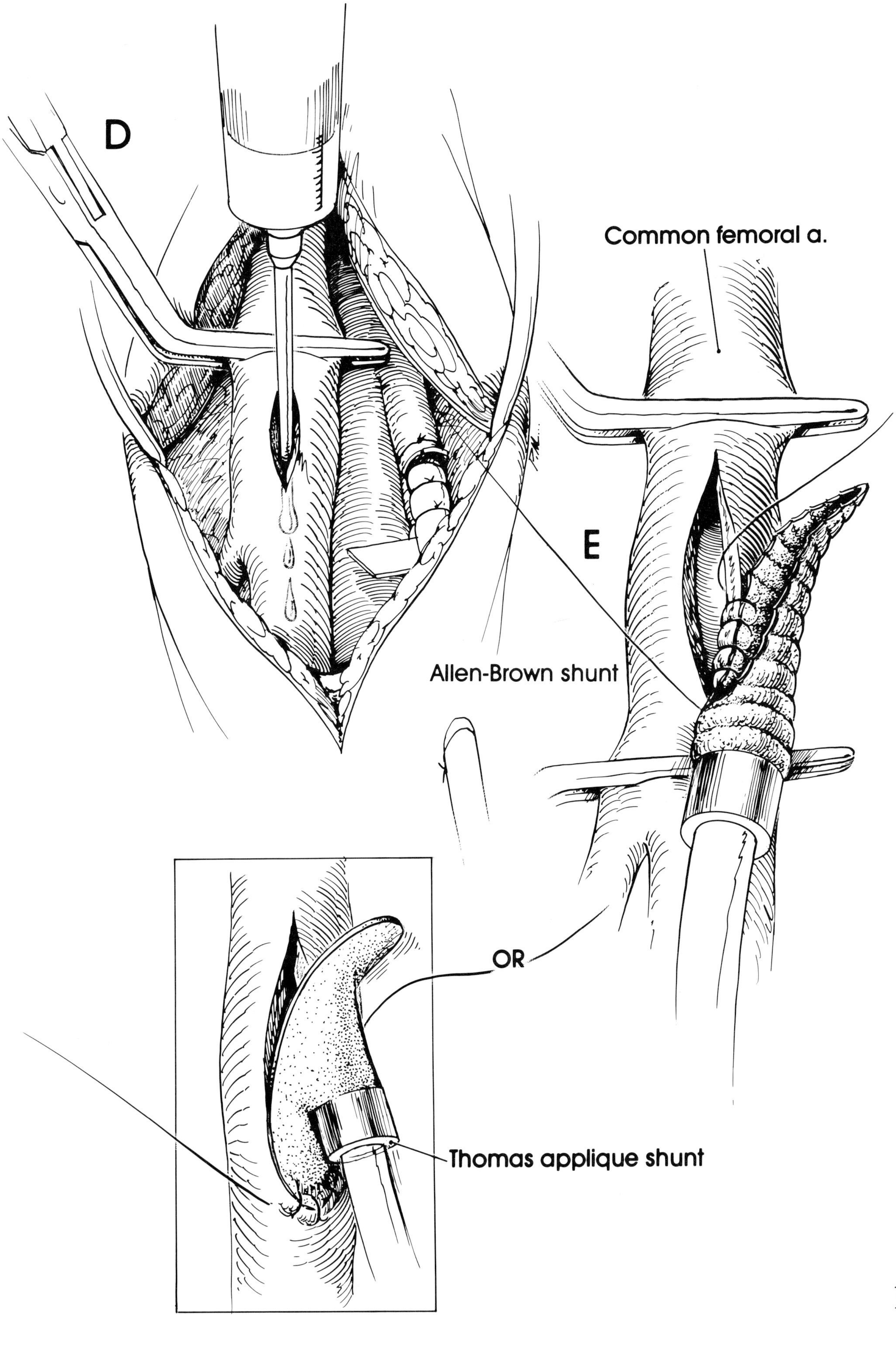
D
Common femoral a.
E
Allen-Brown shunt
OR
Thomas applique shunt

F–G The proximal clamp is removed, and the cannula is allowed to flush, clearing any debris that might be present. The distal vascular clamp is then removed, and the cannula is brought through a stab wound below the skin incision. The arterial limb of the shunt is tested for restriction of flow. The arterial limb is heparinized and a hemostat is placed. The heparin reservoir is connected to the arterial cannula and heparinized. The venous cannula is connected, completing the shunt, and the clamps are removed. The arterial and venous limbs are irrigated in that order, and the heparin lock is primed and positioned perpendicular to the skin. After hemostasis is achieved and the wound has been irrigated with bactericidal solution, the incision is closed with running 3-0 absorbable suture for the subcutaneous tissue and with staples for the skin. The cannulas are anchored at the skin with 3-0 nylon sutures, which are to be removed 10 days after surgery. As with other external indwelling cannulas, routine maintenance irrigation should be done every 3 to 4 hours unless a straight connector is used.

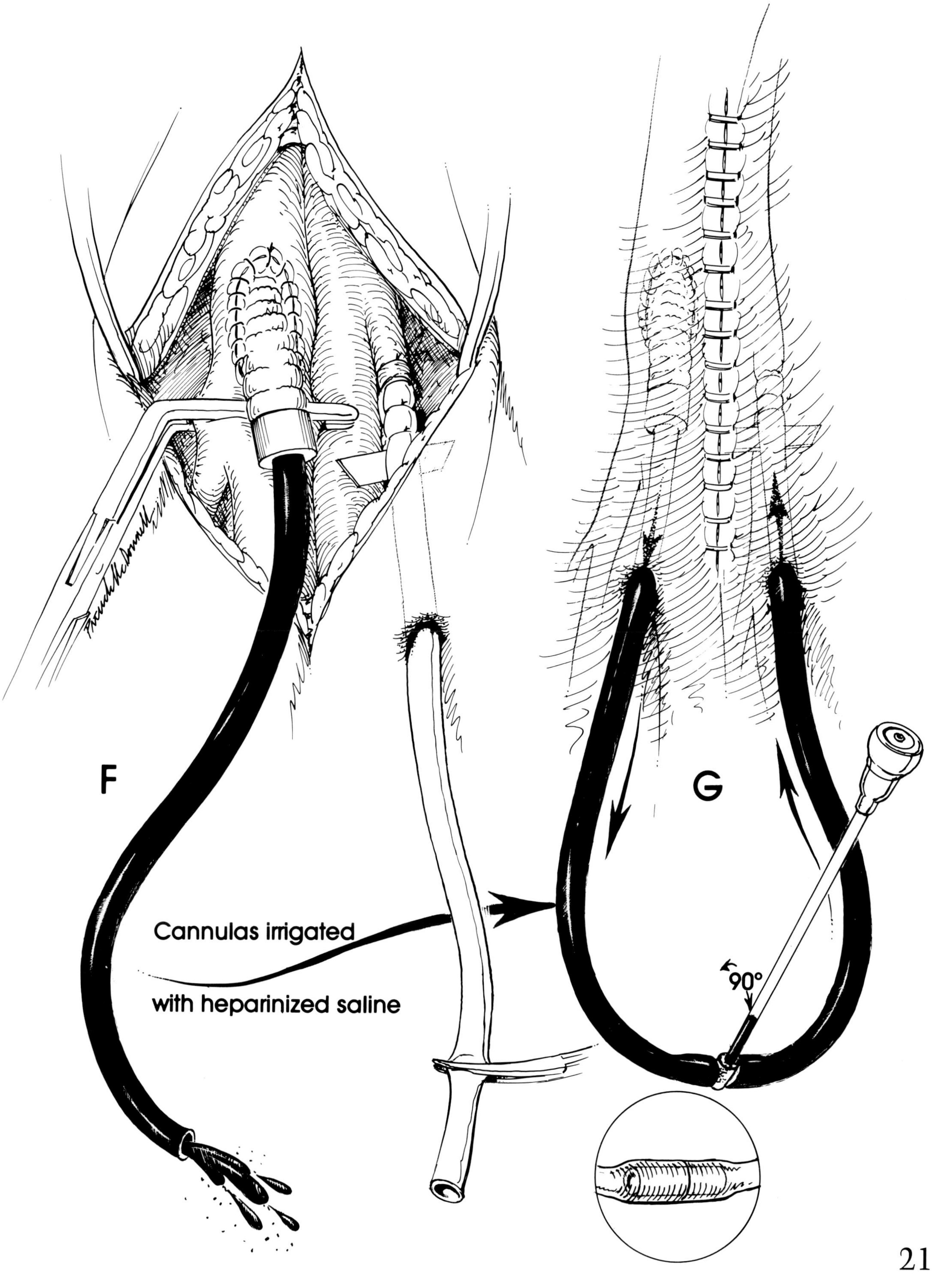
F
G
Cannulas irrigated
with heparinized saline
90°

2

Percutaneous Angioaccess Catheters

Advances in the development of percutaneous angioaccess catheters have limited the indications for the insertion of arteriovenous shunts to obtain temporary vascular access. The Shiley and Sorenson subclavian catheters, which are similar, may be inserted at the bedside and provide good, dependable short-term vascular access. These catheters may be inserted in an operating room where minor variations in technique are permitted that extend their functional life. Their utilization requires the availability of a single needle dialysis machine unless they are used in combination with the Shaldon catheter. The Shaldon femoral catheter allows dependable acute angioaccess but precludes patient ambulation.

Complications associated with the use of these catheters vary, depending on their location. The potential complications of percutaneous subclavian vein catheterization are well known and are directly related to the experience of the individual performing the procedure. The most common complications of femoral catheterization are local hematoma and retroperitoneal bleeding. The latter, which can be serious, may be avoided by not forcing the guide wire against resistance.

Shiley Subclavian Catheter (Short-Term)
Sorenson Subclavian Catheter (Short-Term)

A–C A 14-gauge needle is inserted in the subclavian vein, utilizing the standard infraclavicular approach. As backflow is obtained, the syringe is removed. Occluding the needle with a finger prevents air from entering the vein. The patient is requested to perform a Valsalva maneuver, and the guide wire is positioned in the superior vena cava. We use a portable C-arm fluoroscopy apparatus to confirm proper positioning.

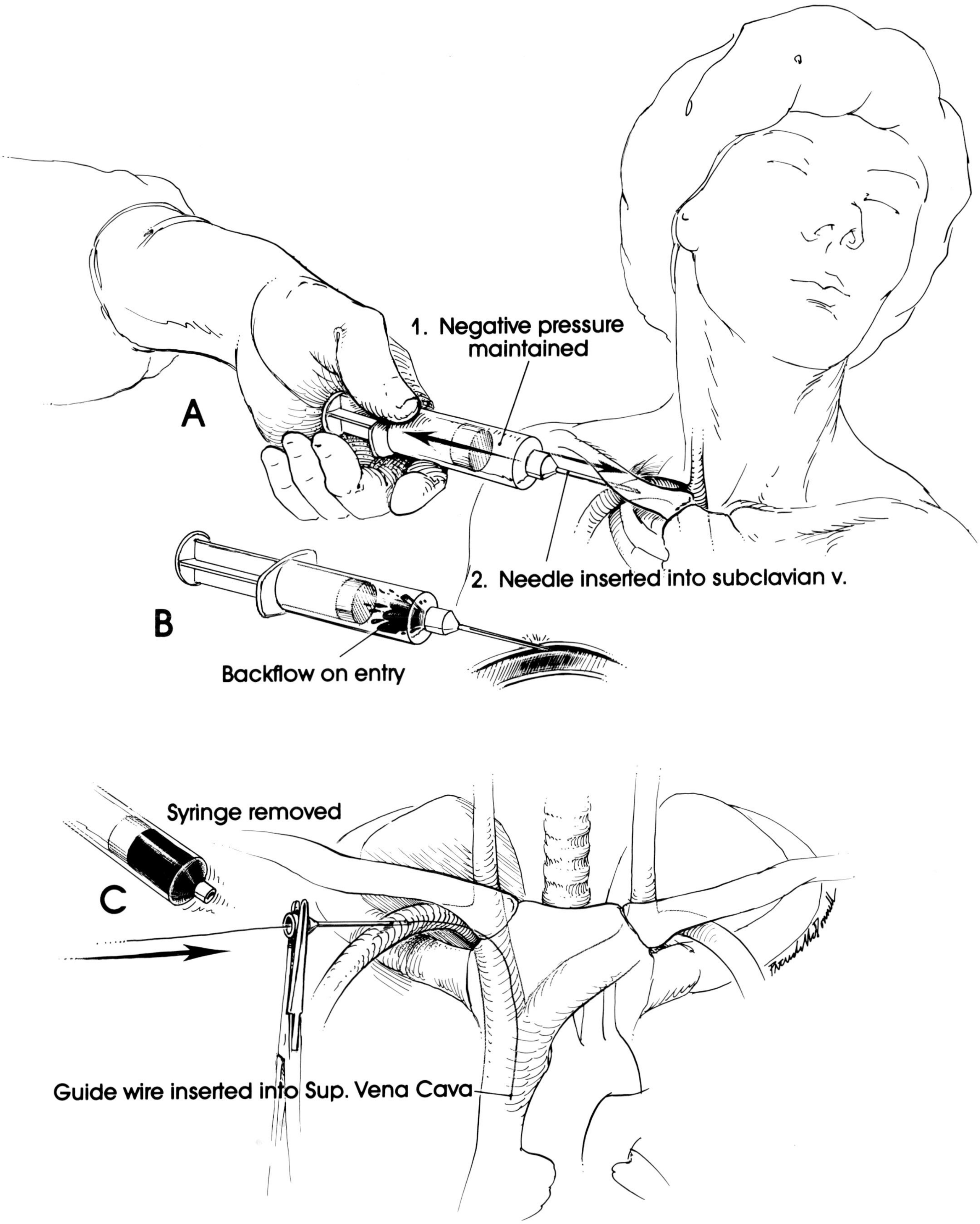
A
1. Negative pressure maintained
2. Needle inserted into subclavian v.
B
Backflow on entry
Syringe removed
C
Guide wire inserted into Sup. Vena Cava

D–I After the needle is removed, the percutaneous catheter is threaded over the guide wire so that the catheter hub is flush with the skin. Then the guide wire is removed and the catheter is tested for backflow, which indicates proper positioning. Both limbs of the connection assembly are heparinized and sealed. An intravenous adapter may be used in lieu of the seal cap. A 3-0 nylon suture is used to anchor the catheter hub in place.

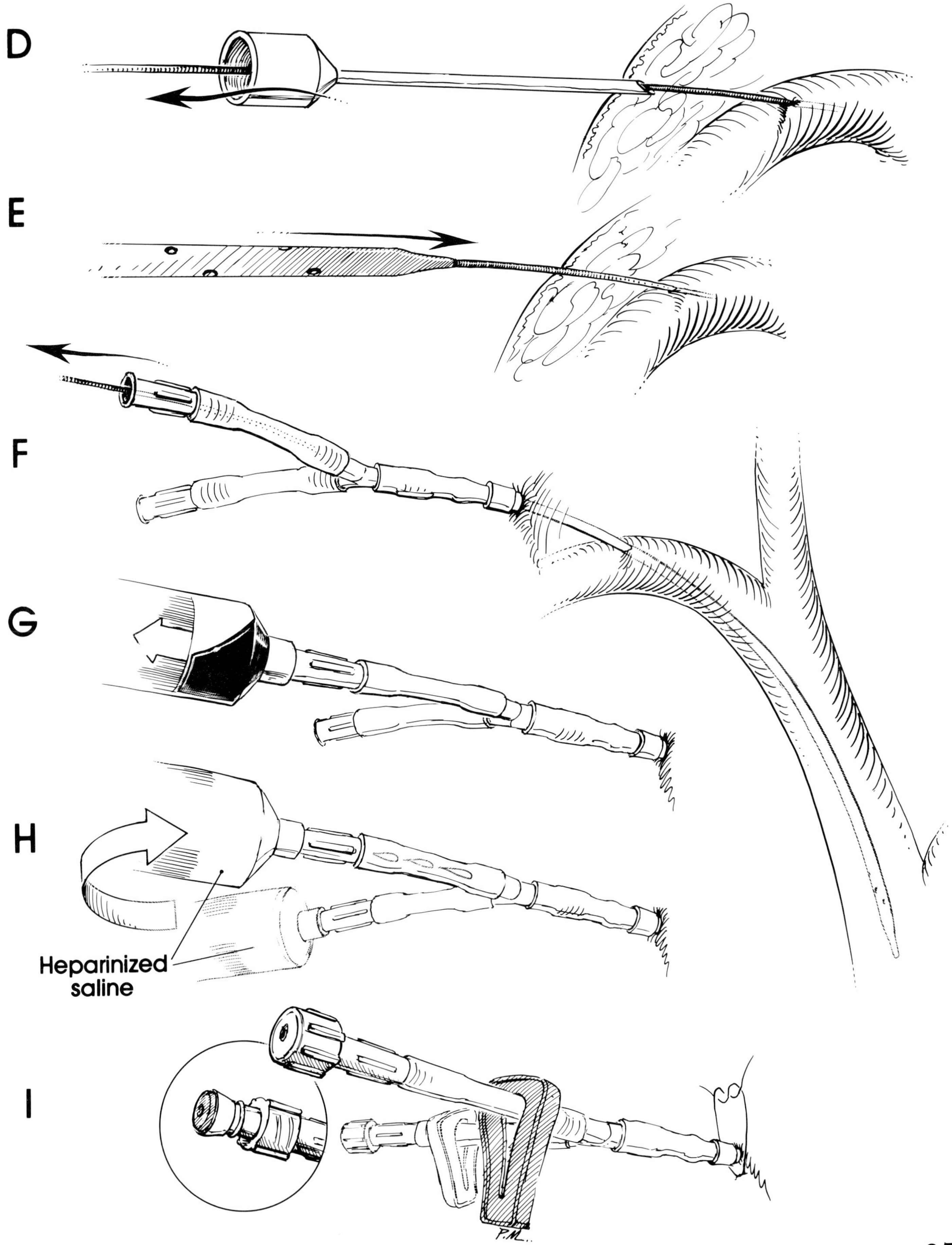
D
E
F
G
H
Heparinized saline
I
P.M.

Shiley Subclavian Catheter (Long-Term)
Sorenson Subclavian Catheter (Long-Term)

A When long-term use of a percutaneous catheter is anticipated, an alternative method of insertion is used. After the guide wire has been inserted and the needle withdrawn, a stab wound is made inferior and lateral to the exit site of the wire.

B A hemostat is introduced into the stab wound, and a tunnel is created up to the wire.

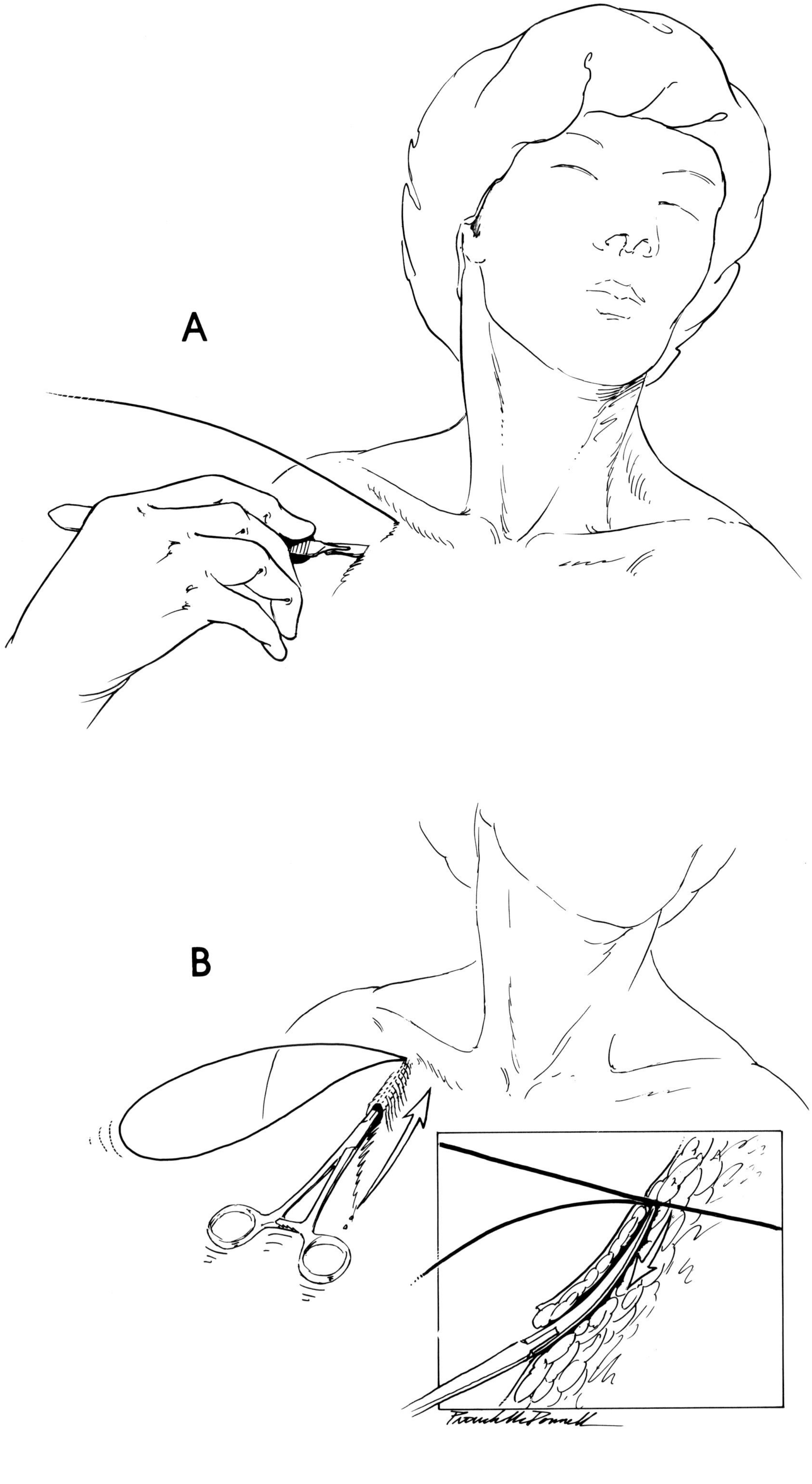
A
B

C The free end of the guide wire is brought through this tunnel and out through the stab wound.

D–E At this point, the catheter is threaded over the wire and advanced until the Y portion of the connection assembly is in the stab wound. The wire is removed, and the catheter is secured with 3-0 nylon suture.

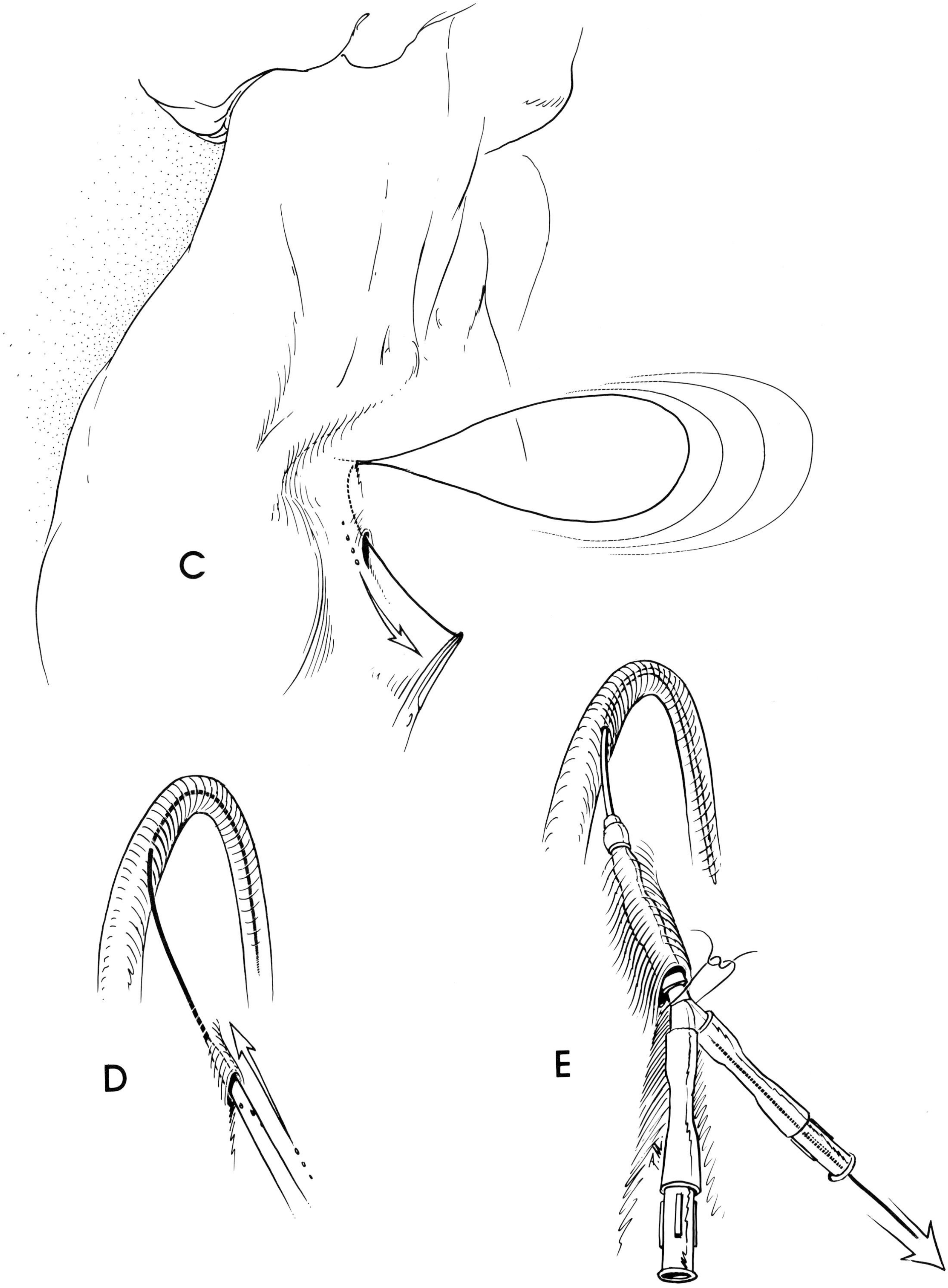
C
D
E

F–H Both limbs of the connection assembly are irrigated and capped, as previously described (p. 26). This procedure reduces the possibility of infection and accidental dislodgment; however, in contrast to the first method described in this chapter (p. 23), we prefer to do it in the operating room and not at the patient's bedside.

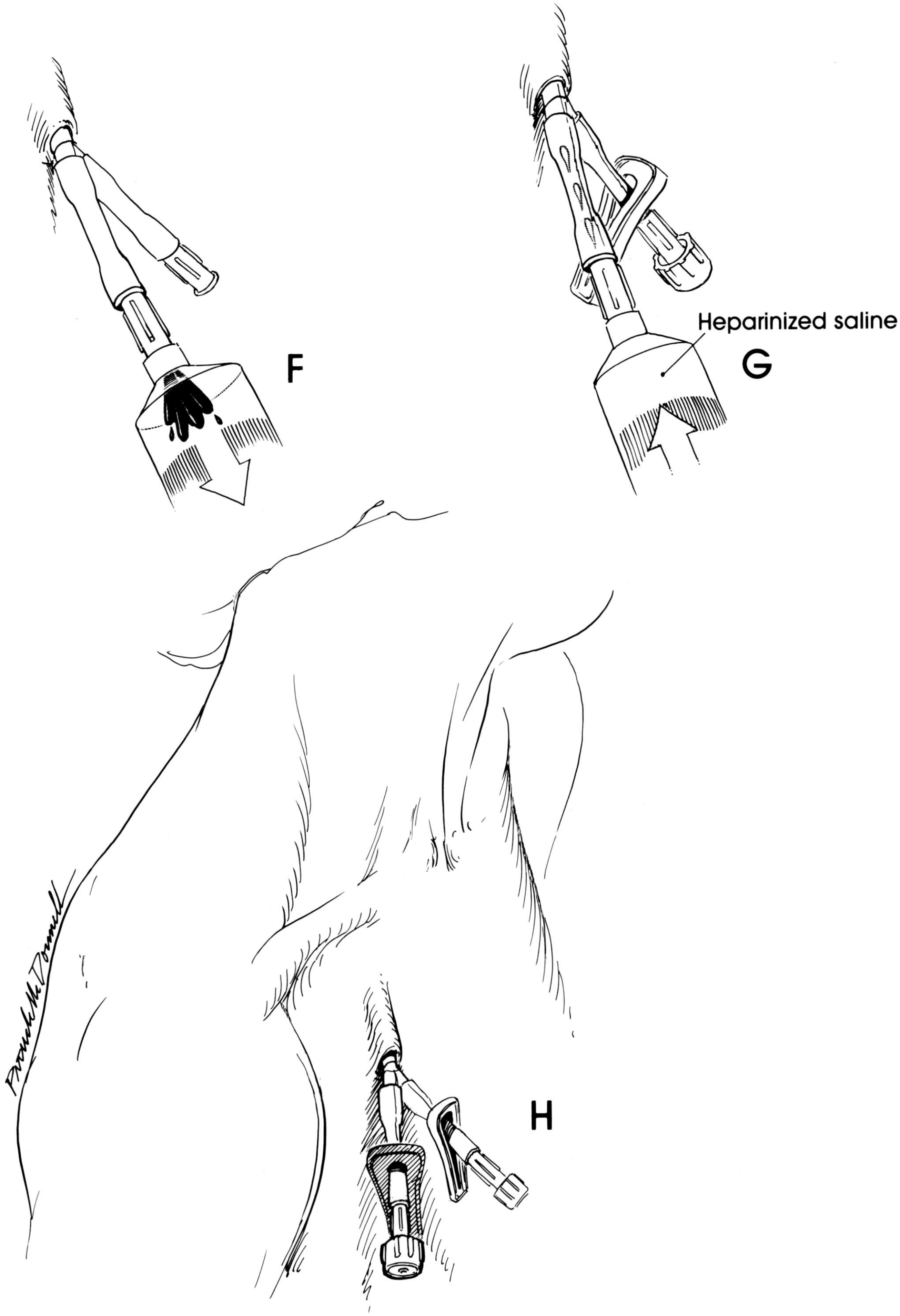
Heparinized saline
F
G
H

Shaldon Femoral Catheter

A A 16-gauge needle and cannula are inserted perpendicularly in the femoral vein immediately below the inguinal ligament. Negative pressure is maintained on the syringe to allow aspiration of blood on entry.

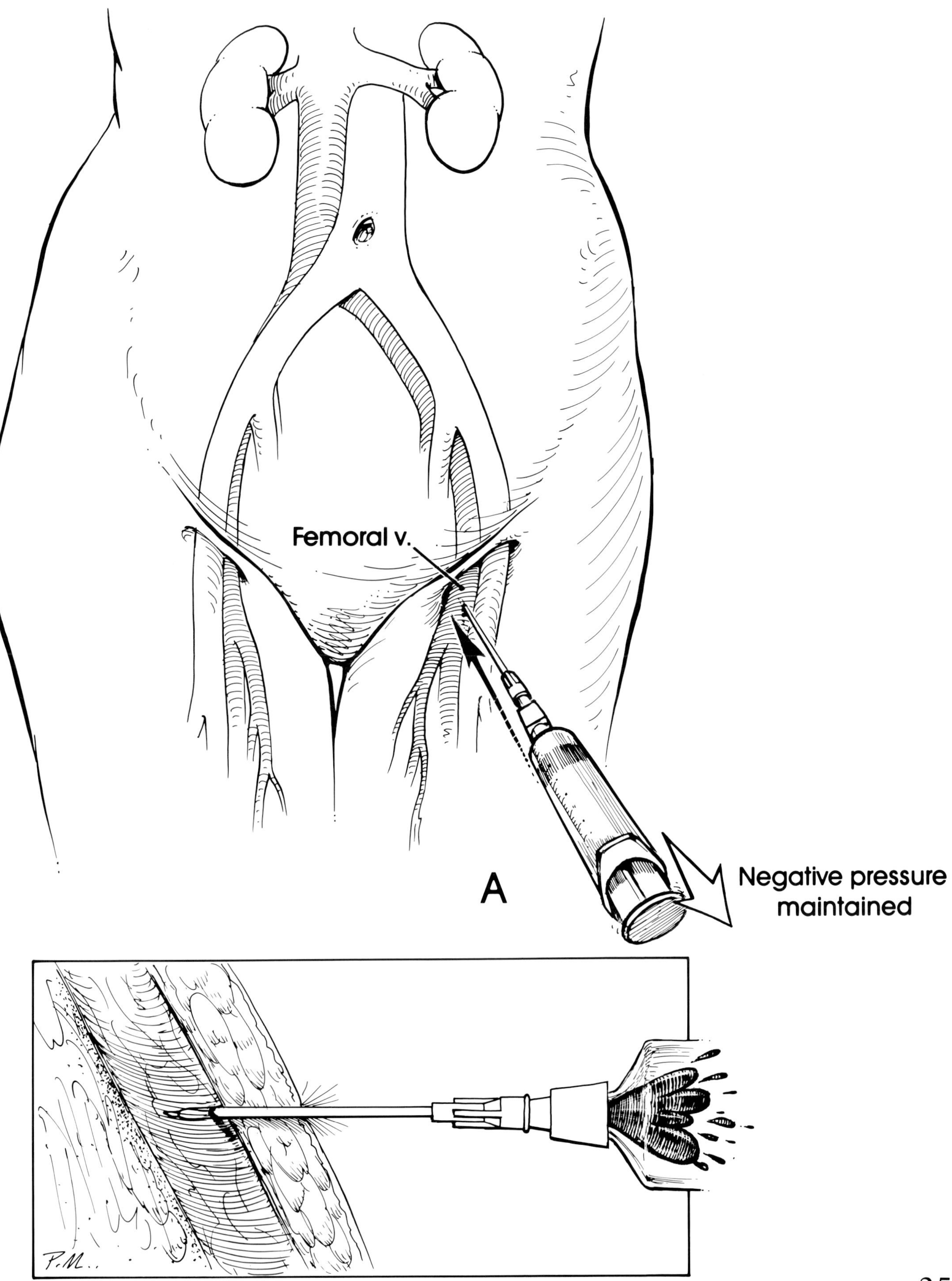
Femoral v.
A
Negative pressure
maintained
P.M.

B–D Once proper positioning has been confirmed, the needle portion of the catheter assembly is withdrawn. The flexible end of a guide wire is then inserted through the cannula and advanced into the inferior vena cava.

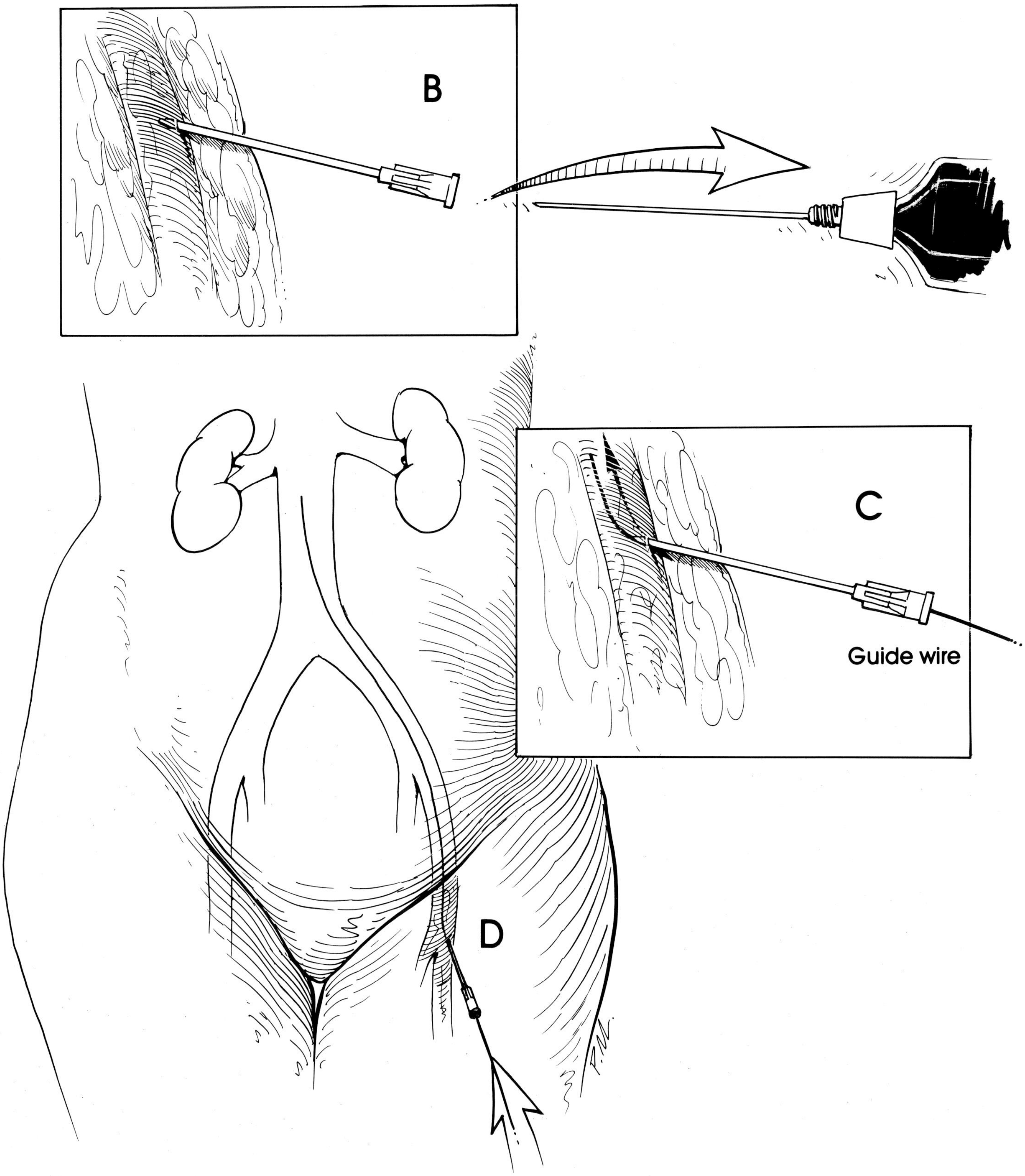
B
C
Guide wire
D

E–G After the cannula is withdrawn, a no. 11 blade is used to enlarge the needle puncture site. The catheter is threaded over the guide wire and advanced until the hub is at skin level.

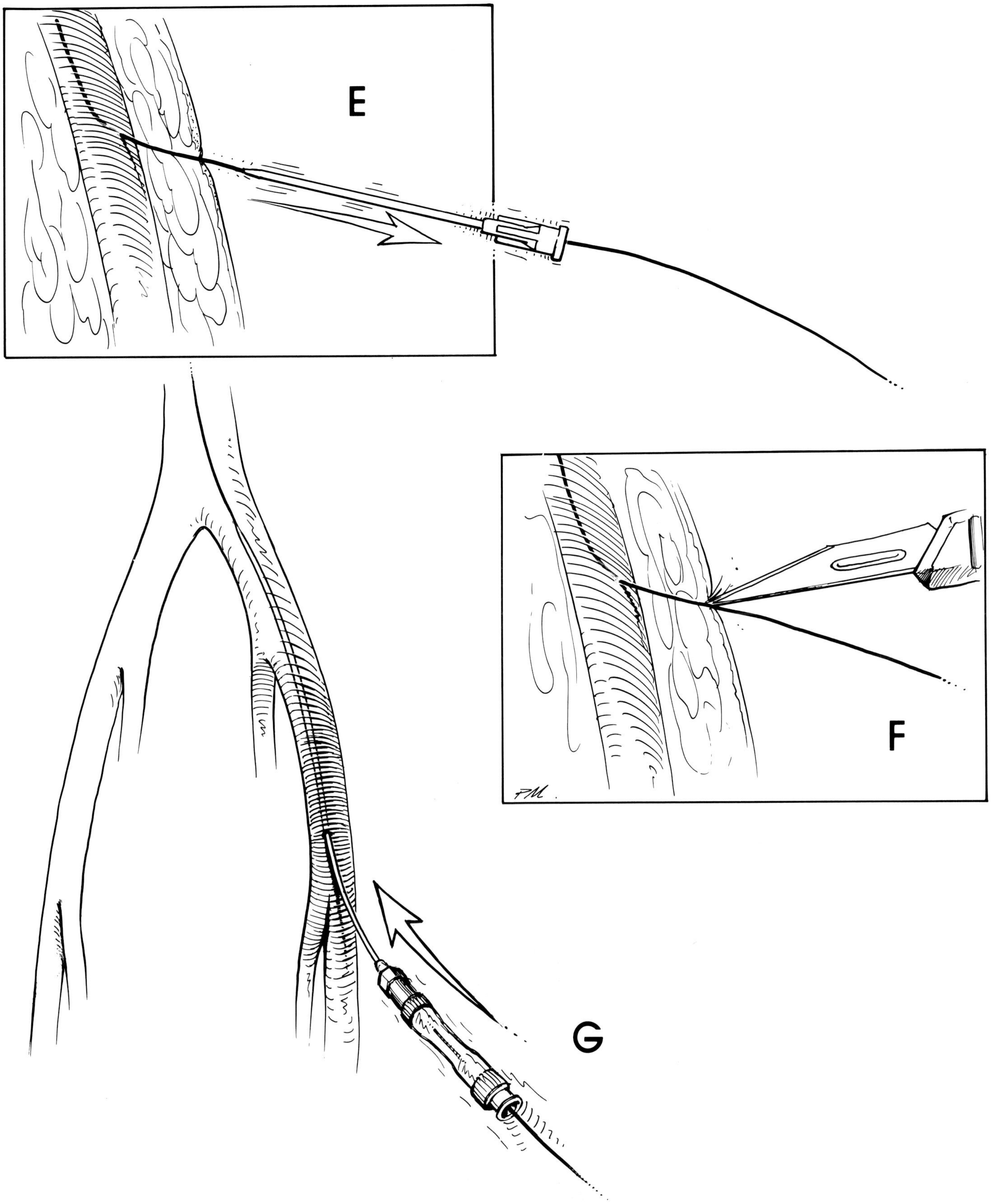
E
F
G
PM

H–K The guide wire is removed, and aspiration of blood confirms proper positioning of the catheter. The heparin lock is filled, and the catheter hub is secured in place with a 3-0 nylon stitch.

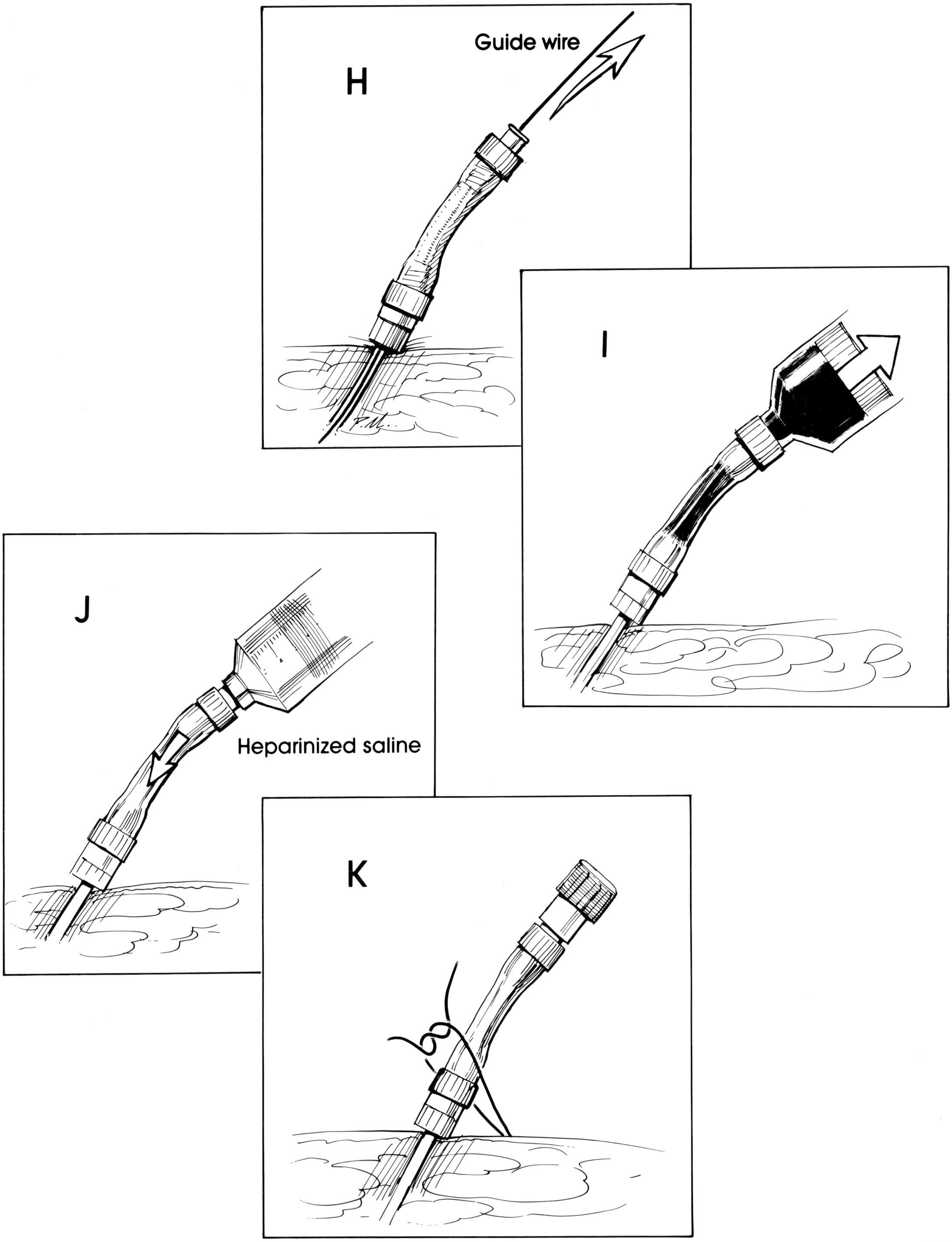

H
Guide wire
I
J
Heparinized saline
K

L The two percutaneous femoral catheters, properly positioned, procure an effective venovenous angioaccess circuit. The technique is particularly valuable in patients with congestive heart failure, since it entails no additional cardiac loading.

When a single needle technique is preferred, the Shaldon catheter positioned in the inferior vena cava provides excellent access.

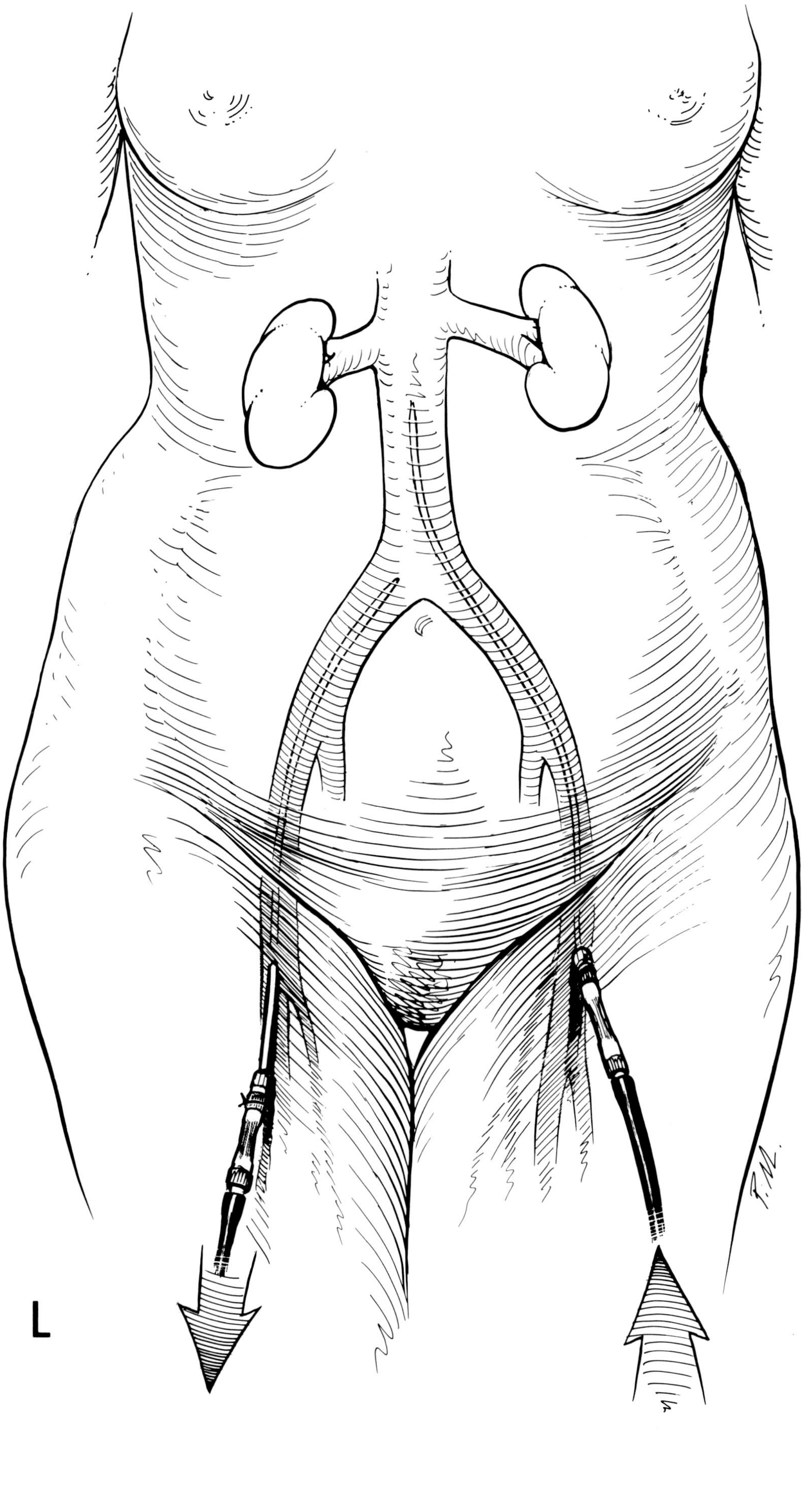

L

M Use of a subclavian catheter as one limb of the venovenous circuit is an alternative to the bilateral femoral vein technique. The method is liable to all the potential complications associated with subclavian vein catheterization.

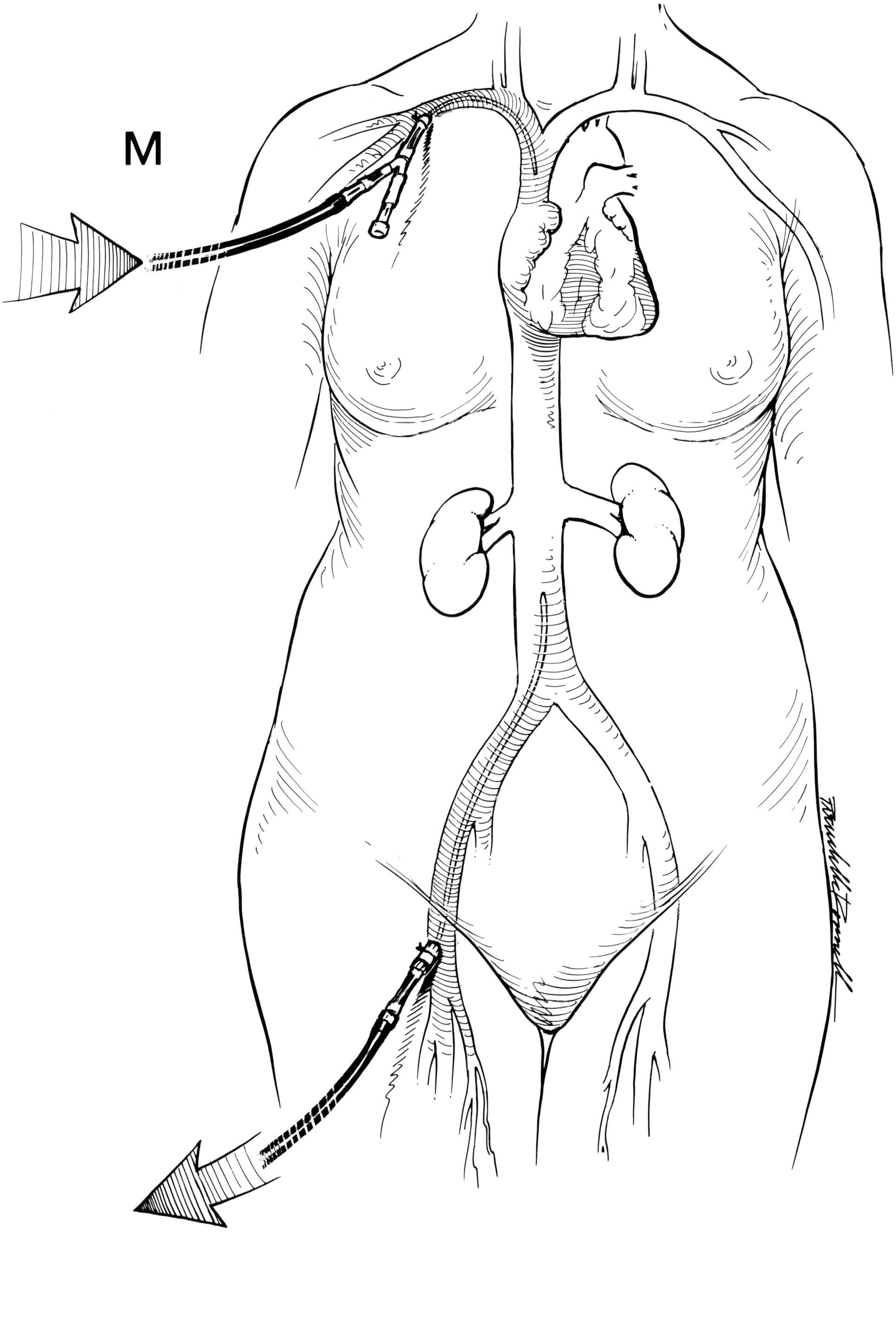
M

Primary Arteriovenous Fistulas

3

USE of a primary arteriovenous fistula eliminates the problems of potential hemorrhage from dislodgment and the restricted mobility associated with external prosthetic devices. These fistulas have also significantly reduced the number of thrombotic and infectious complications associated with external indwelling cannulas. A primary arteriovenous fistula is ideal in patients who have adequate peripheral vasculature to support arterialization of the forearm veins. However, a primary fistula cannot be used immediately prior to venipuncture and so should be constructed several weeks in advance to allow for maturity. If this is not possible, the patient should be maintained with a temporary access device until the fistula matures.

The major technical decision to be made in the construction of primary arteriovenous fistulas is the type of radial artery–cephalic vein anastomosis to be used. The original side-to-side Brescia-Cimino fistula functions satisfactorily in most patients; however, it is associated with complications that are not a problem with other configurations. Use of an end-to-side radial artery–cephalic vein anastomosis precludes arterialization of the veins of the hand, and the anastomosis can be constructed with the same degree of technical ease as the side-to-side configuration. An end-to-end anastomosis avoids the development of both arterial and venous complications in the hand but is technically more difficult to construct. Thus, the ideal anastomosis would offer the hemodynamic configuration of an end-to-end fistula with the technical ease of the end-to-side variety. This can be achieved by constructing an end-to-side anastomosis and ligating the distal artery.

Side-to-Side Fistula

A Once radial and ulnar artery competency has been determined with an Allen test, the patency of the forearm veins can be assessed by applying a pneumatic tourniquet to the upper arm.

B An incision approximately 5 cm long is made midway between the courses of the radial artery and the cephalic vein in the wrist.

C The vessels are identified and mobilized. Mobilization must be sufficient to allow the construction of the side-to-side anastomosis without tension.

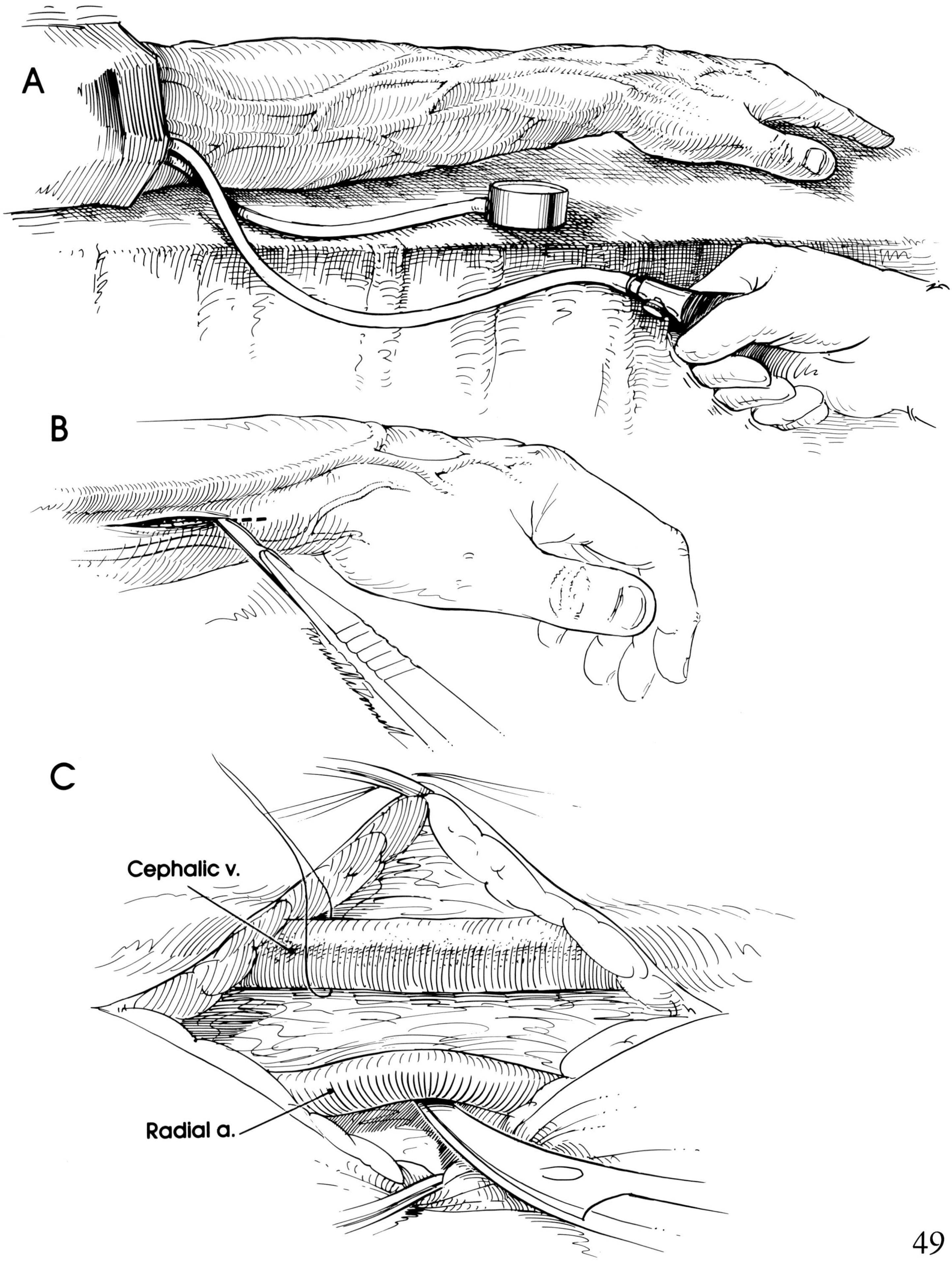
A
B
C
Cephalic v.
Radial a.

D The cephalic vein is occluded distally with a microvascular bulldog clamp. An incision is begun with a no. 11 blade along the medial side of the vein so that it will not be necessary to rotate the vessel to construct the anastomosis.

E The venotomy is extended with Potts scissors until it is approximately one and one-half times the diameter of the radial artery.

D

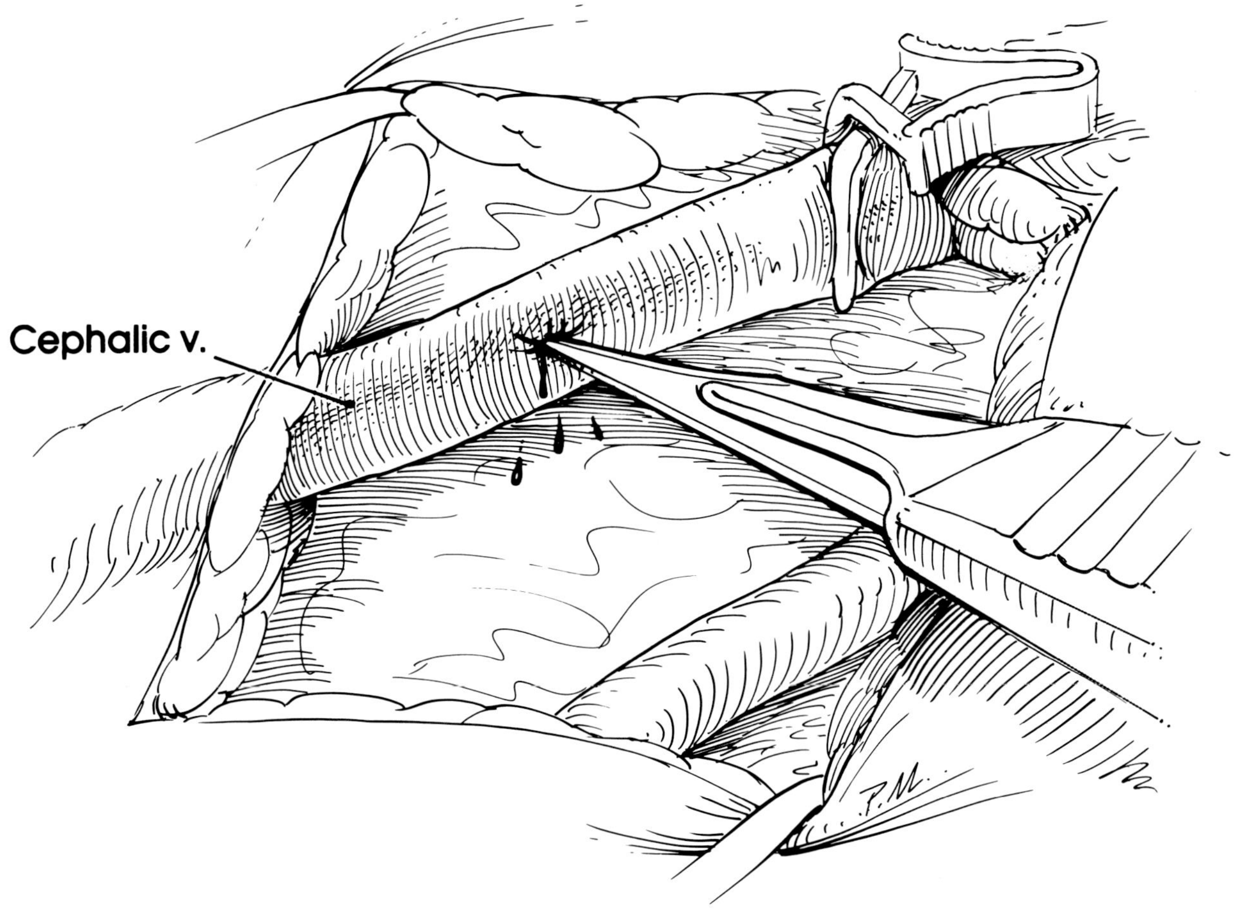

E

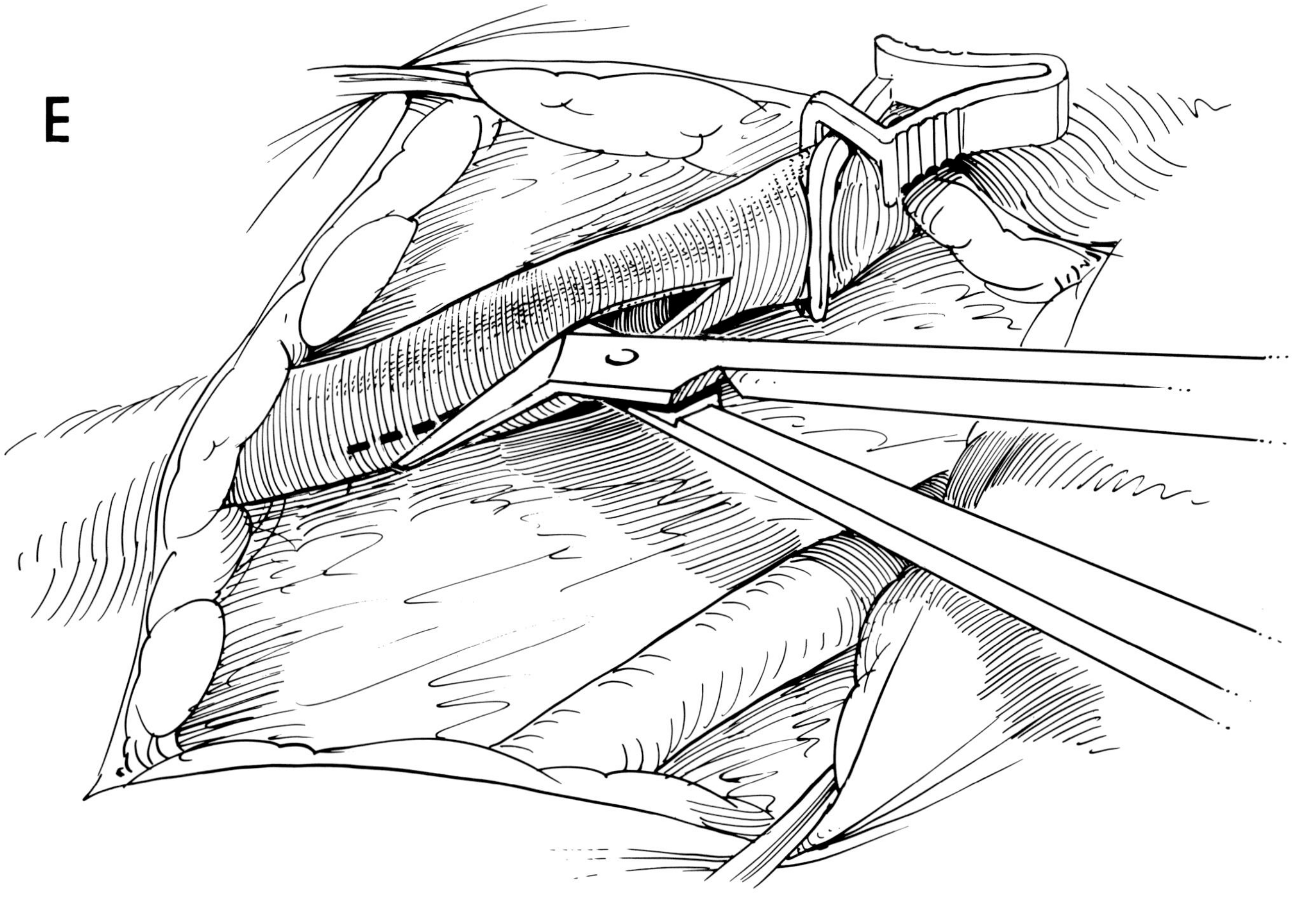

F Heparinization is performed, and a second bulldog clamp is placed on the vein.

G A microvascular bulldog clamp is placed proximally on the radial artery, with care taken not to fracture the intima. Then an arteriotomy incision is made that is identical in size and position to the venotomy incision.

F

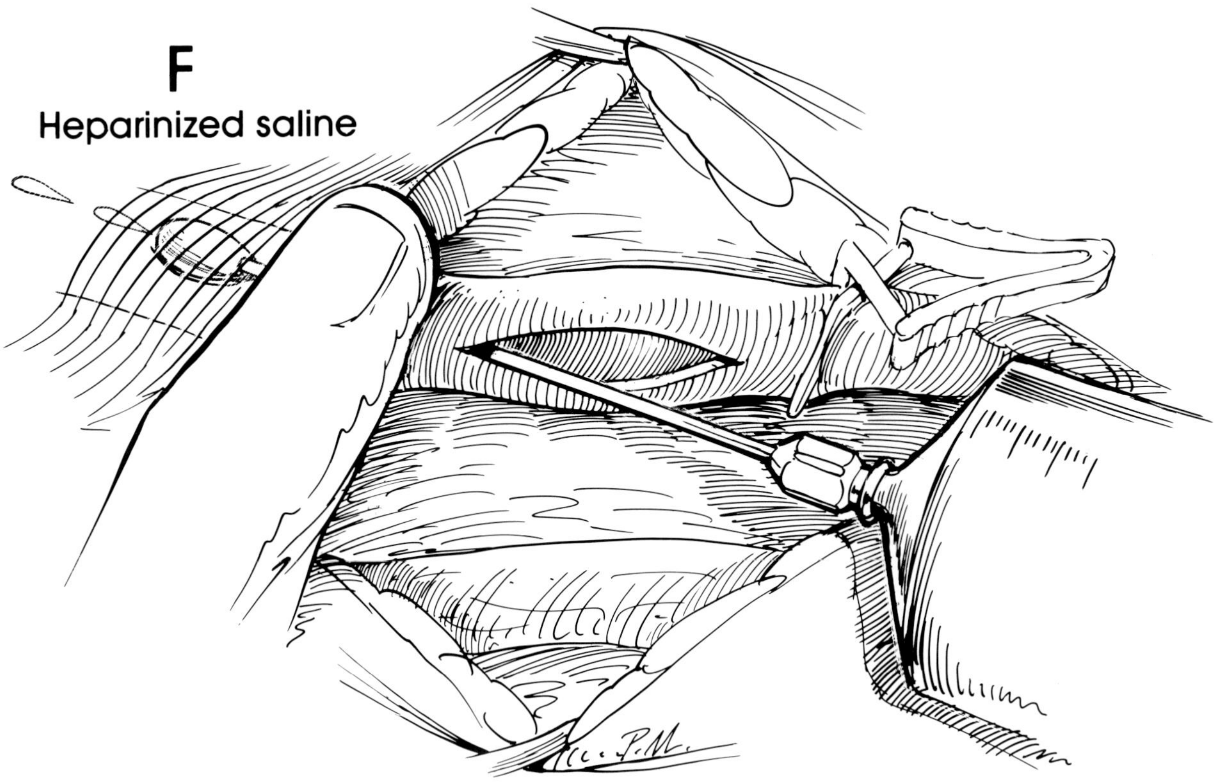

G

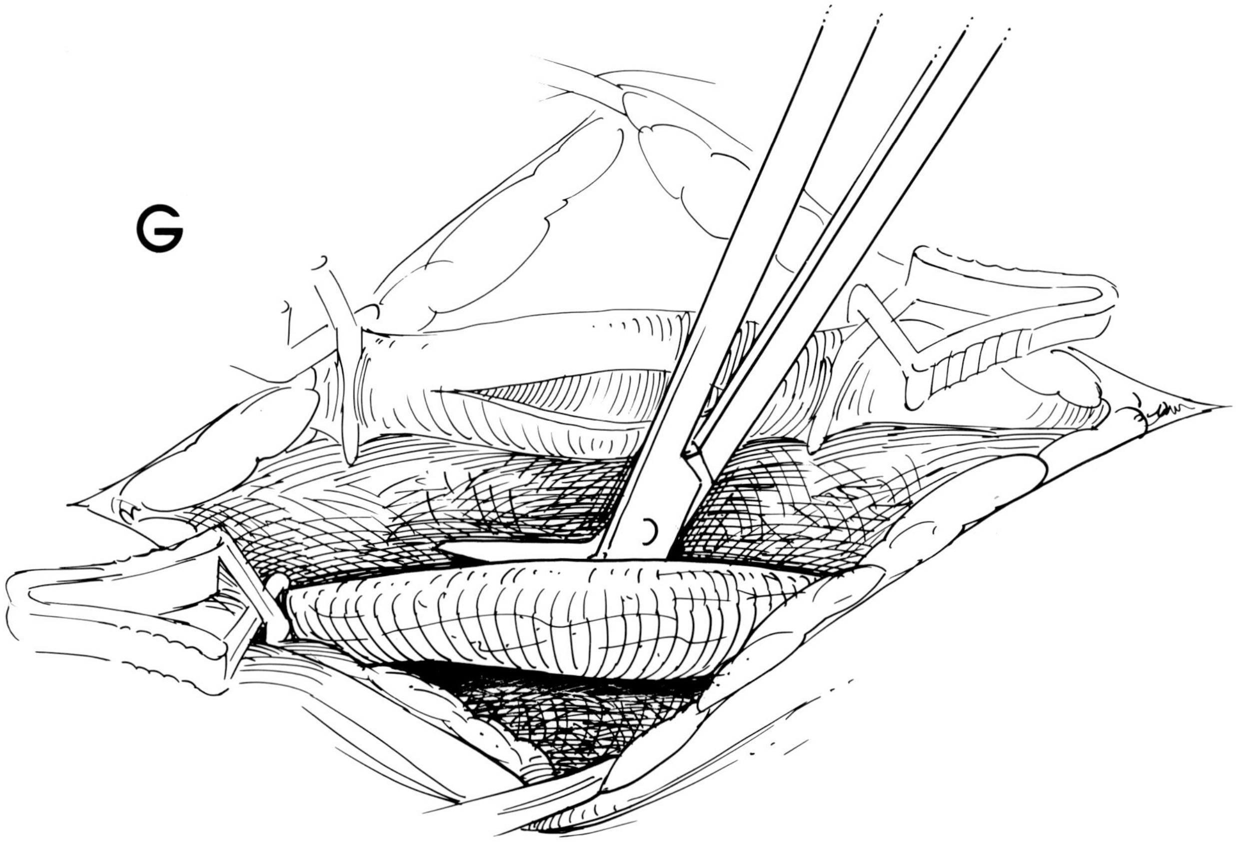

H A running 7-0 double-armed polypropylene vascular suture is used to anastomose the inferior borders of the arteriotomy and venotomy.

I After the underside of the anastomosis has been completed, the superior aspect is closed in an identical fashion and the suture is tied.

H

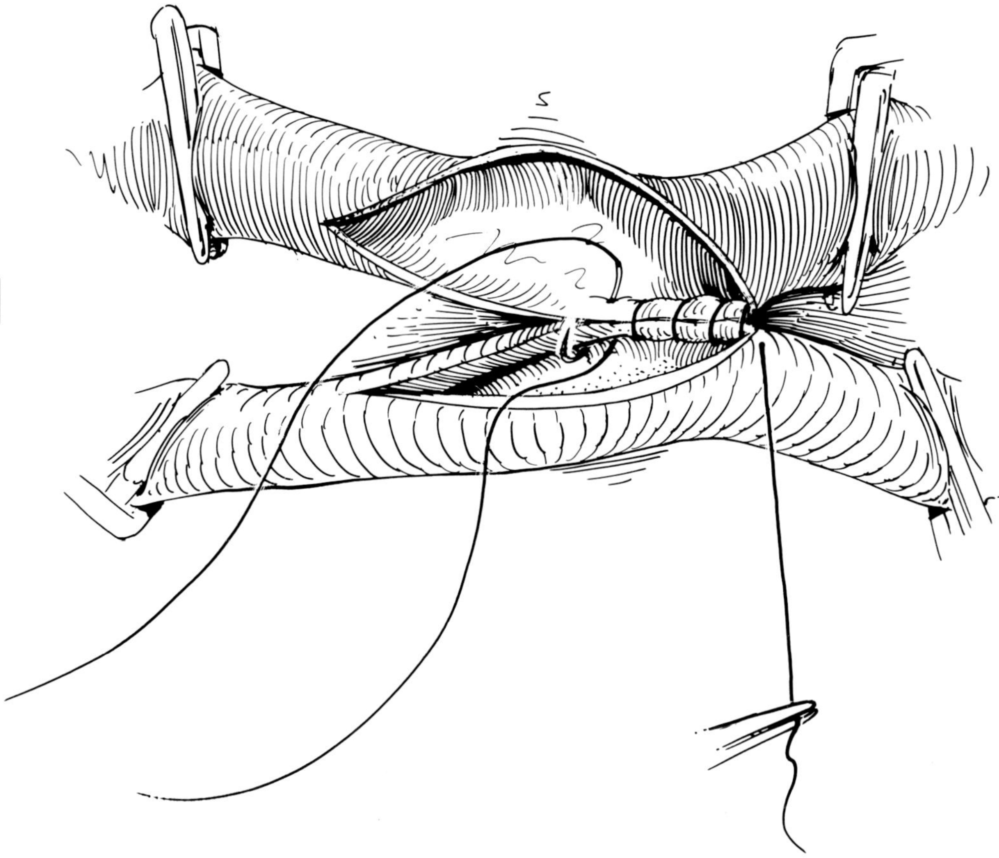

I

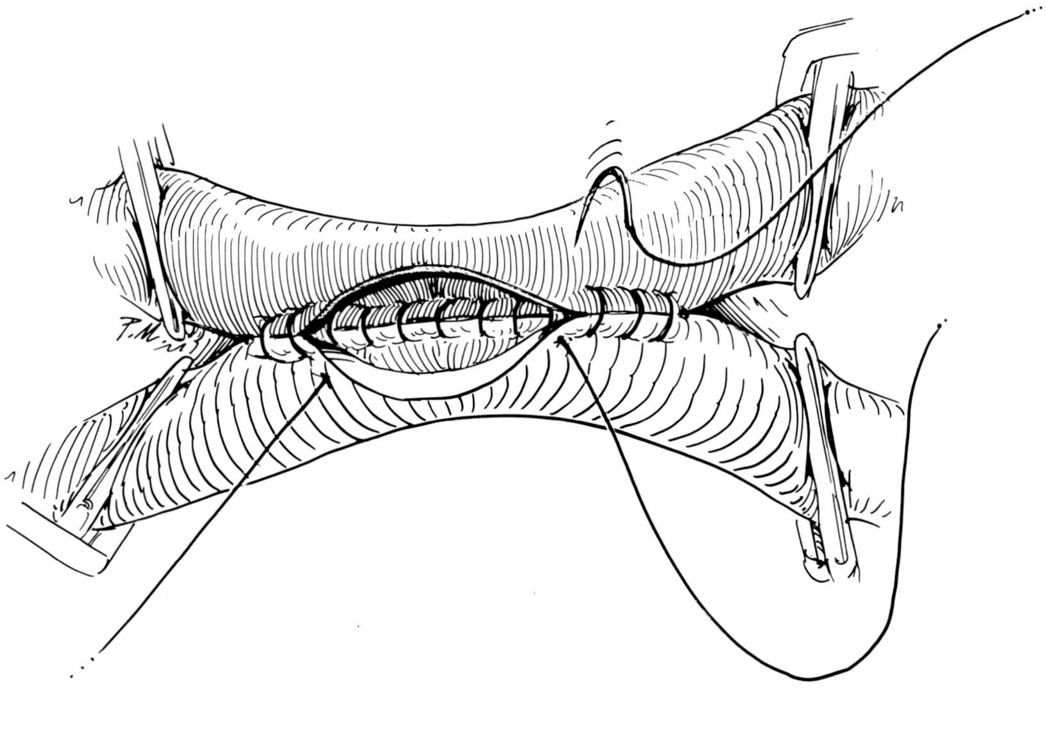

J Clamps are removed, and the fistula is allowed to fill. The anastomosis is inspected for leaks. The vessels should lie without tension or kinks.

K A palpable pulse and thrill indicate adequate function of the fistula. The incision is closed with a single layer of 3-0 absorbable suture for the subcutaneous tissue and with staples for the skin.

J

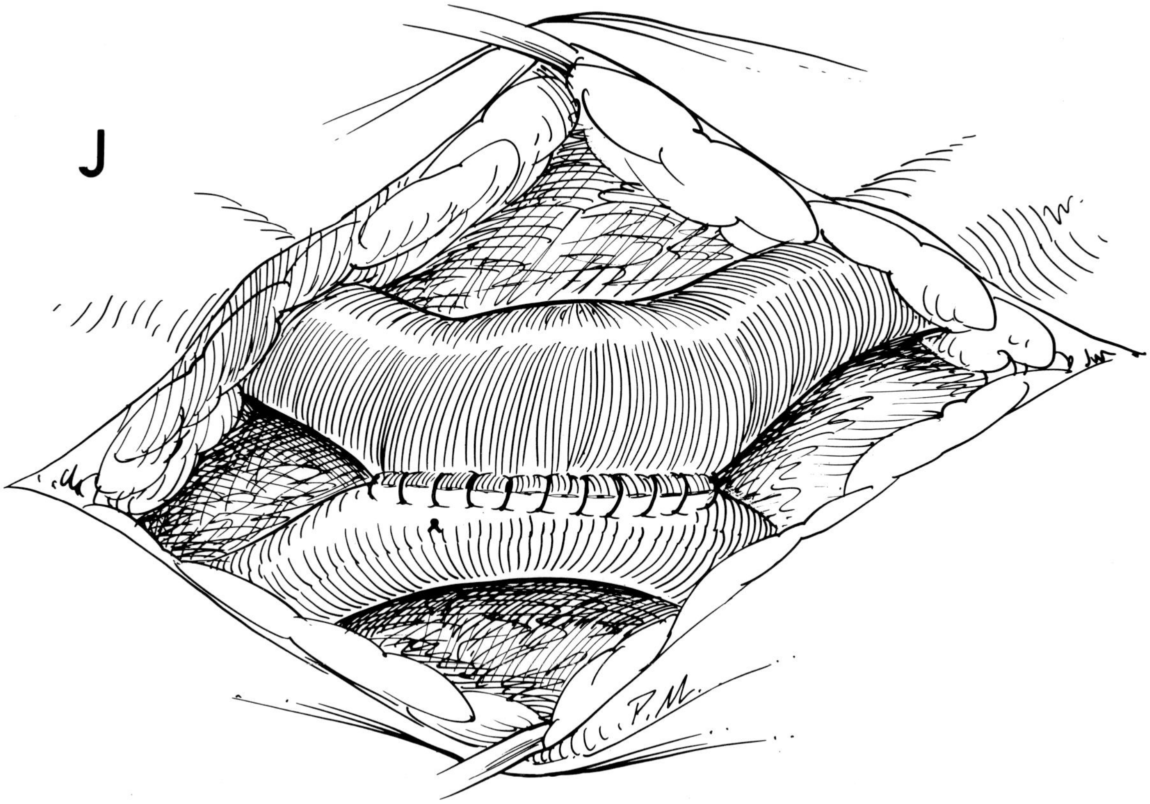

K

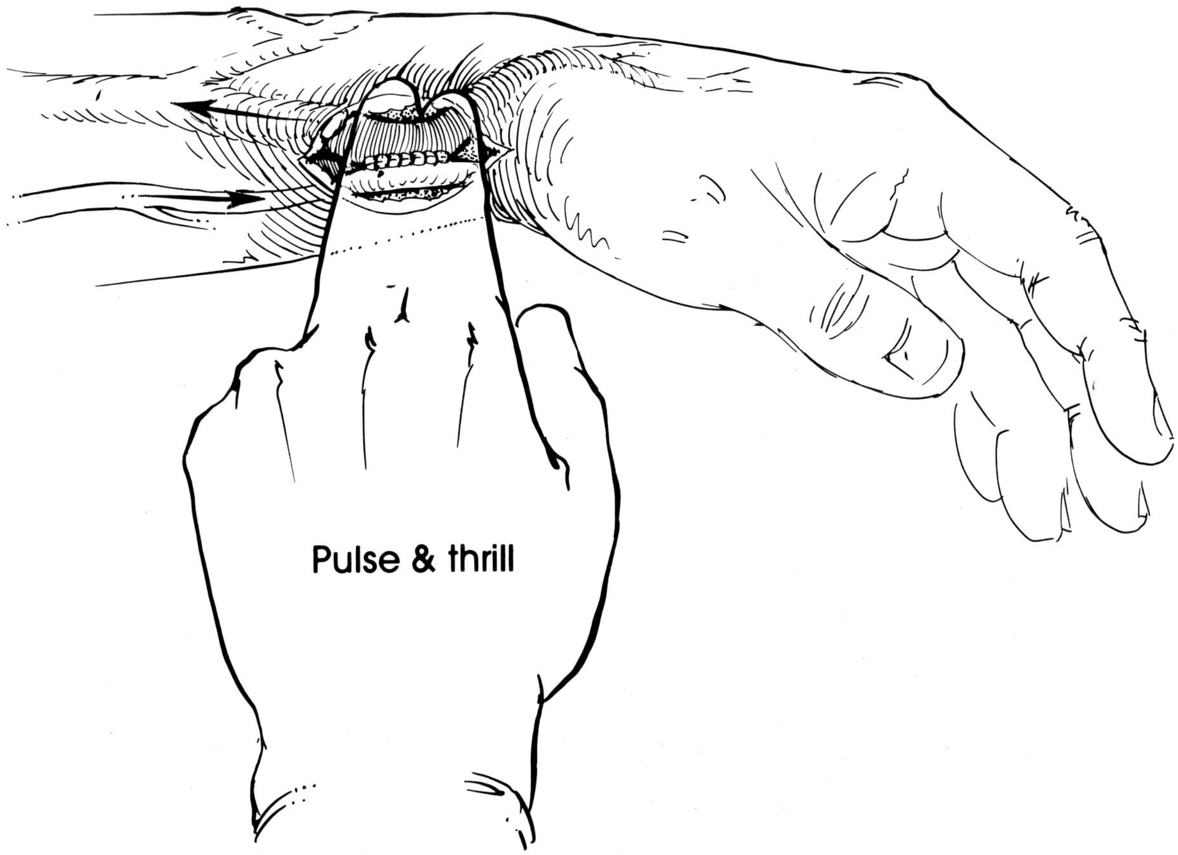

End-to-Side Fistula

A A skin incision is made, and the cephalic vein and radial artery are identified and mobilized. A distal ligature is placed on the vein.

B The cephalic vein is then divided immediately proximal to the ligature to allow adequate vessel length for construction of the flared end-to-side anastomosis.

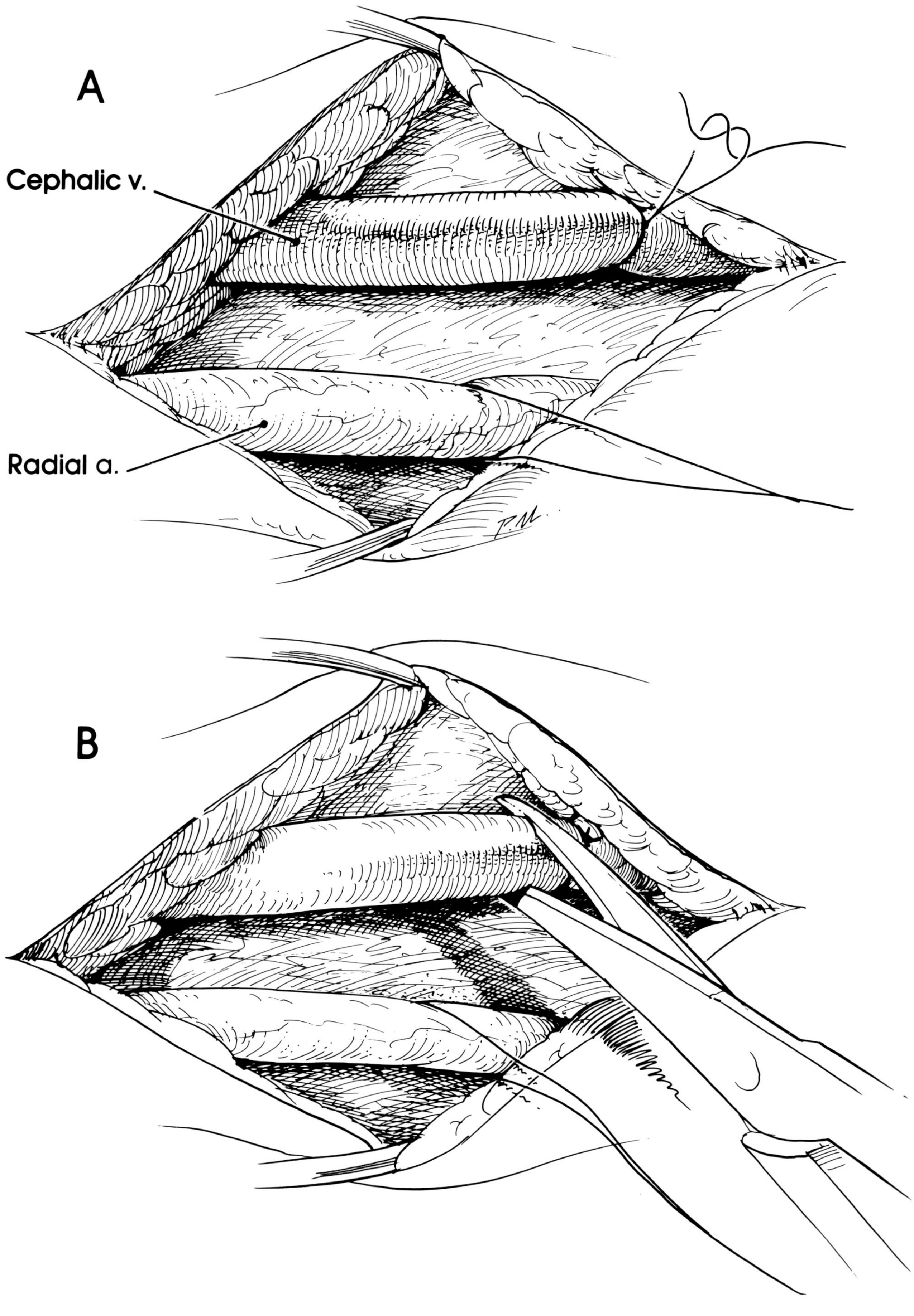
A
Cephalic v.
Radial a.
B

C The vein is irrigated with heparinized saline and clamped.

D A microvascular bulldog clamp is used to stop the arterial inflow, and an arteriotomy is made with a no. 11 blade. The arteriotomy is made along the medial aspect of the vessel to avoid kinking at the anastomosis.

C

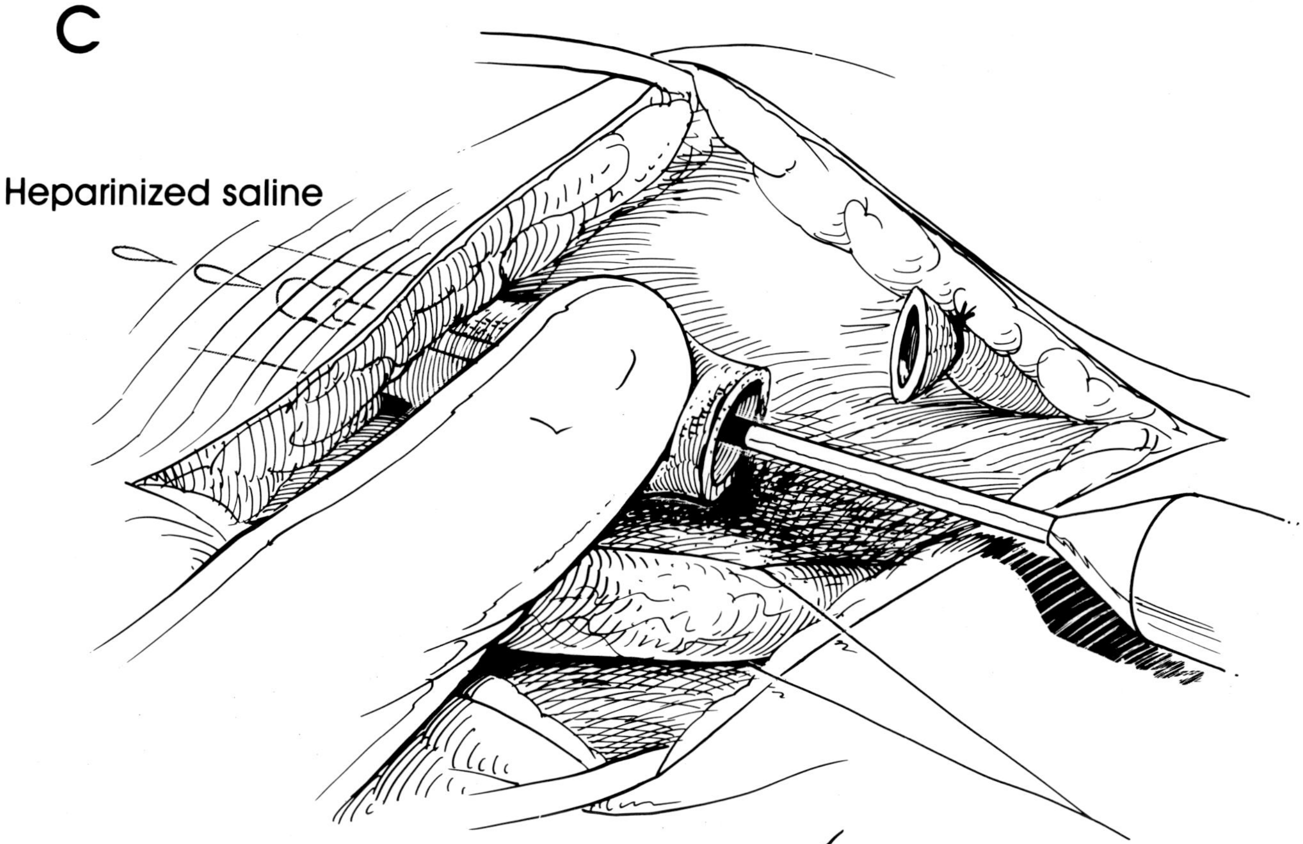

D

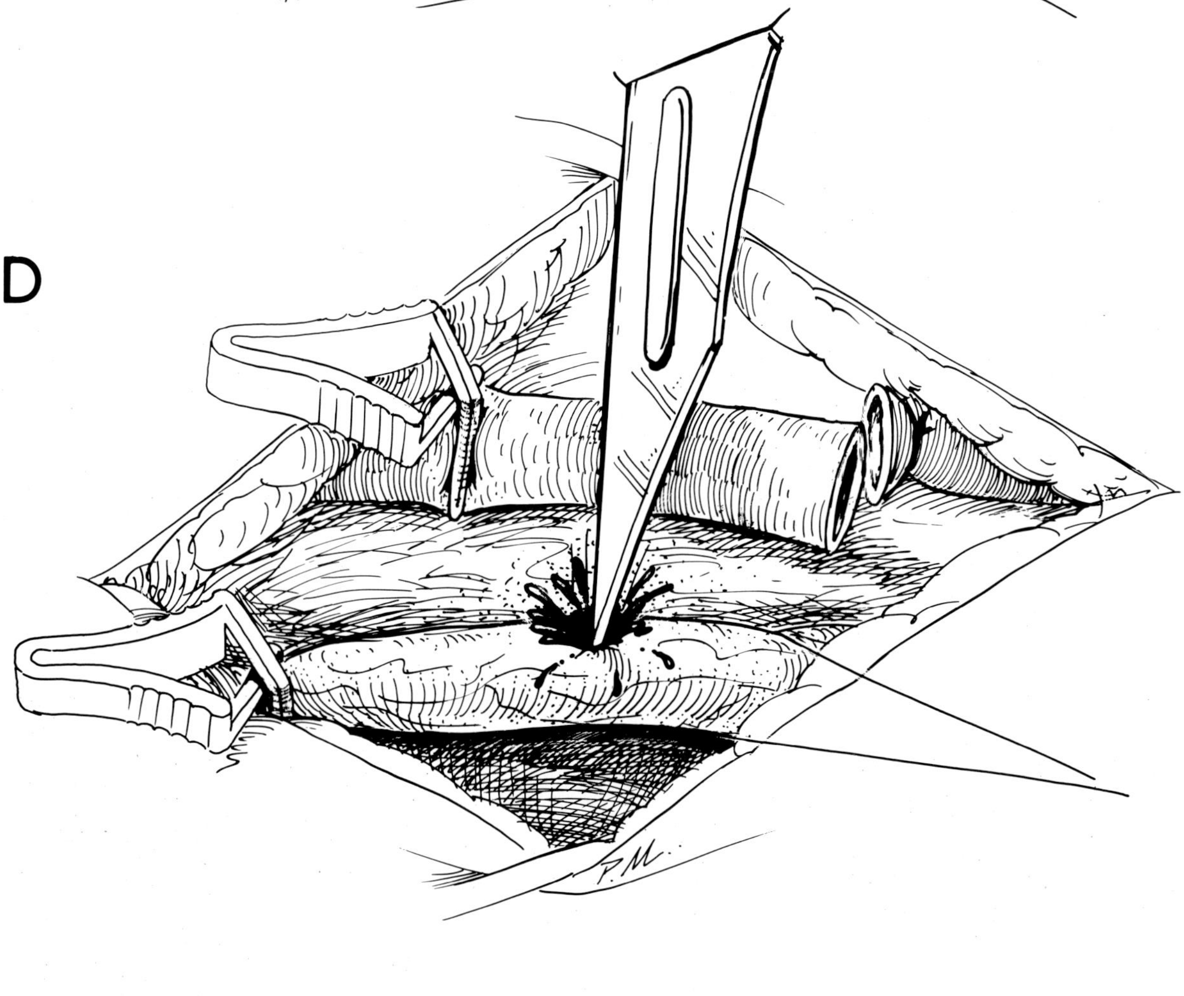

E The arteriotomy is extended to one and one-half times the vessel diameter.

F The radial artery is heparinized distally.

E

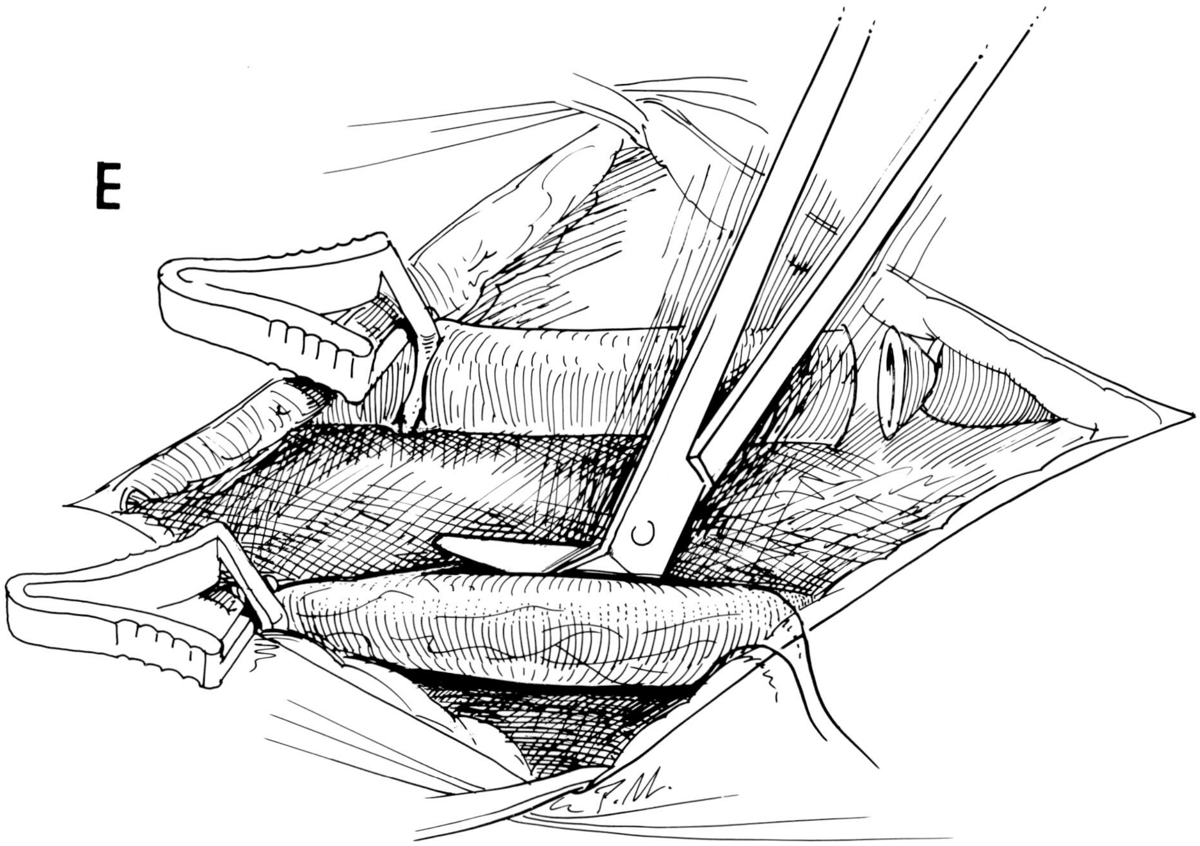

F

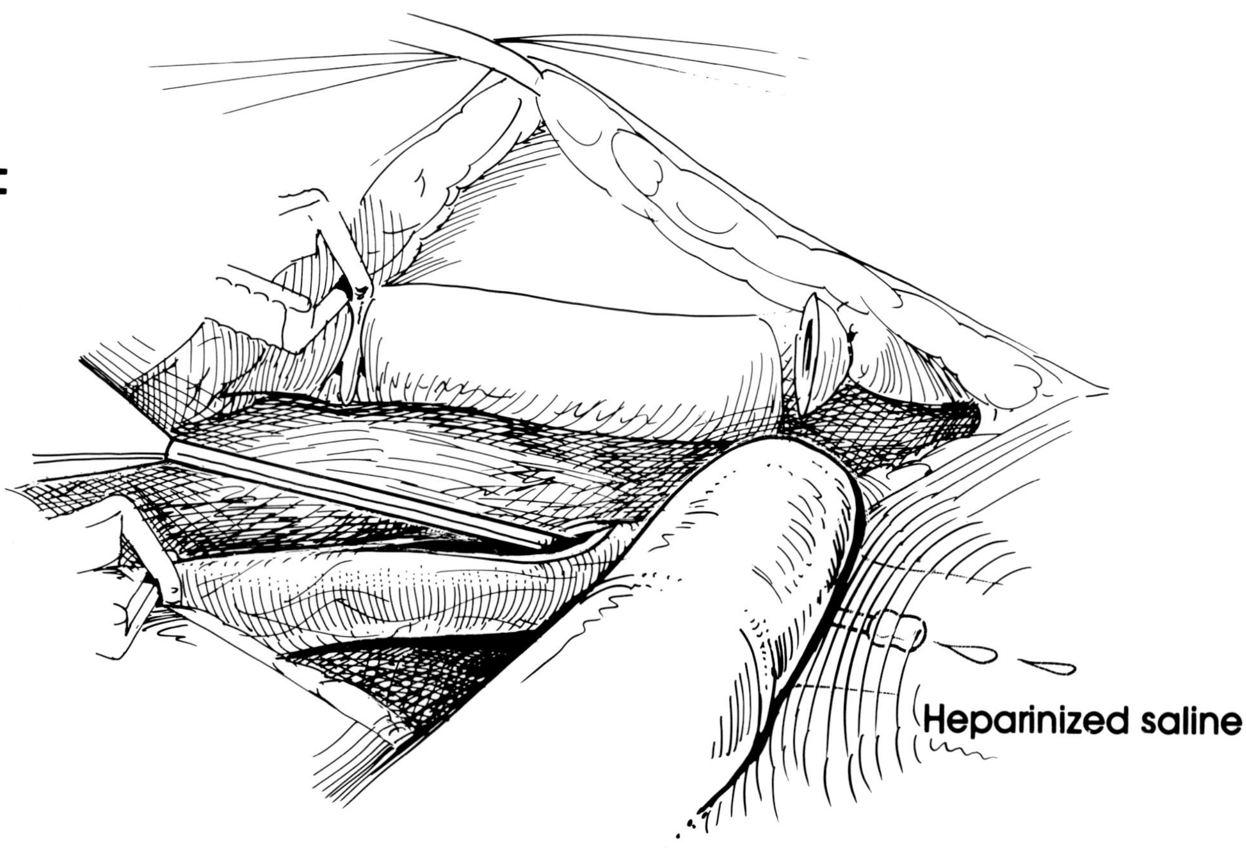

G The cephalic vein is tapered to accommodate the length and position of the arteriotomy.

H The inferior side of the anastomosis is constructed with running 7-0 polypropylene suture.

G

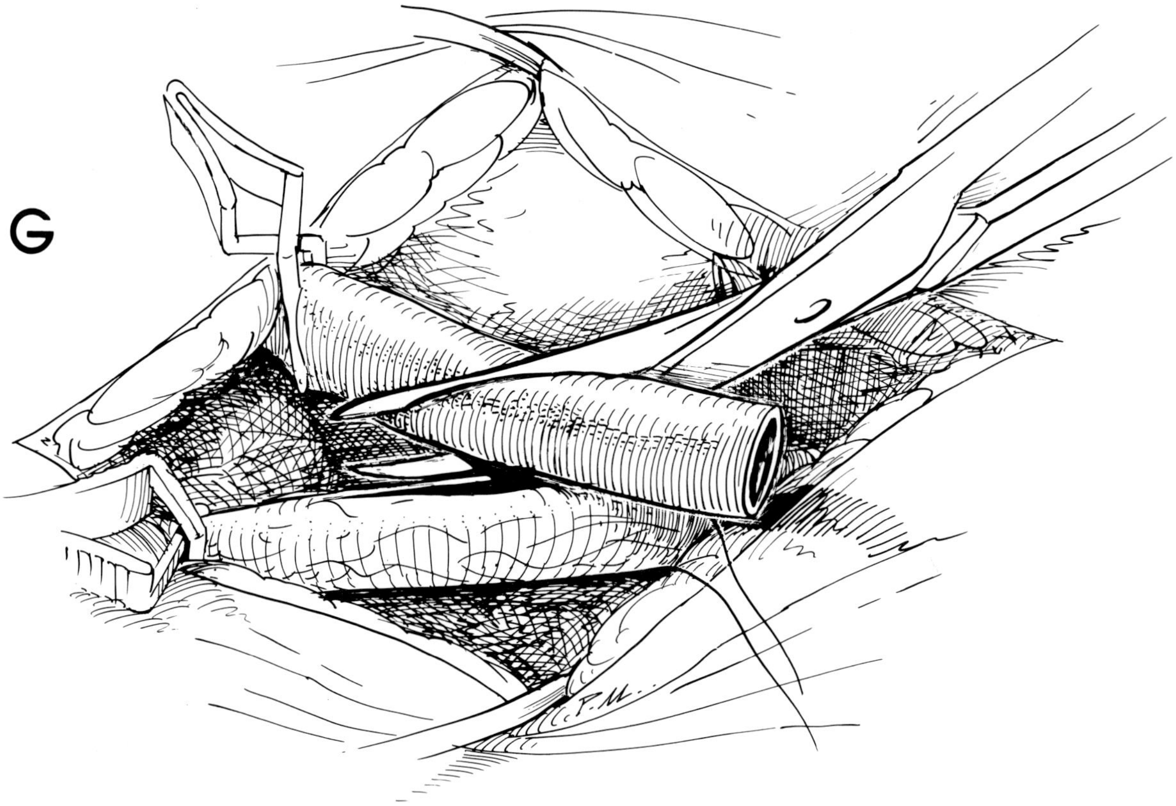

H

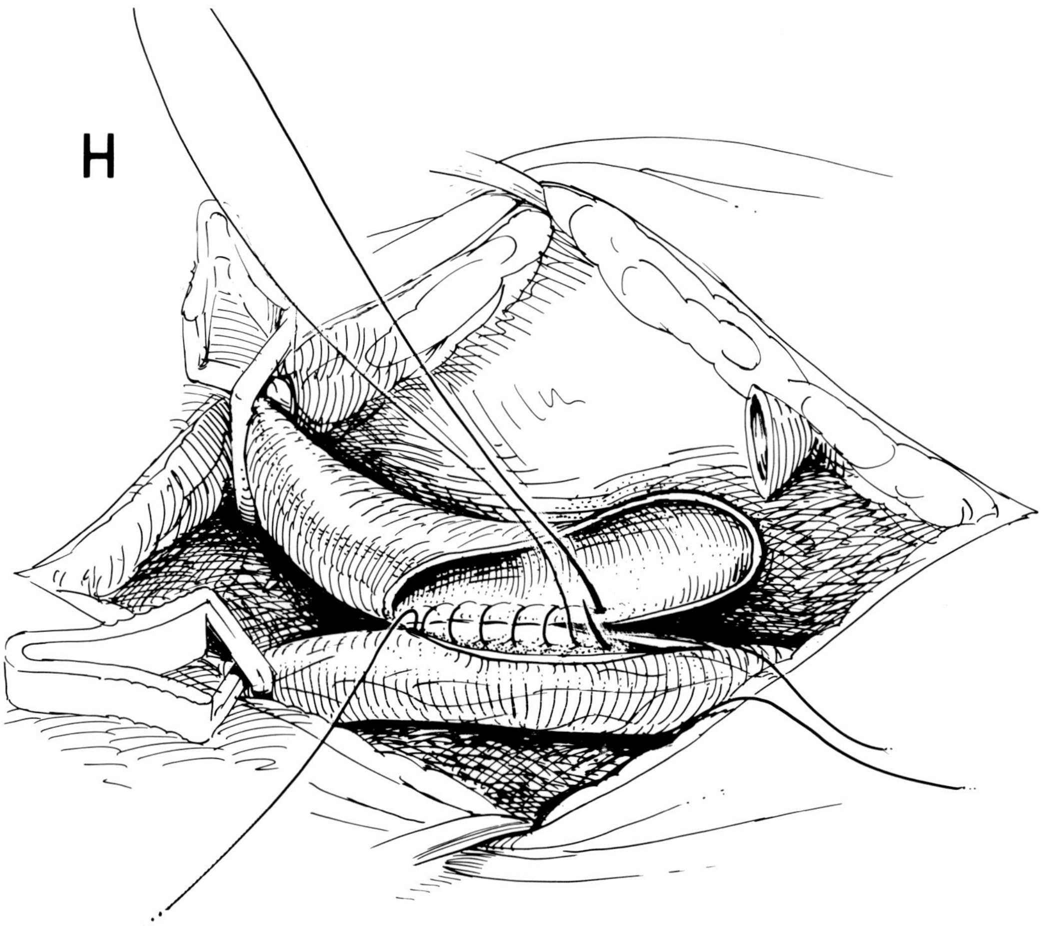

I Once the anastomosis is completed, the clamps are removed, allowing the end-to-side fistula to fill.

J We recommend that the radial artery be tied with a 3-0 silk ligature immediately distal to the anastomosis, thereby converting the end-to-side fistula into a functional end-to-end configuration.

I

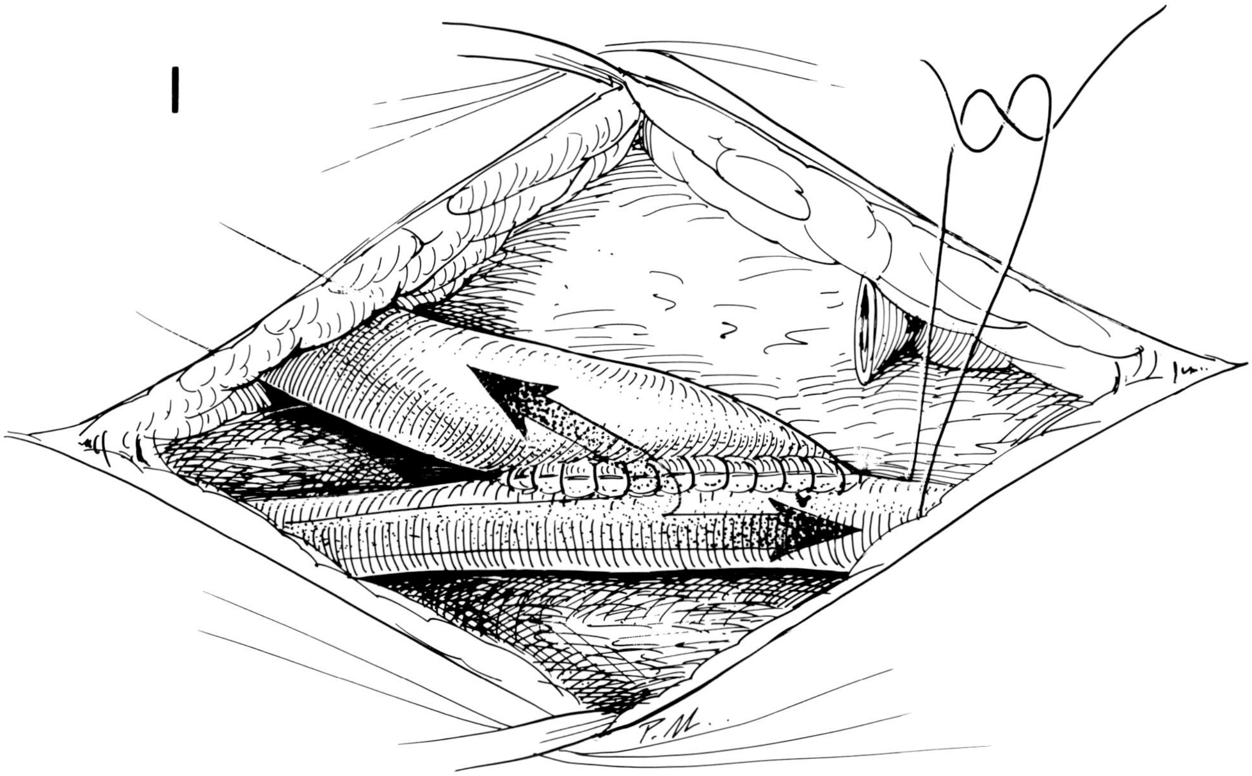

J

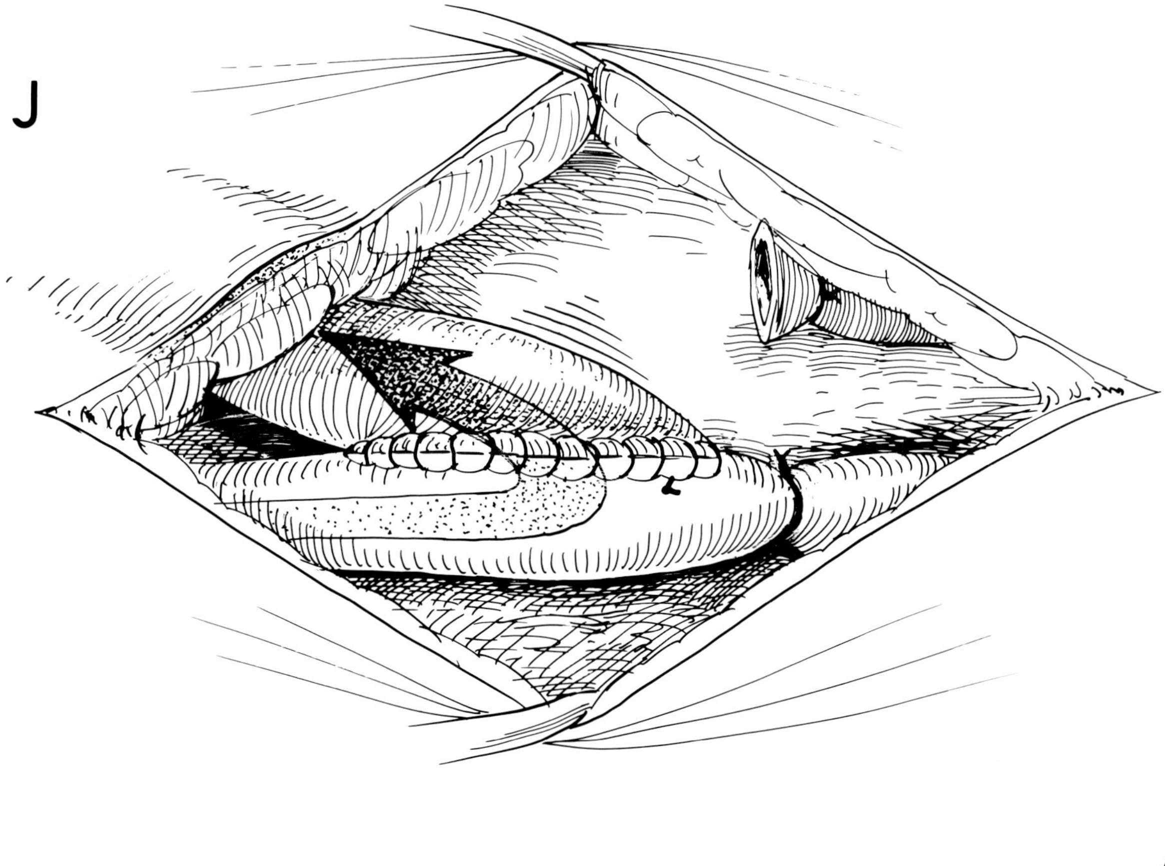

K A palpable pulse and thrill confirm appropriate function of the fistula. The incision is reapproximated in the standard fashion.

This end-to-side fistula can be constructed with the technical ease of an end-to-side anastomosis while procuring the preferable hemodynamics of the more technically difficult, true end-to-end configuration.

K

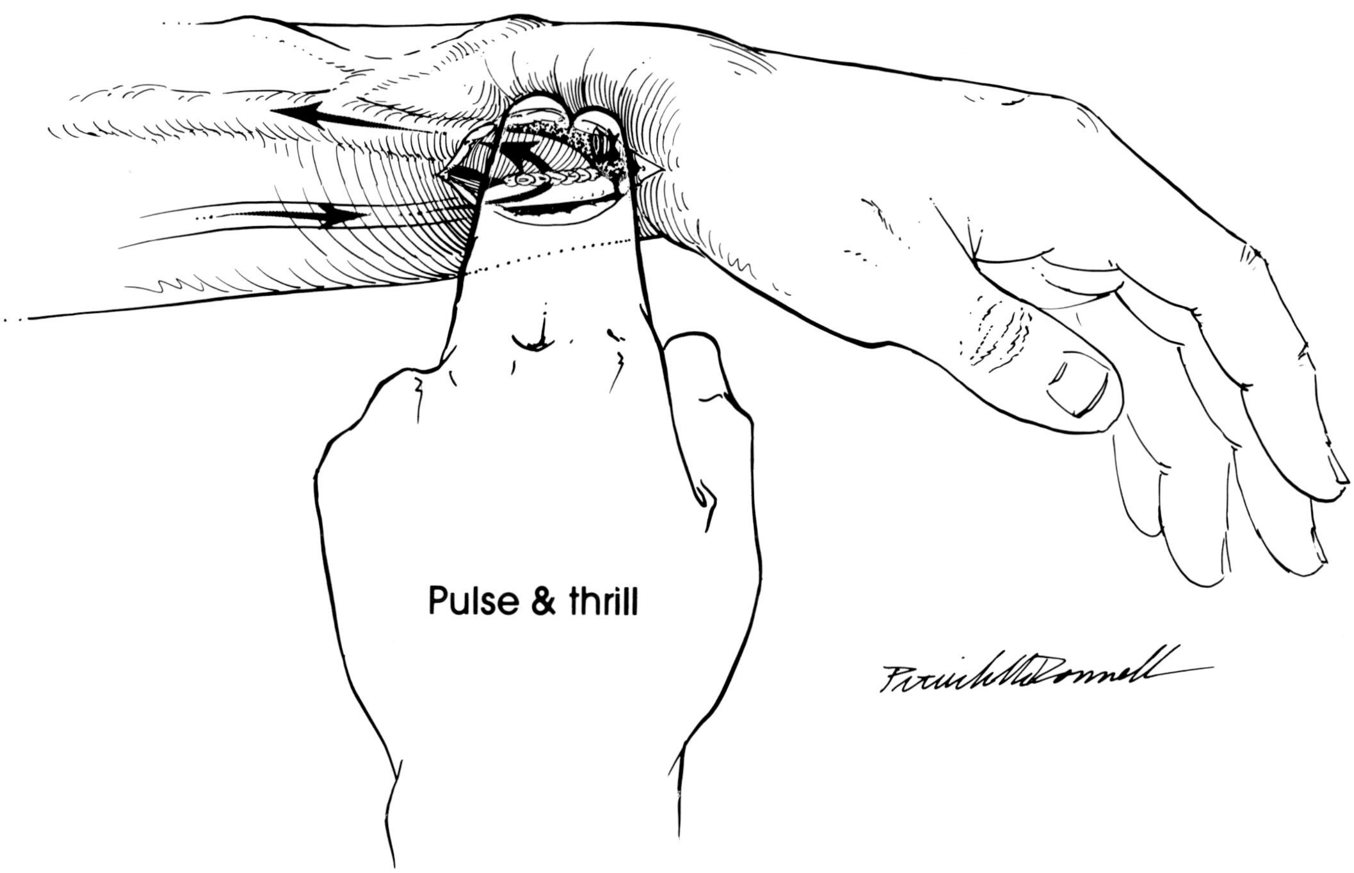

End-to-End Fistula

A The cephalic vein and radial artery are mobilized sufficiently for the end-to-end anastomosis, and both vessels are encircled with 3-0 silk ligatures.

B The venous ligature is tied.

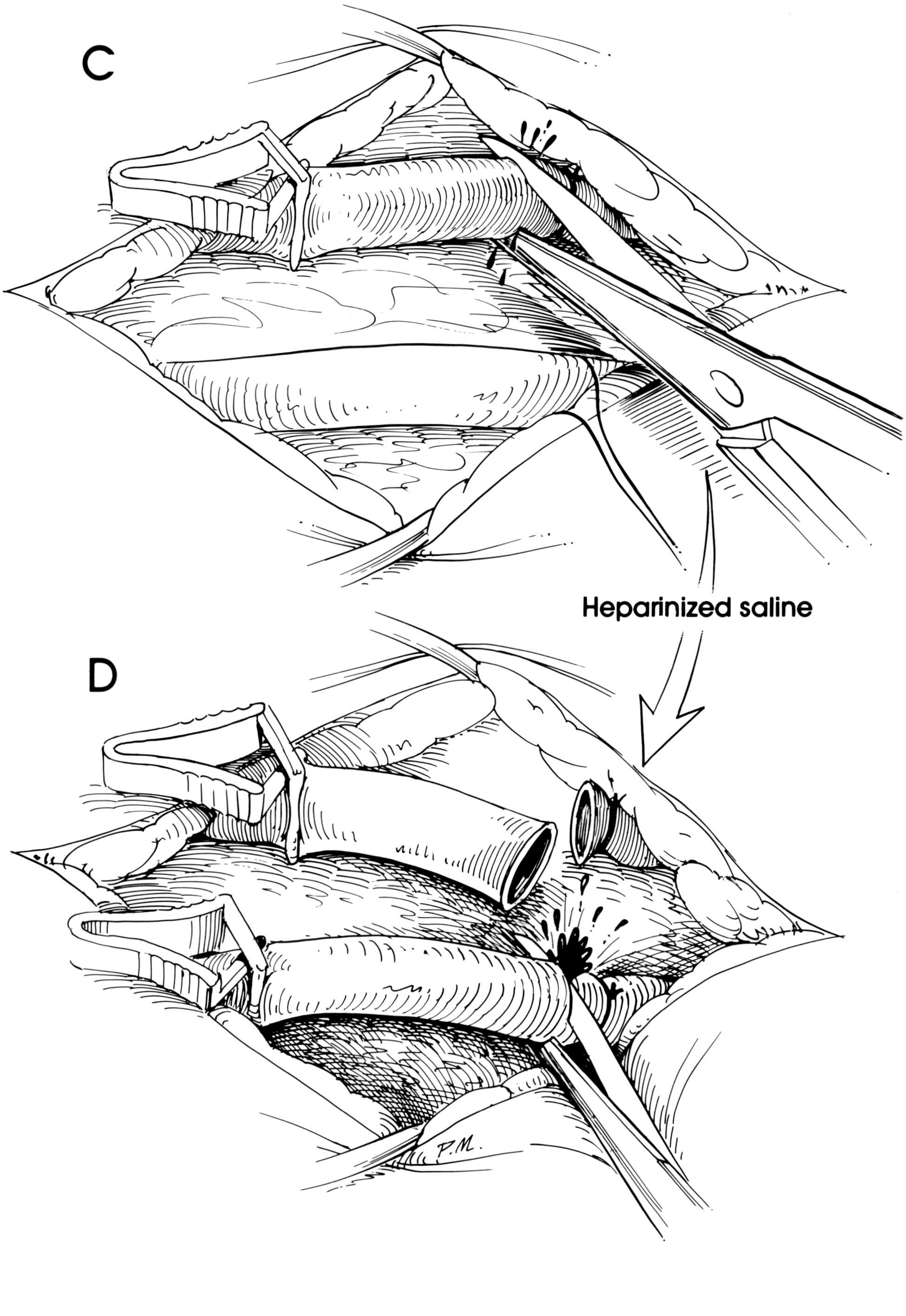
C
Heparinized saline
D
P.M.

E The arterial clamp is removed, the vessels are heparinized, and the clamp is replaced.

F The vessels are tapered to accommodate the flared end-to-end anastomosis.

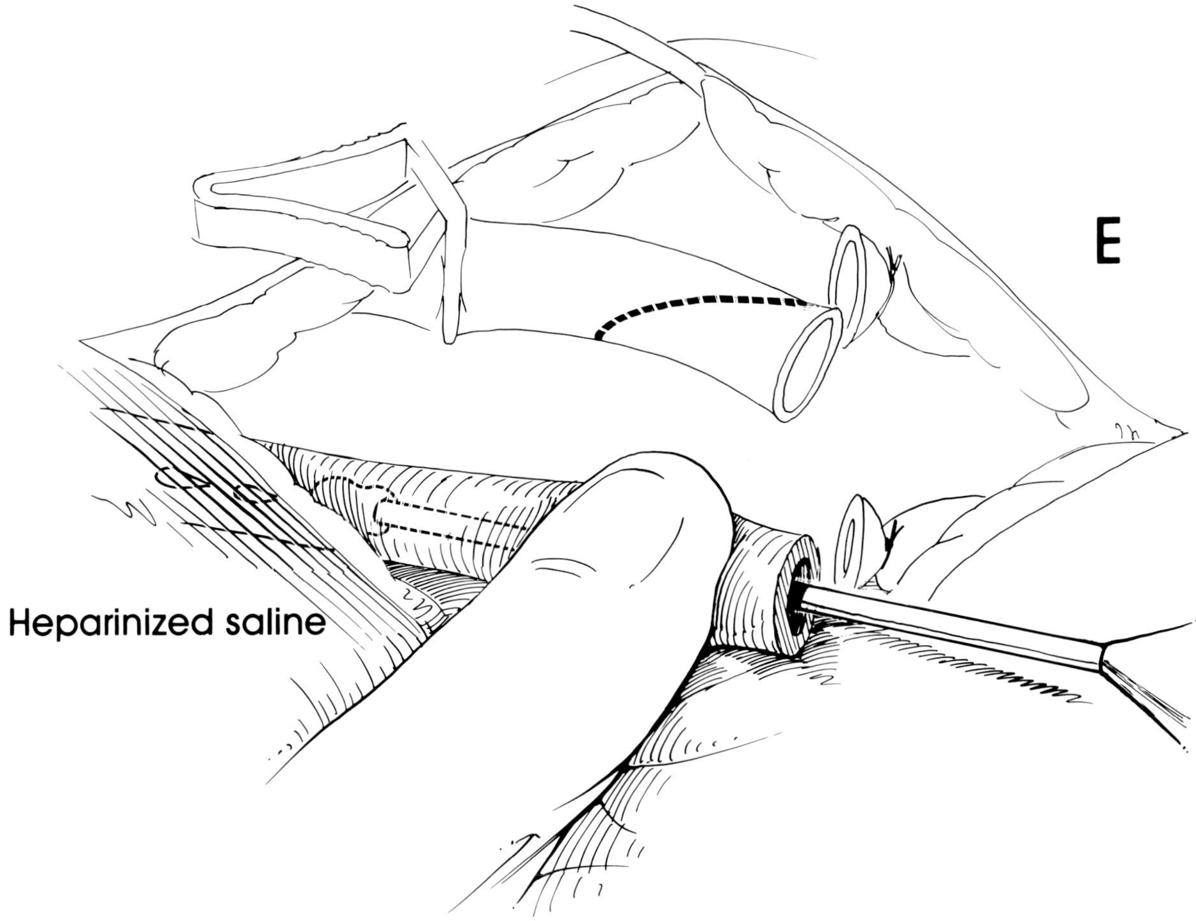

E

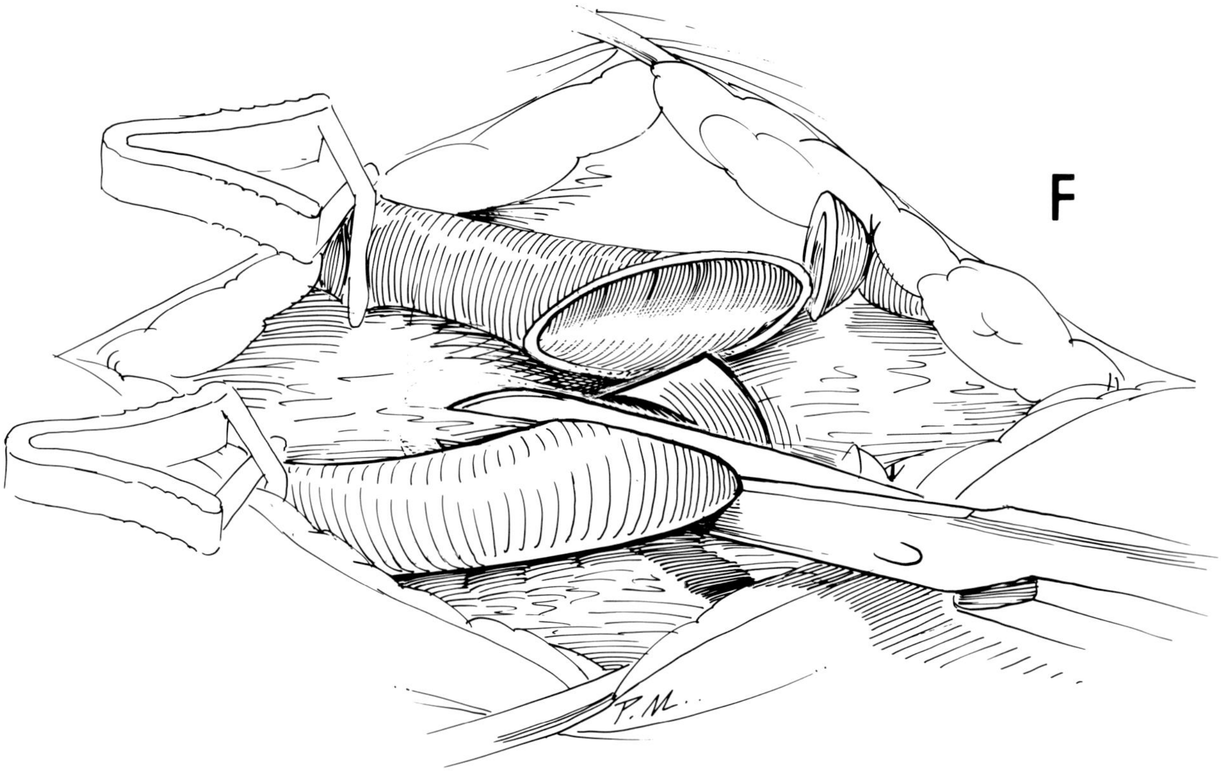

F

G The superior portion of the anastomosis is constructed with running 7-0 sutures, starting with the heel.

H The vessels are then rolled over so that their undersides are exposed. Starting from the heel, the rest of the fistula is constructed.

G

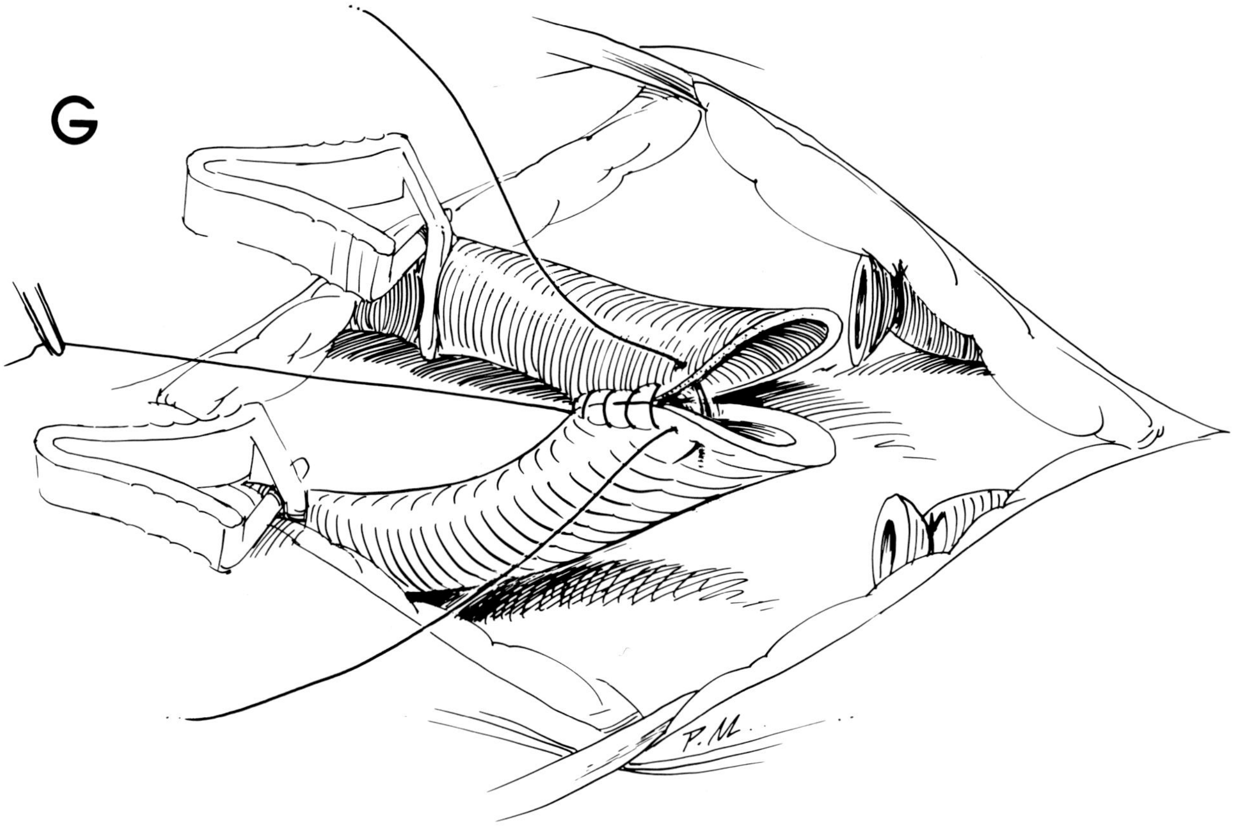

H

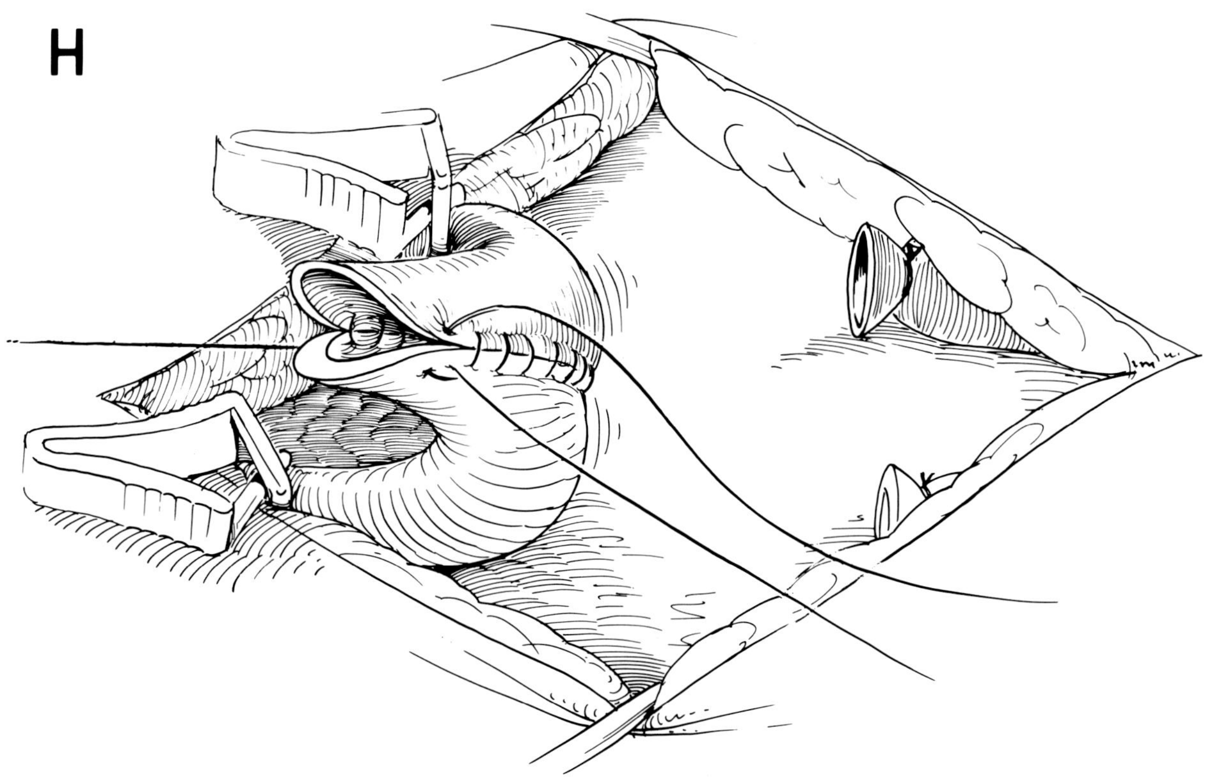

I Clamps are removed, and the anastomosis is inspected. The fistula is secured in place with a single 6-0 polypropylene stitch.

J A palpable pulse and thrill confirm function. The subcutaneous tissue and skin are reapproximated in routine fashion.

The true end-to-end anastomosis provides a fistula which is hemodynamically superior to the side-to-side variety, although its construction is technically more difficult than the functional end-to-end fistula.

I

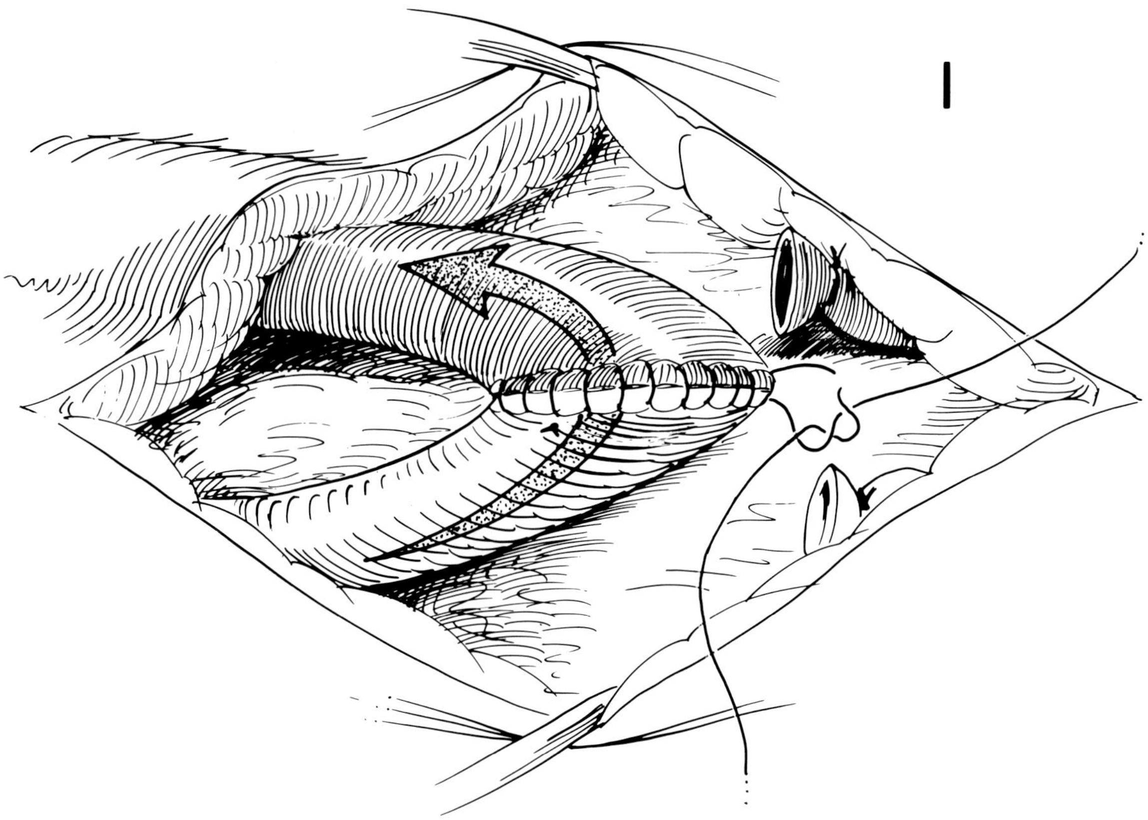

J

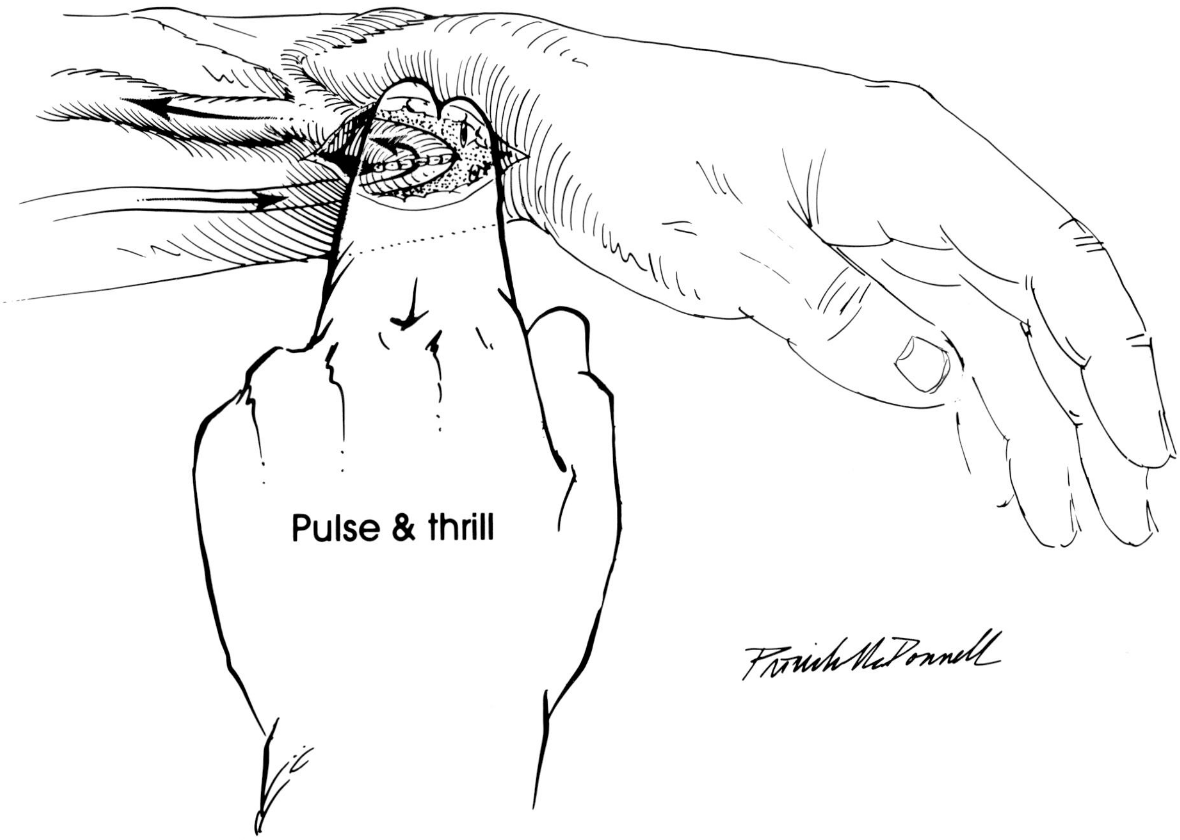

Complications of Primary Arteriovenous Fistulas

4

THE HEMODYNAMIC COMPLICATIONS associated with a Brescia-Cimino fistula can be attributed to the side-to-side configuration of the anastomosis. First, a steal syndrome may develop because of continuity between the radial and ulnar arteries after construction of the fistula. The flow through the fistula is such that blood from the palmar arch is drawn retrograde through the distal radial artery. Because of this phenomenon, digital arteries do not fill adequately and symptoms develop.

The other major hemodynamic complication is venous hypertension or arterialization of the hand. This "sore thumb" syndrome, as it is also known, is caused by the retrograde diversion of arterial flow into the distal cephalic vein. Such retrograde diversion is usually secondary to venous hyperplasia proximal to the fistula, but it can occur primarily. Correction of outflow tract obstruction secondary to venous hyperplasia is approached according to the length of the obstruction and availability of accessory veins in the vicinity of the fistula. Vein patch venoplasty works well in cases of short lesions; however, in the case of longer obstructions, a venovenous anastomosis is preferable to a long vein patch. Several modifications of the Brescia-Cimino fistula have been introduced to avoid these problems.

Arterial Steal Syndrome

A An incision approximately 5 cm long is made overlying the previously constructed fistula.

B The side-to-side radial artery–cephalic vein fistula is identified and mobilized. A 3-0 silk ligature is placed around the radial artery distal to the fistula, and the suture is tied. The subcutaneous tissue is closed with 3-0 absorbable suture, and the skin is reapproximated with staples.

C The distal radial artery ligature eliminates retrograde flow, thus allowing the ulnar artery to fill the palmar arch and digital branches.

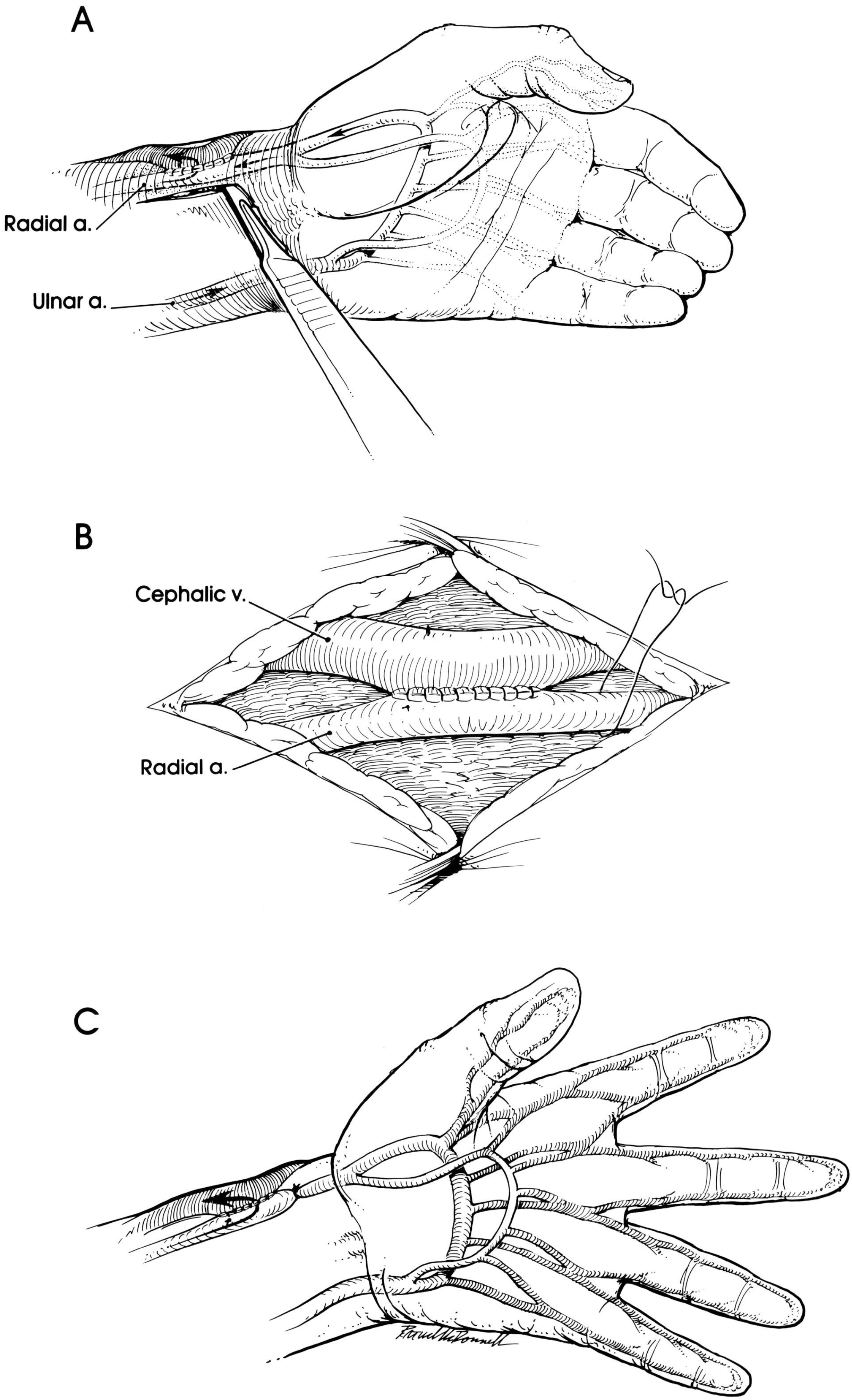
A
Radial a.
Ulnar a.
B
Cephalic v.
Radial a.
C

Outflow Tract Obstruction

Patch Graft Angioplasty

A An incision is made overlying the previously constructed primary fistula.

B The fistula, radial artery, and cephalic vein are identified and mobilized. The cephalic vein immediately distal to the fistula is tied with a 3-0 silk suture.

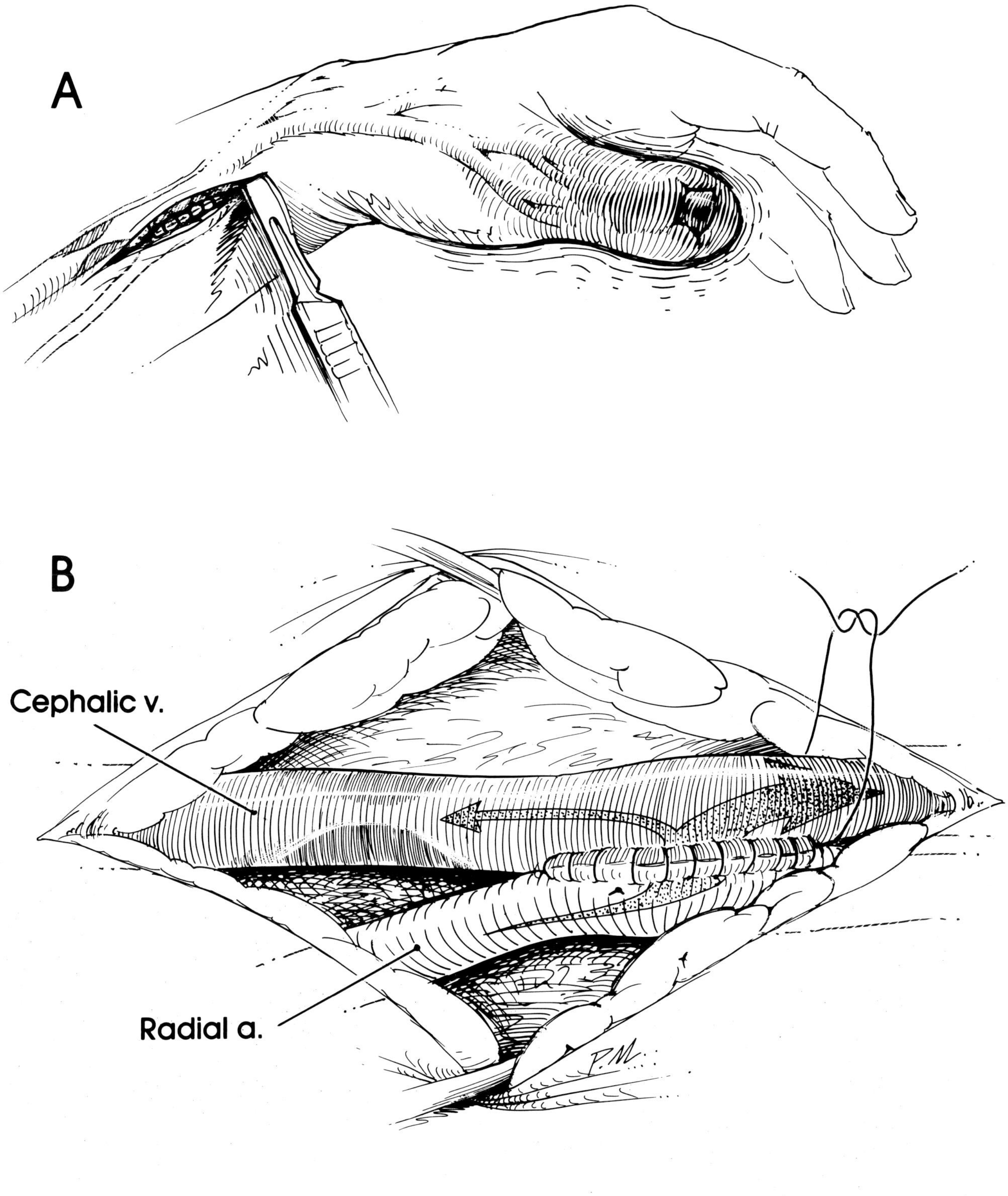
A
B
Cephalic v.
Radial a.

C The vein proximal to the fistula is opened at the level of the stenosis previously identified on angiography.

D A microvascular bulldog clamp is placed immediately proximal to the fistula, and the venotomy is extended to points proximal and distal to the stenotic lesion.

C

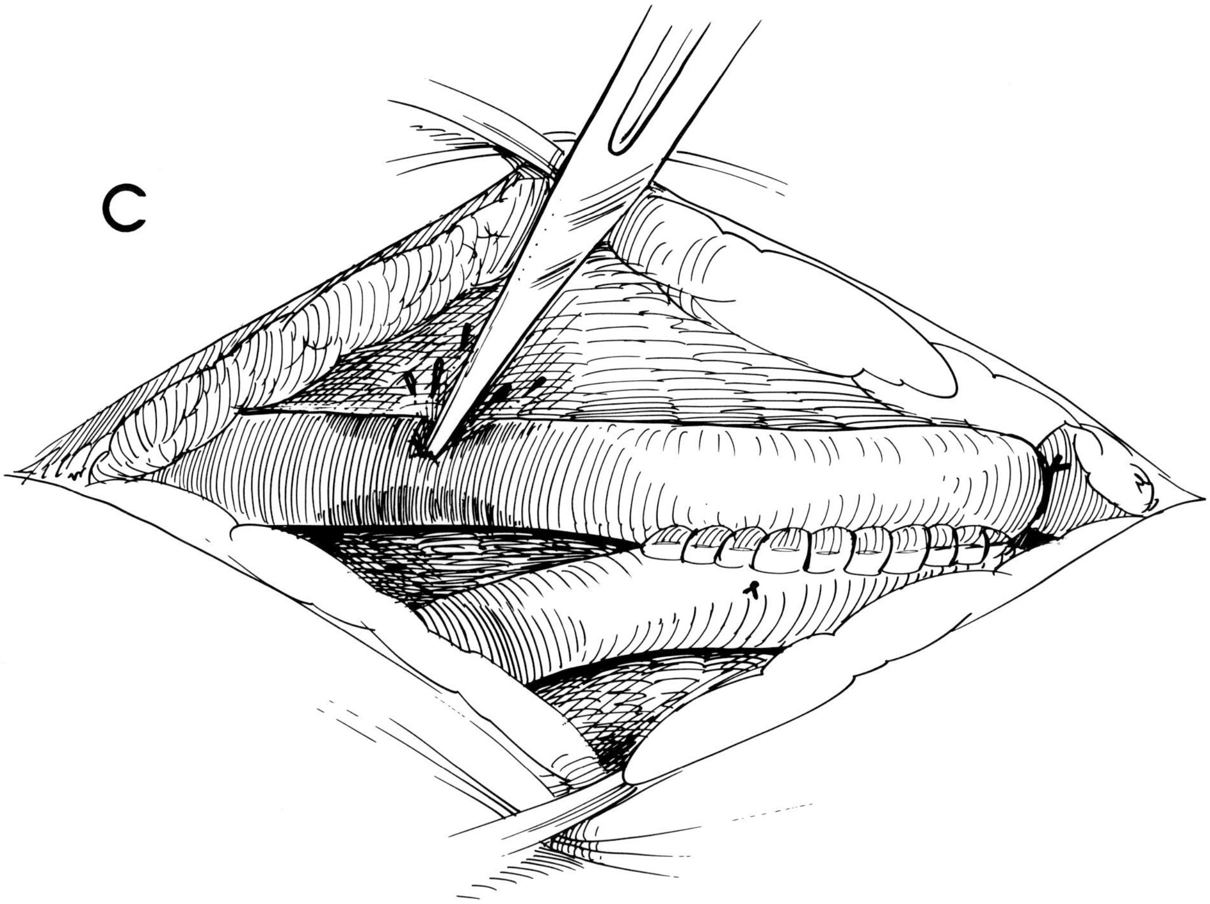

D

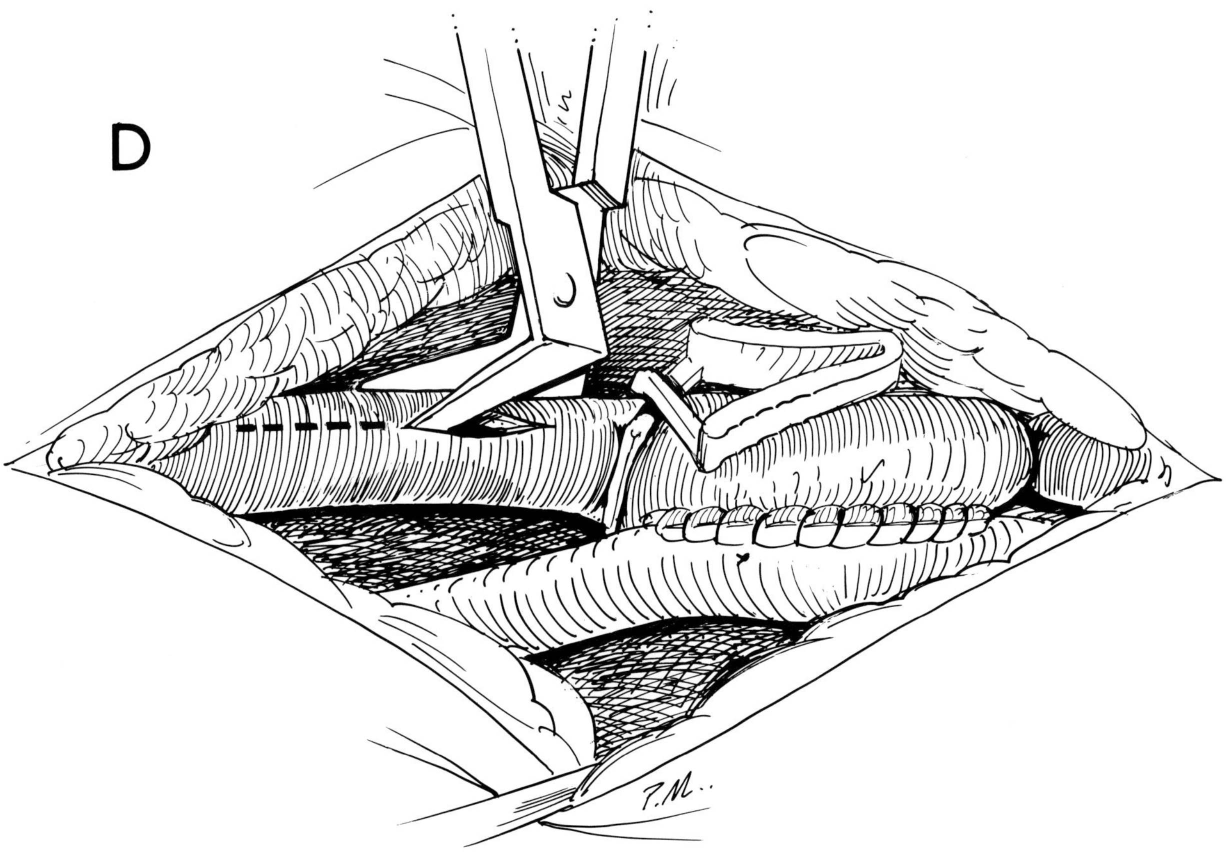

E The bulldog clamp is removed, the fistula and radial artery are heparinized, and the clamp is replaced. The vein is then heparinized.

F The distal cephalic vein is exposed and mobilized. A 3-0 silk ligature is tied, and the venous segment between the two ties is removed and prepared as a vein patch.

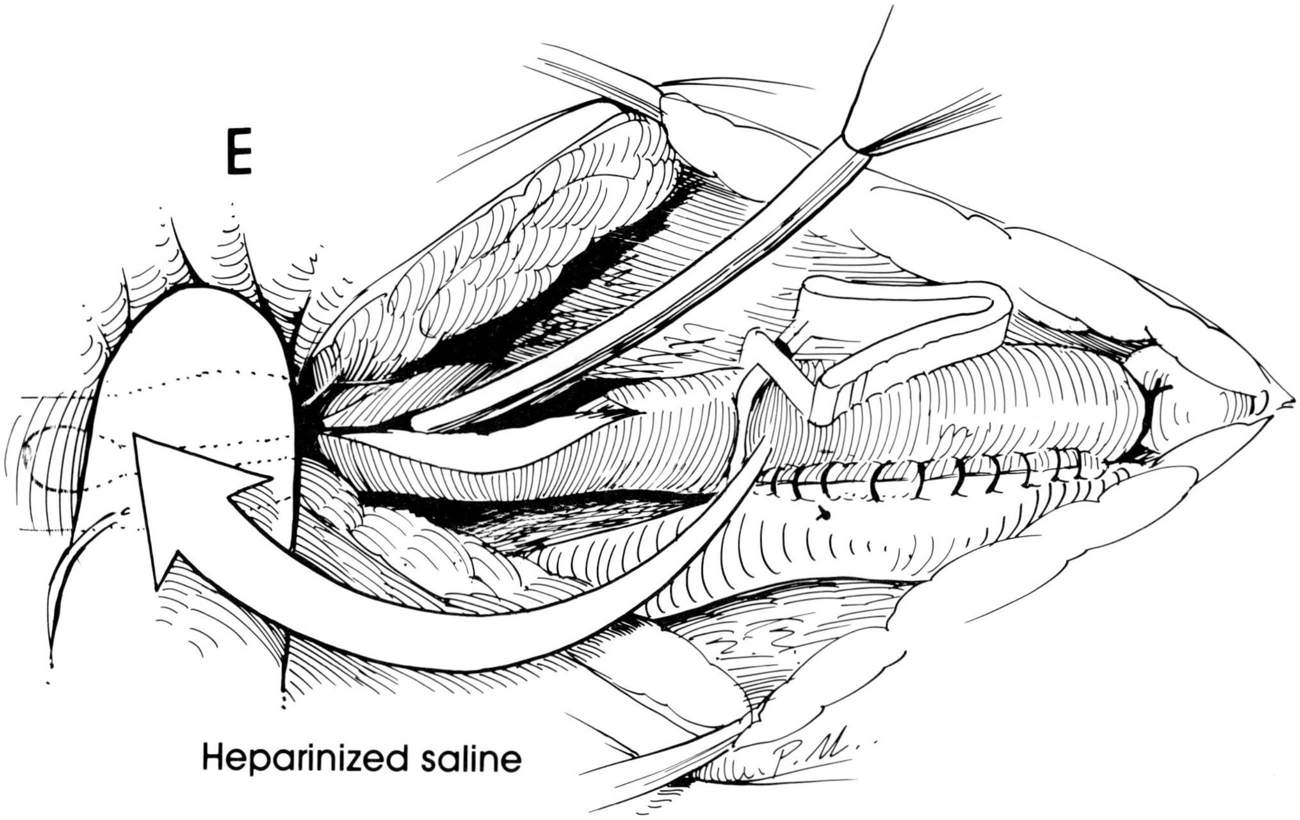
E
Heparinized saline

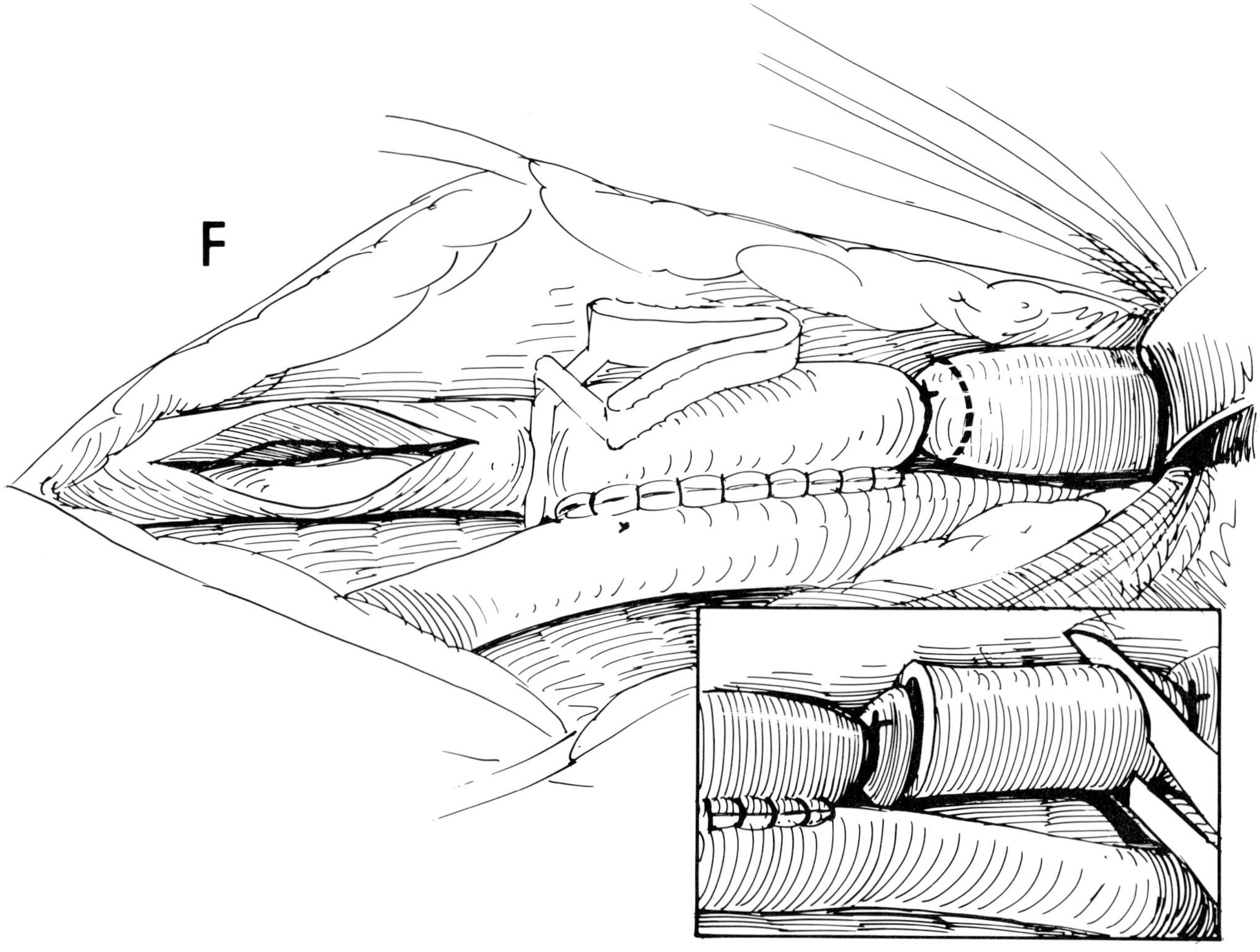
F

G The vein patch is incorporated into the venotomy with running 7-0 polypropylene suture, and the clamp is removed.

H A palpable pulse and thrill confirm adequate outflow tract enlargement with the patch graft venoplasty. The incision is closed in the usual fashion.

Hypertension of the hand has been corrected by ligation of the distal cephalic vein, which eliminates retrograde flow.

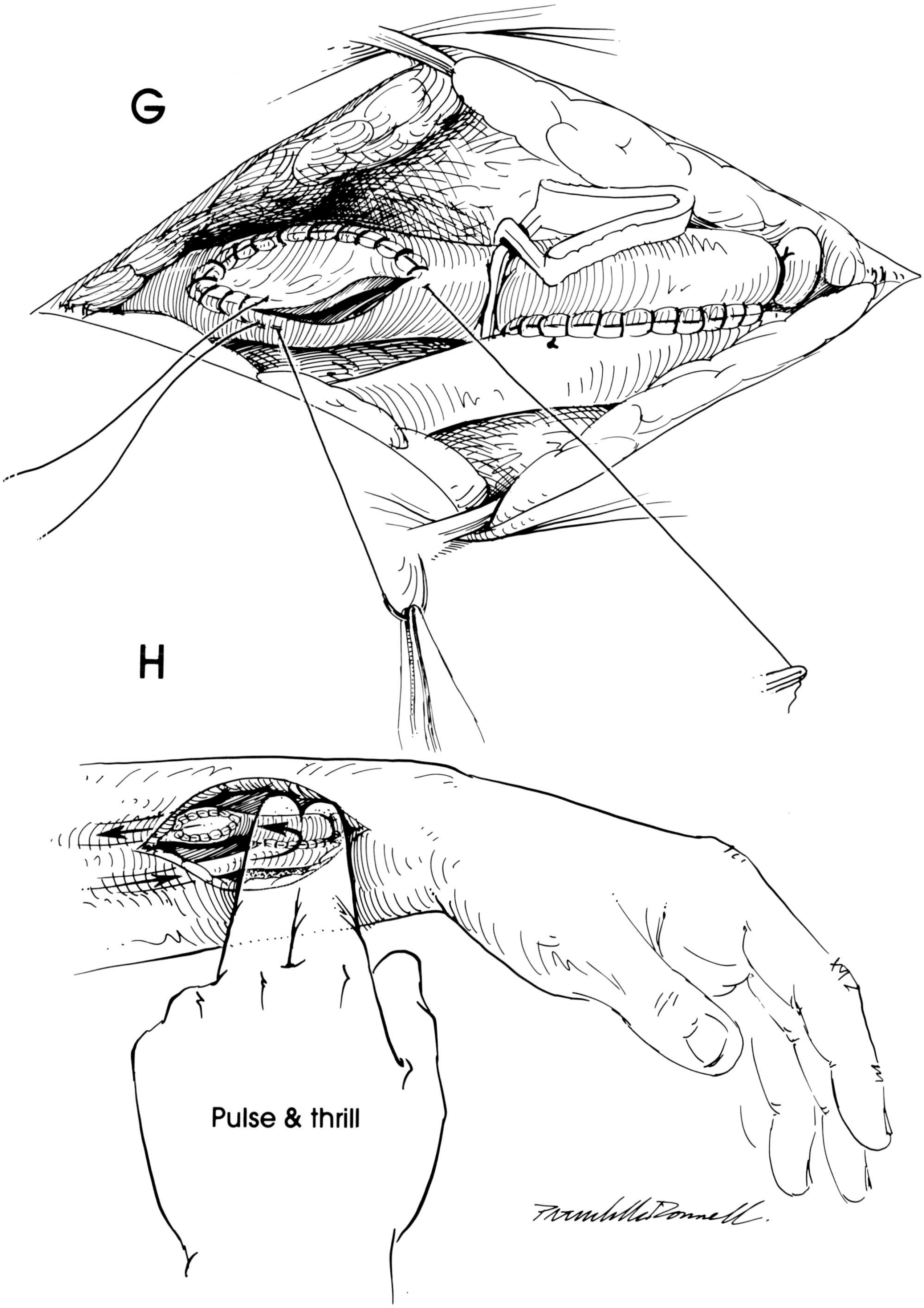
G
H
Pulse & thrill

Outflow Tract Obstruction

Venovenous Anastomosis

A A skin incision is made overlying the malfunctioning fistula.

B The radial artery–cephalic vein fistula and the large accessory vein previously identified on angiography are mobilized sufficiently to allow an end-to-side anastomosis to be constructed.

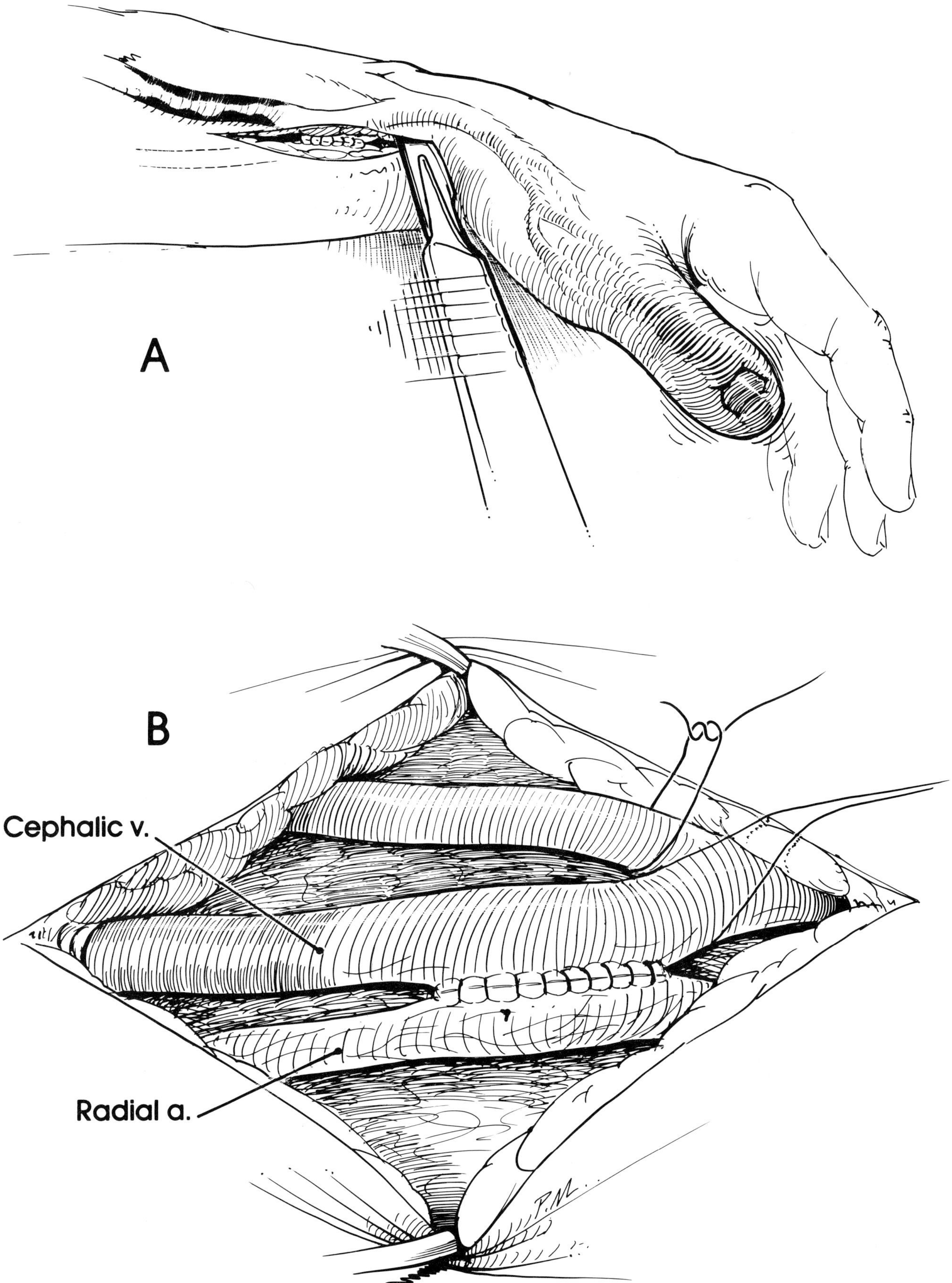
A
B
Cephalic v.
Radial a.

C The accessory vein is ligated at its origin and divided just proximal to the ligature.

D The vein is heparinized and then clamped.

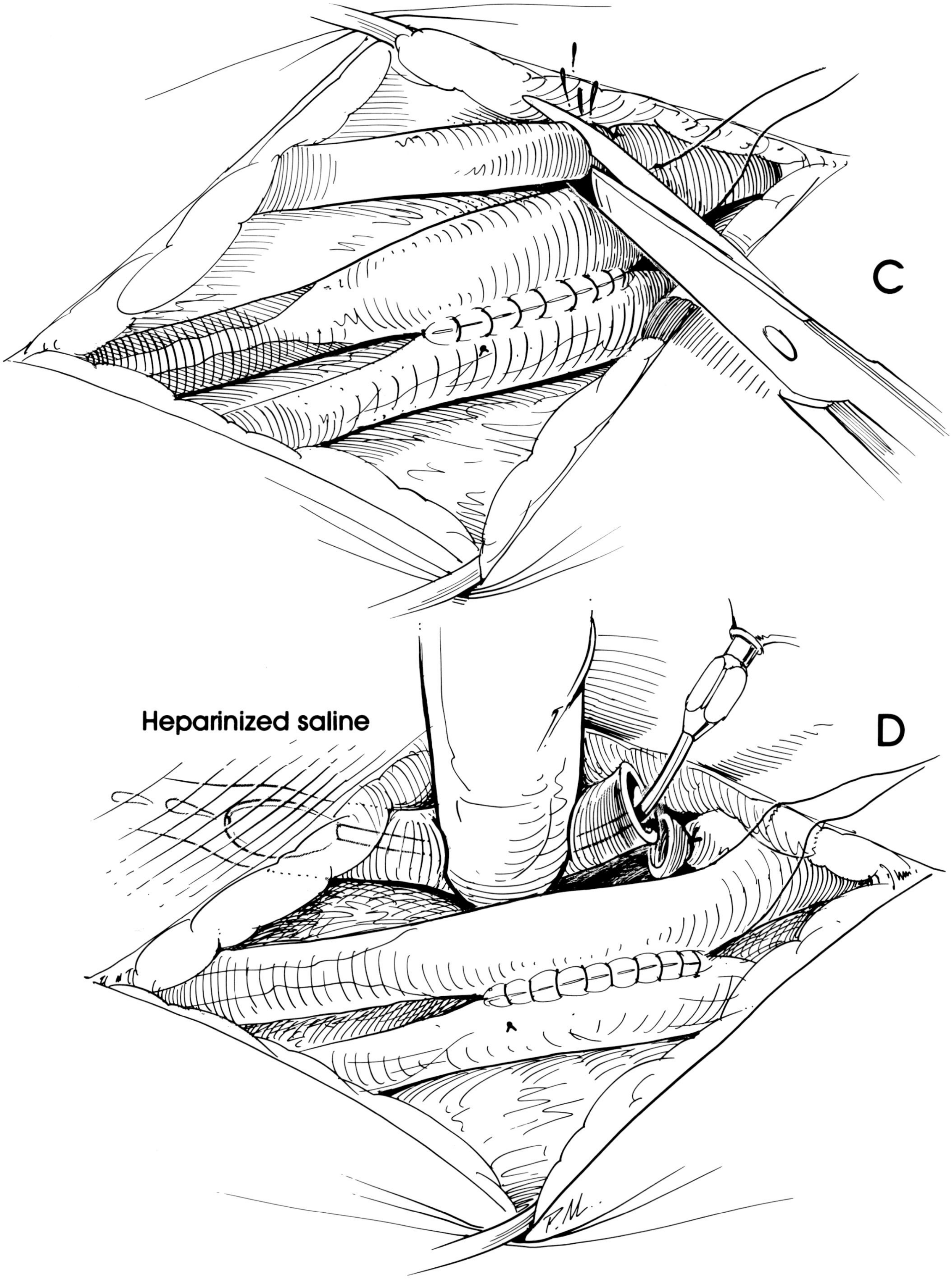
C
Heparinized saline
D

E Clamps are placed on the radial artery proximal and distal to the fistula. A lateral venotomy is then made immediately opposite the radial artery–cephalic vein anastomosis. The radial artery and cephalic vein are heparinized, and the clamps are replaced.

F The accessory vein is tapered to allow construction of the end-to-side anastomosis without tension or kinking secondary to redundancy. The venovenous anastomosis is completed with 7-0 polypropylene suture.

E

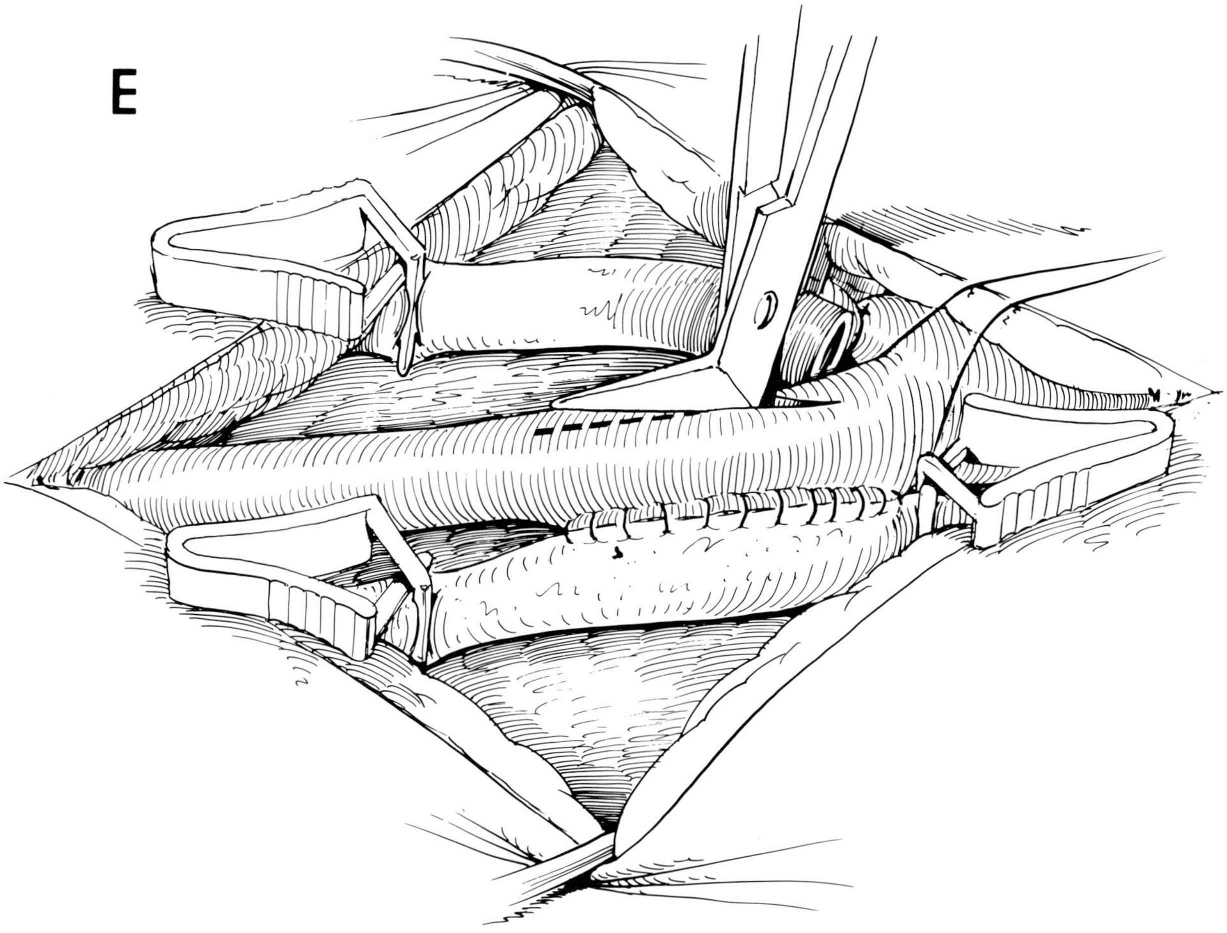

F

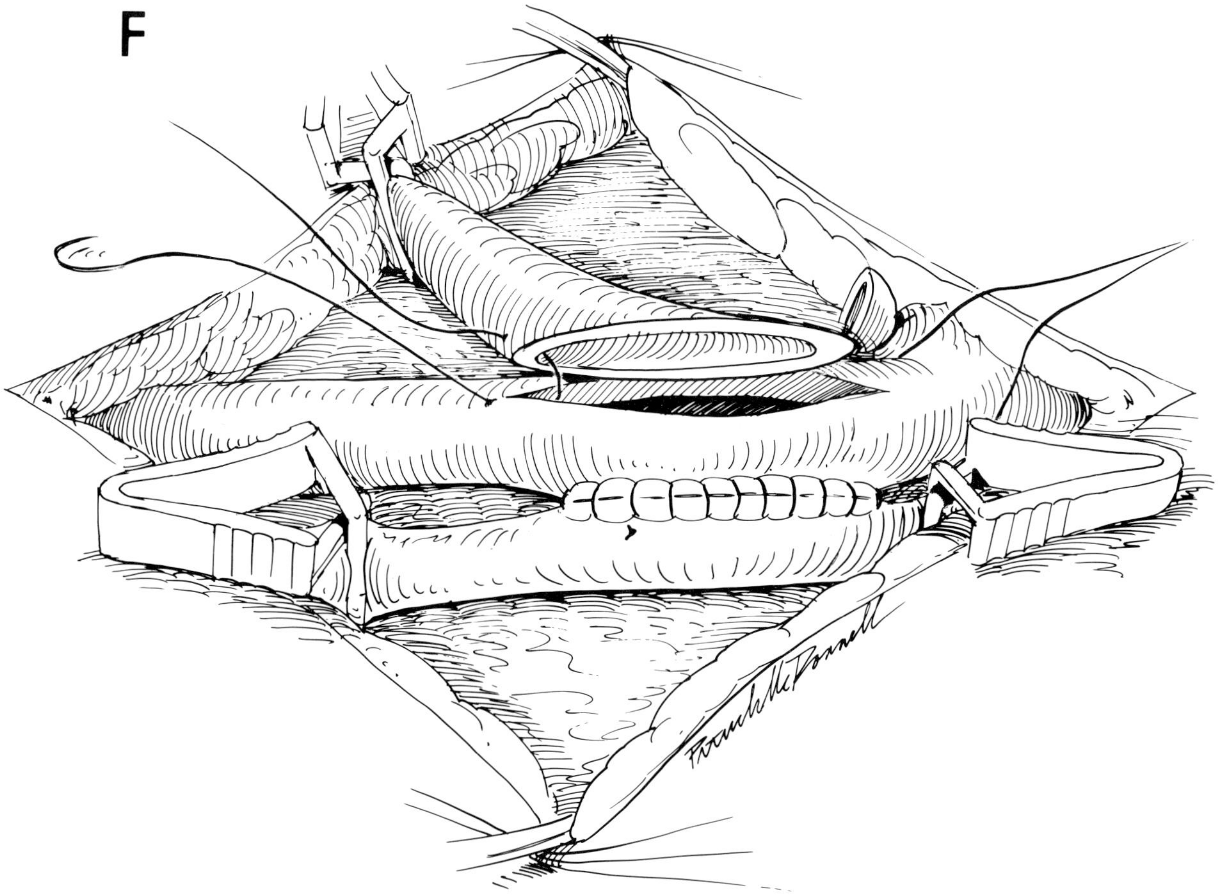

G Clamps are removed, and the suture line is inspected. The cephalic vein immediately distal to the fistula is ligated to ensure correction of the venous hypertension.

H A palpable pulse and thrill confirm correction of the outflow obstruction.

G

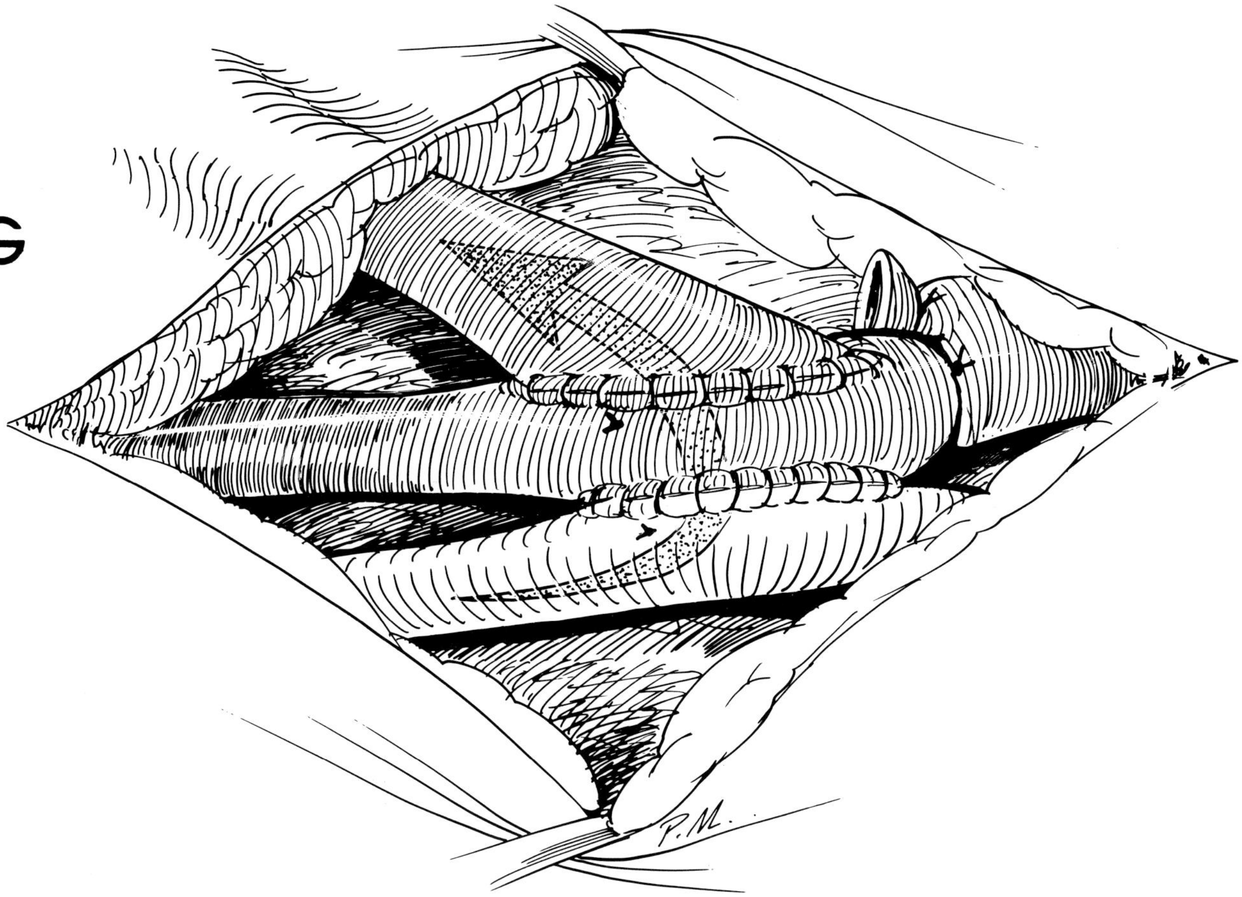

H

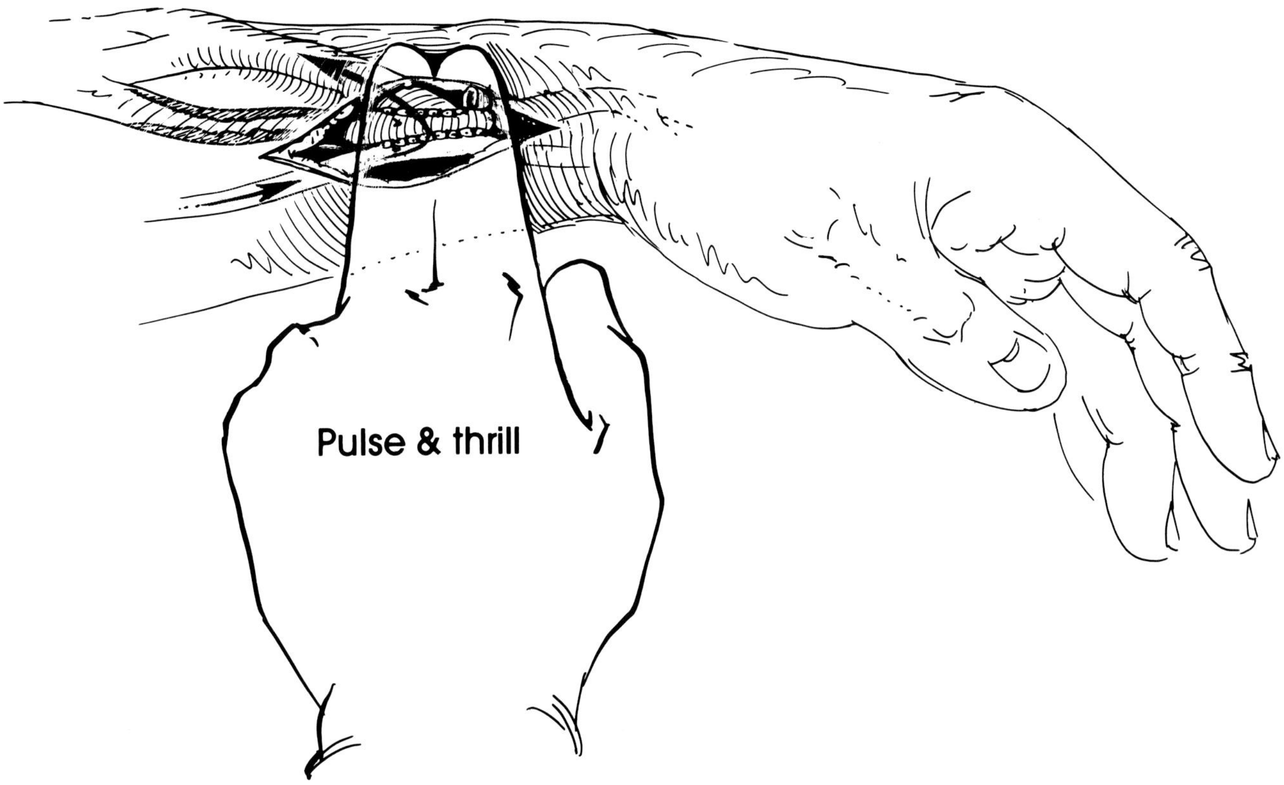

Graft Arteriovenous Fistulas

5

GRAFT ARTERIOVENOUS FISTULAS are indicated in patients who do not have vessels of the caliber or quality necessary to support the construction of a primary fistula. Various graft materials have been used, with varying degrees of success. Materials that have been used include autogenous saphenous vein, Dacron velour, modified bovine carotid xenograft, expanded polytetrafluoroethylene, and, most recently, modified human umbilical vein.

We recommend that looped forearm grafts be used as the initial approach in patients needing a graft arteriovenous fistula. The forearm location allows ready access and the looped configuration provides excellent flow while maximizing the area available for cannulation. To reduce inconvenience for the patient, the nondominant forearm should be used when possible. If a looped forearm graft cannot be used, other sites must be found, and some alternative sites and methods are described in this chapter. Regardless of location, graft fistulas should not be punctured before the third postoperative week. Earlier puncture risks hematoma formation in the subcutaneous tunnel following needle withdrawal, which will result in further delay in healing.

Looped Forearm Graft Fistula

A A transverse incision approximately 8 cm long is made 4 cm below the skin crease in the antecubital fossa.

B–C The cephalic vein and brachial artery are identified and mobilized. The basilic vein and concomitant brachial vein are alternatives if the cephalic vein is not satisfactory. The vessels should be mobilized sufficiently so that clamps may be placed away from the area of intended anastomosis. Then the brachial artery is clamped proximally, and an arteriotomy is begun.

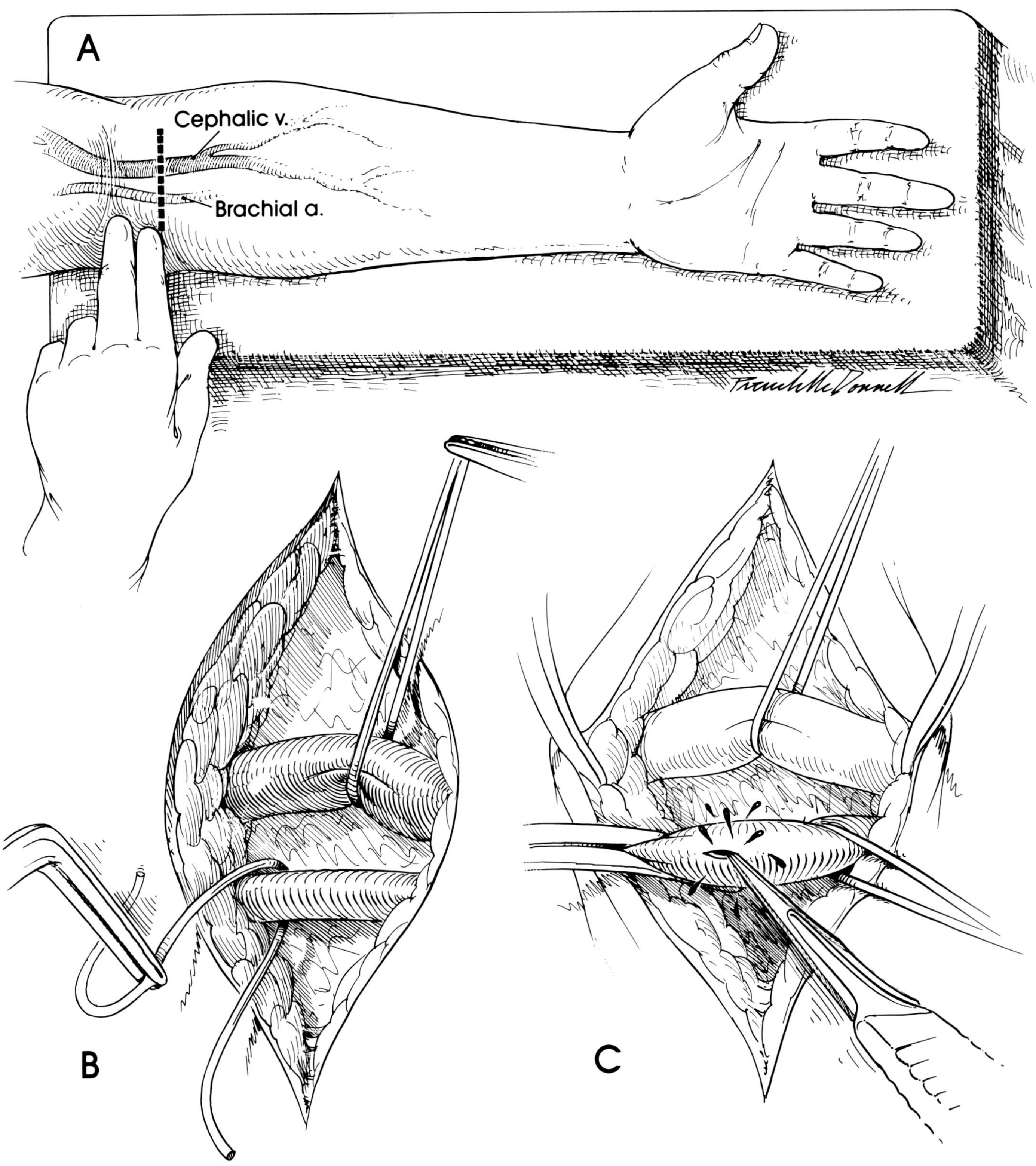
A
Cephalic v.
Brachial a.
B
C

D–G The arteriotomy is extended to approximately one and one-half times the diameter of the graft to be used, and heparinization is performed. The graft is tapered appropriately, and the end-to-side anastomosis is constructed with running 6-0 polypropylene sutures. When the arterial anastomosis is completed, the proximal clamp is opened, allowing the graft to flush. After any debris has been evacuated, the graft is heparinized and a distal clamp is placed.

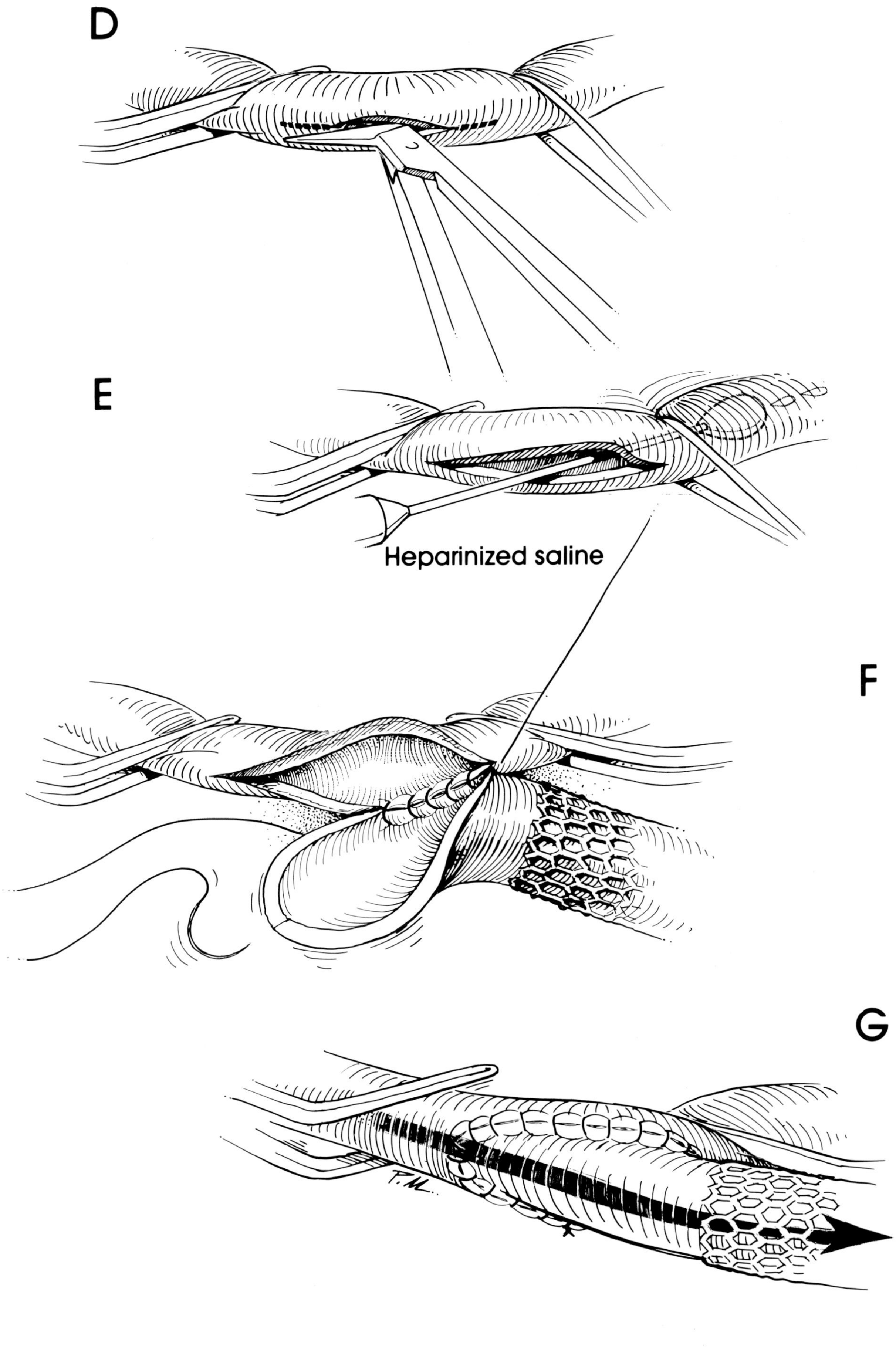
D
E
Heparinized saline
F
G
P.M.

H The graft is placed on the skin in the looped configuration that it will occupy in the subcutaneous tissue. The graft should be positioned carefully in a gently curved loop without twists or kinks and then placed in its subcutaneous tunnel so that this orientation is maintained. A counterincision approximately 3 cm long is made 2 cm below the most inferior portion of the looped graft.

I The clamp is placed immediately distal to the arterial anastomosis, and the graft is decompressed.

J–K The medial tunnel is created by inserting a curved spongestick into a cleavage plane between the forearm fistula and the subcutaneous tissue. The shape of the tunnel should conform to the position of the graft. The depth of the tunnel must be sufficient to prevent devascularization of overlying skin but should not be so deep as to interfere with palpation and cannulation of the graft. The free end of the graft is then grasped by the jaws of the spongestick, with care taken to maintain proper orientation of the graft.

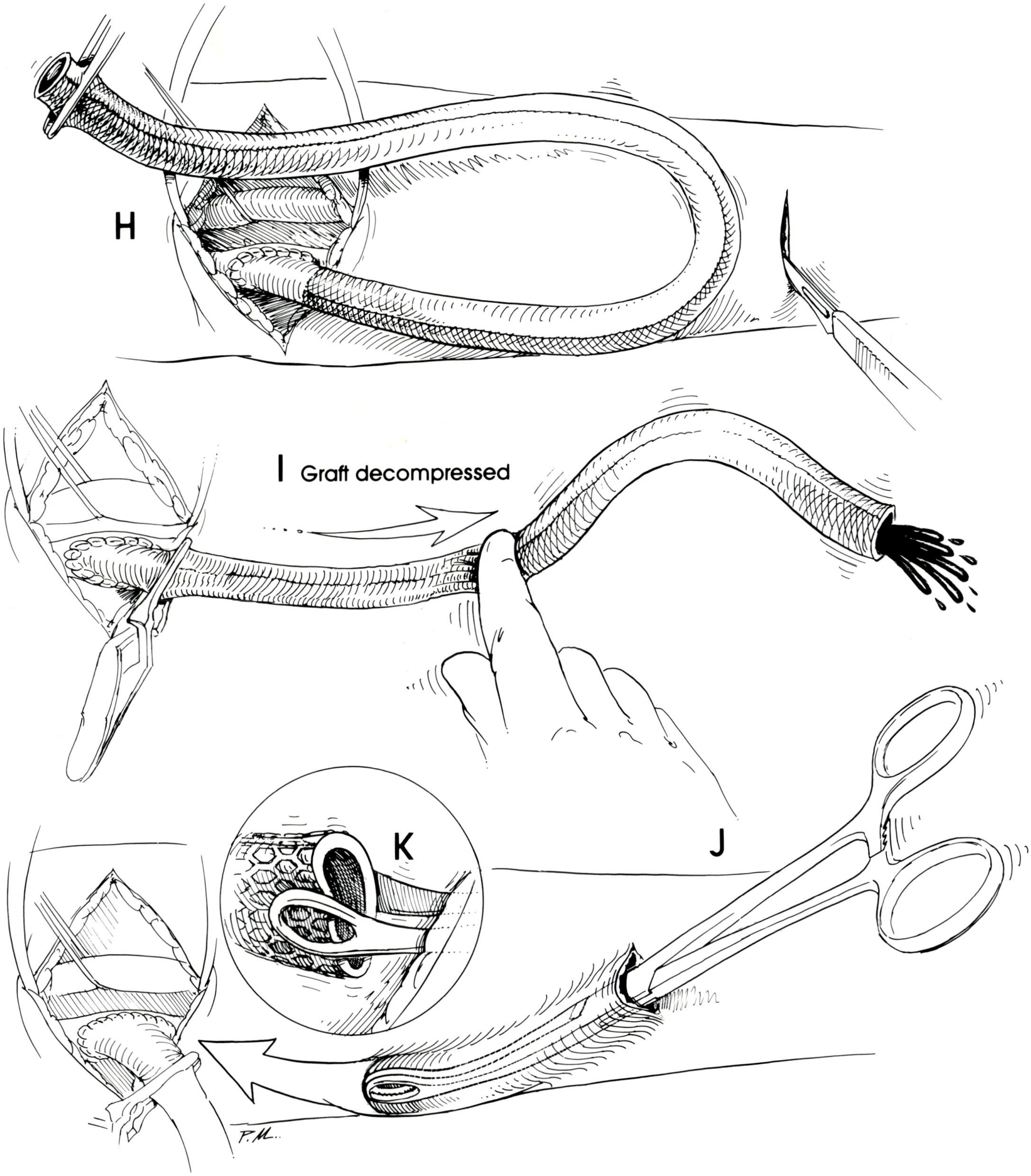
H
I Graft decompressed
J
K
P.M.

L The decompressed graft is delivered through the counterincision. A forceps handle is used to prevent rolling of the skin's free edge with traction of the graft.

M–N The graft is flushed and then filled with heparinized saline. The position of the arterial limb of the fistula within the tunnel should be checked at this point.

O The clamp is placed at the level of the counterincision, and the portion of the graft distal to the clamp is decompressed. The lateral return tunnel is constructed through the subcutaneous tissue, as described previously (Fig H).

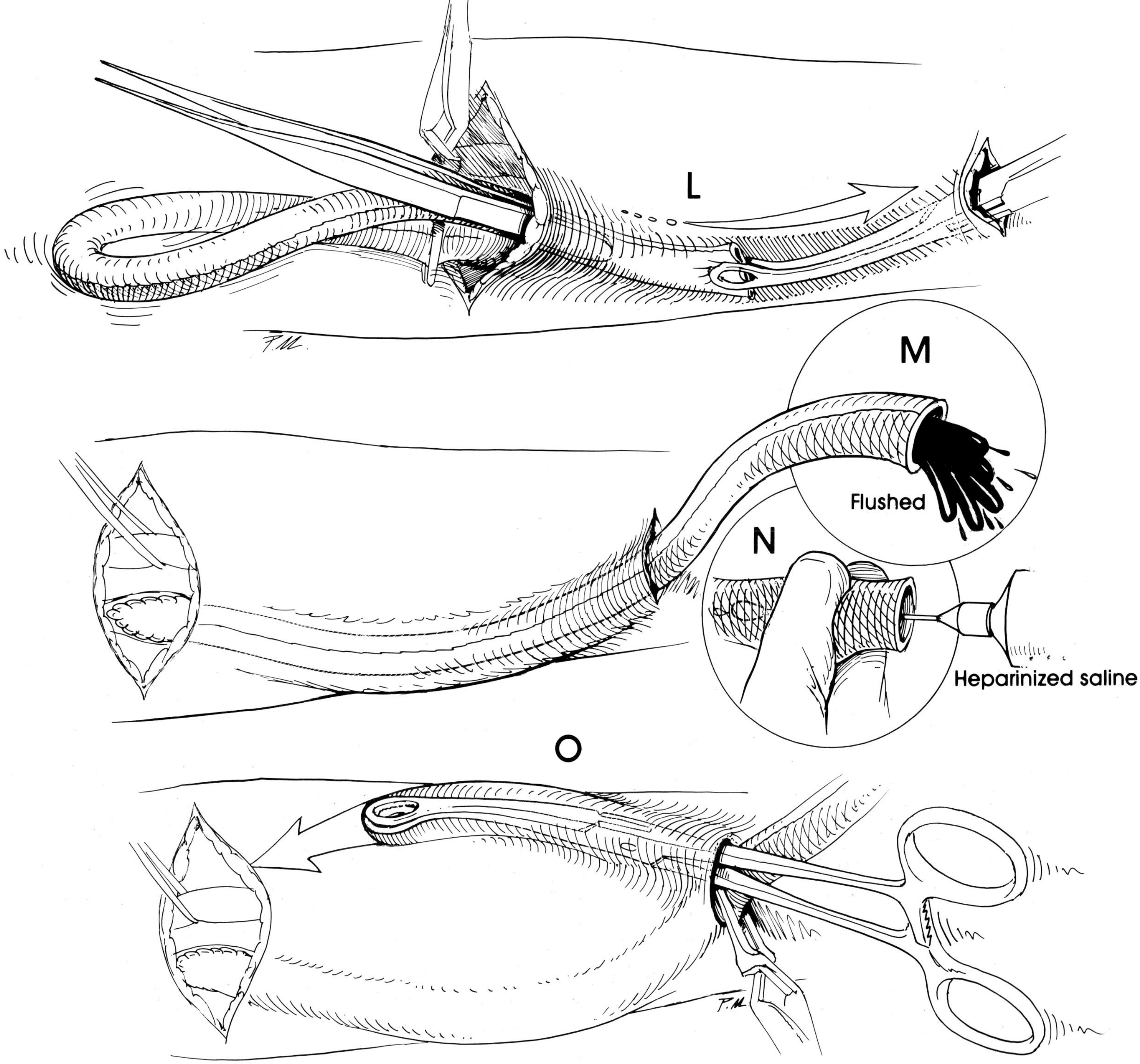
L
M
Flushed
N
Heparinized saline
O

P The venous limb of the graft is brought through the return tunnel and the antecubital incision.

Q–R The graft is flushed, filled with heparinized saline, and clamped. Positioning of the graft within its tunnel should be reconfirmed.

S–T Proximal and distal clamps are placed on the cephalic vein, and the venotomy is extended to one and one-half times the graft diameter. After the proximal clamp has been placed, the graft is tapered for construction of the end-to-side venous anastomosis, which is then done with running 7-0 polypropylene suture.

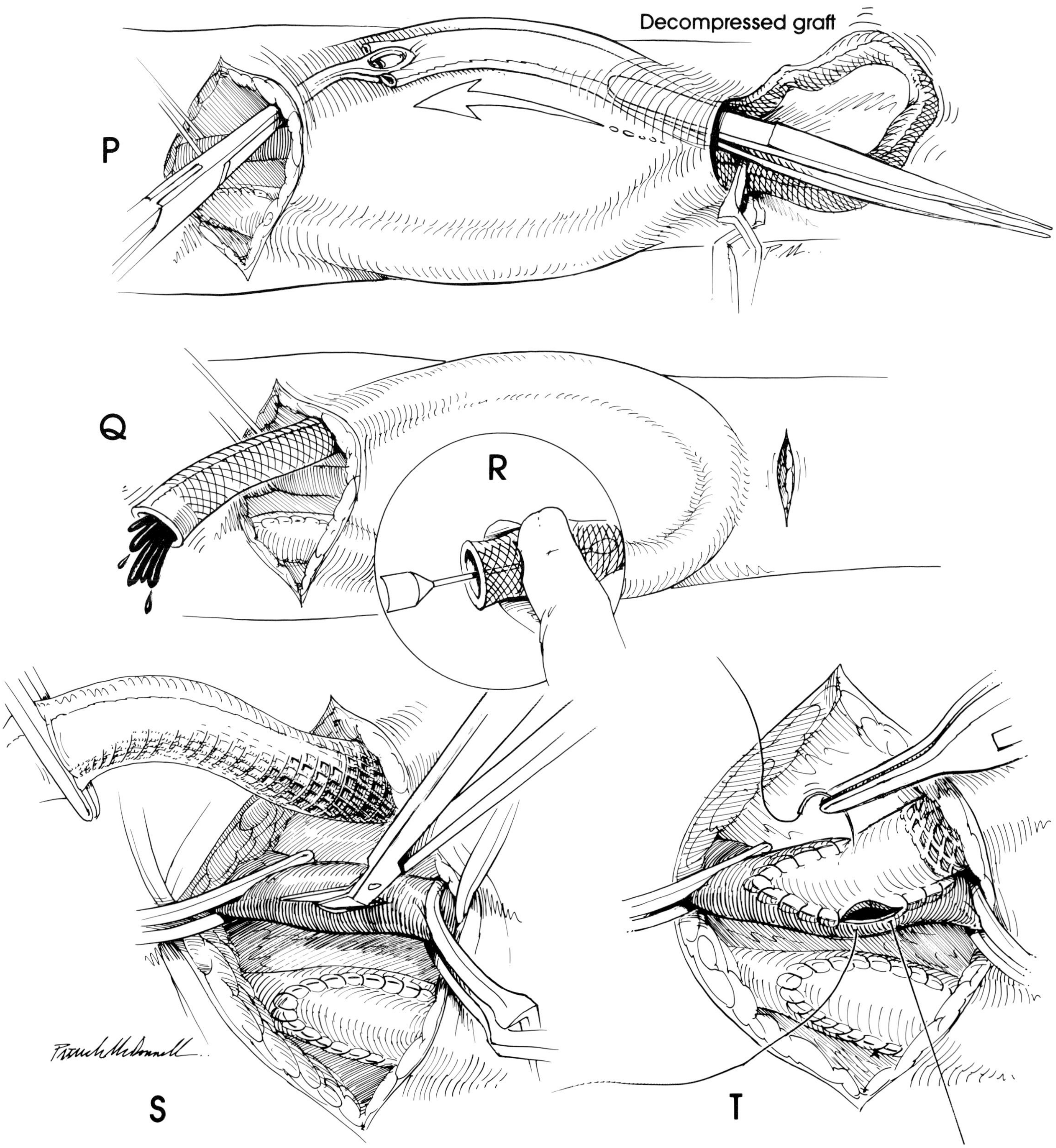
Decompressed graft
P
Q
R
S
T

U The graft fistula is allowed to fill, and the anastomoses are inspected. A single layer of 3-0 absorbable suture is used for closure of the subcutaneous tissue, and staples are used for the skin.

V A palpable pulse and thrill confirm adequate function.

W The position of the graft relative to the elbow joint is such that flexion of the arm does not compromise blood flow through the fistula.

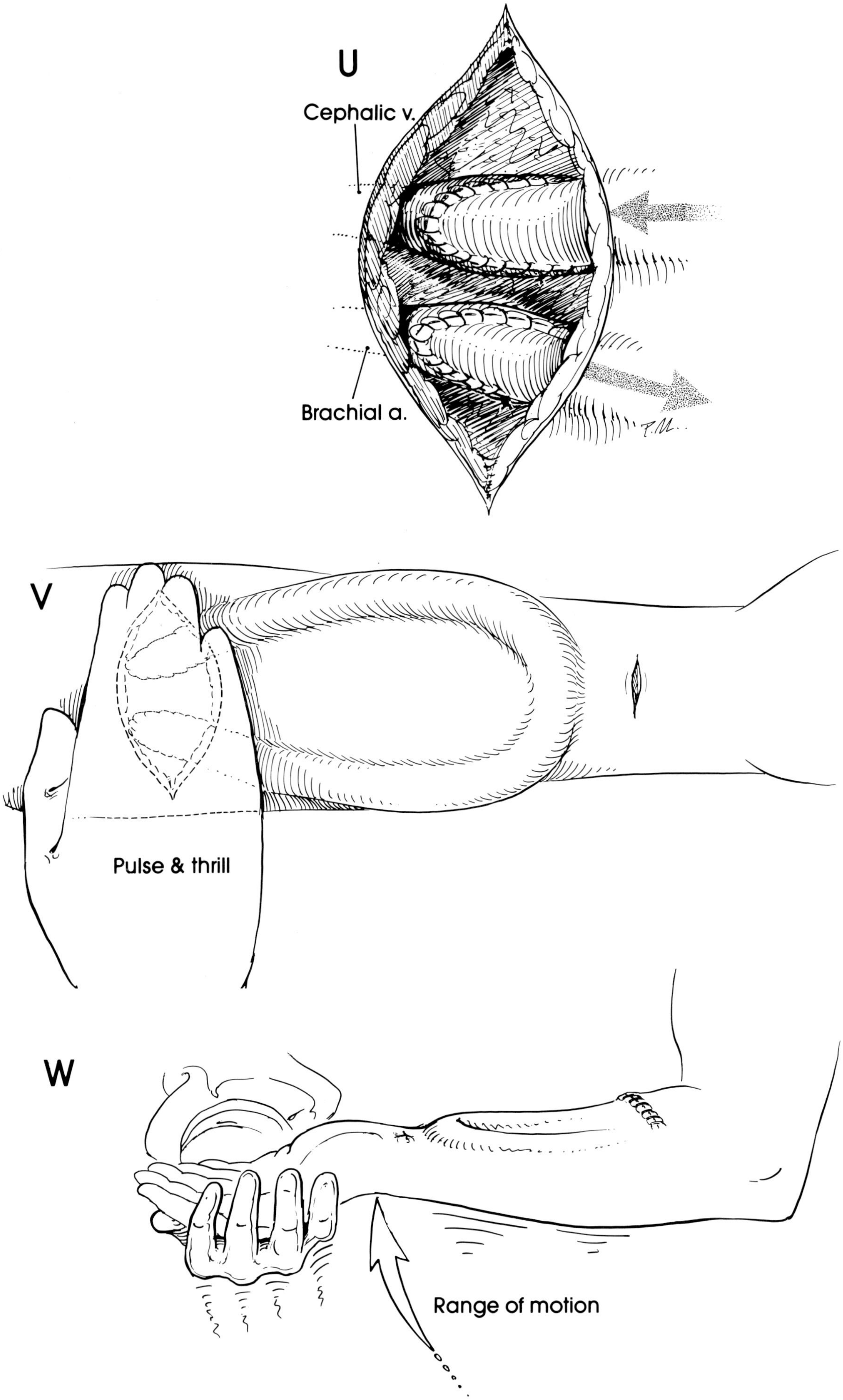
U
Cephalic v.
Brachial a.
V
Pulse & thrill
W
Range of motion

Straight Forearm Graft Fistula

A A transverse incision approximately 6 cm long is made 4 cm below the antecubital skin crease. The cephalic vein is identified and mobilized. The basilic vein and corresponding brachial vein are alternative sources of venous runoff for the graft fistula. The radial artery is then exposed through a 5-cm longitudinal incision.

B Microvascular bulldog clamps are placed proximally and distally on the radial artery, and the arteriotomy is begun.

C The arteriotomy is extended to a length one and one-half times the graft diameter.

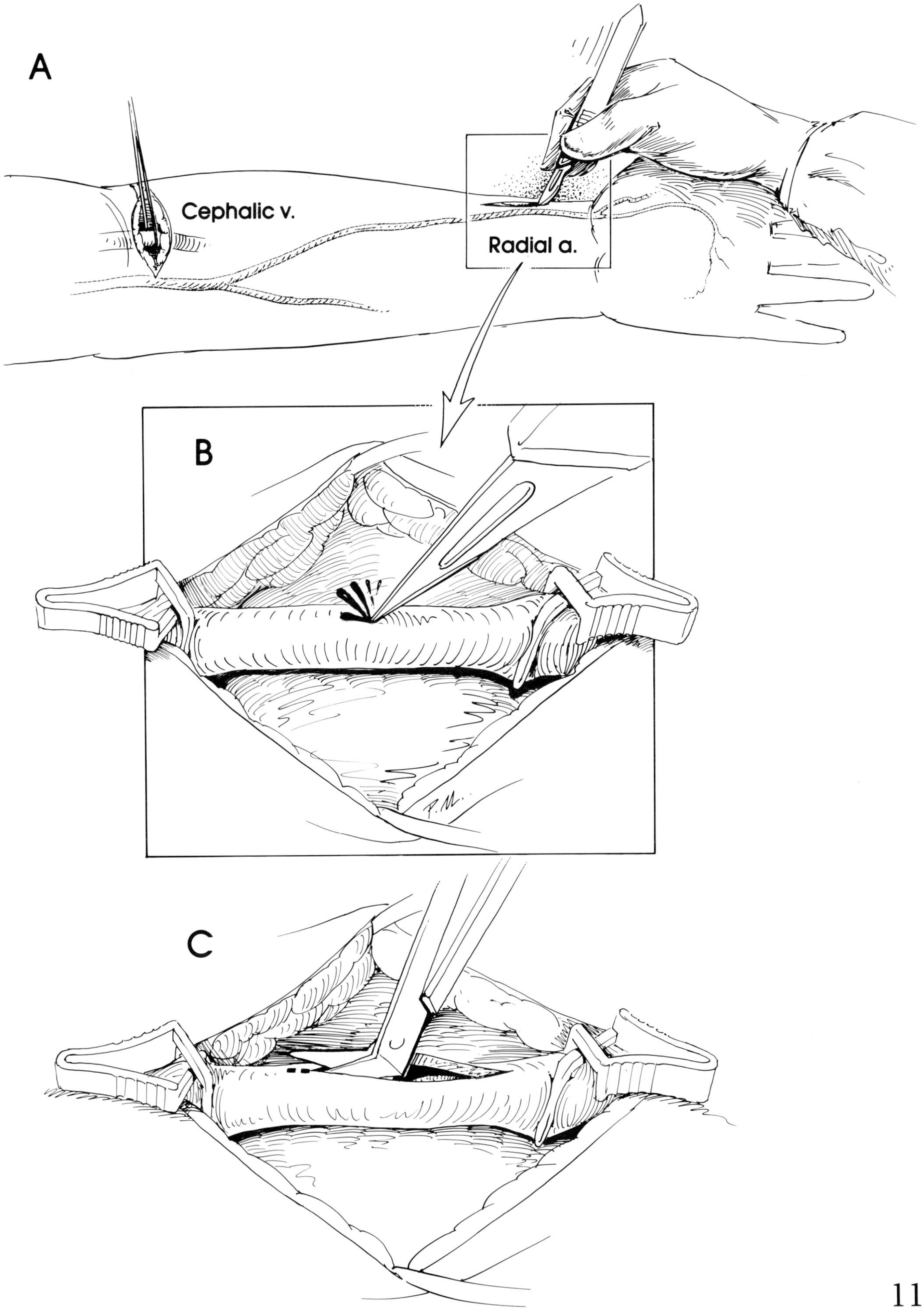
A
Cephalic v.
Radial a.
B
C

D The radial artery is heparinized, and the vascular clamps are replaced.

E The graft is tapered appropriately to allow construction of a low-profile, flared end-to-side anastomosis. Running 6-0 polypropylene suture is used to incorporate the graft with the artery.

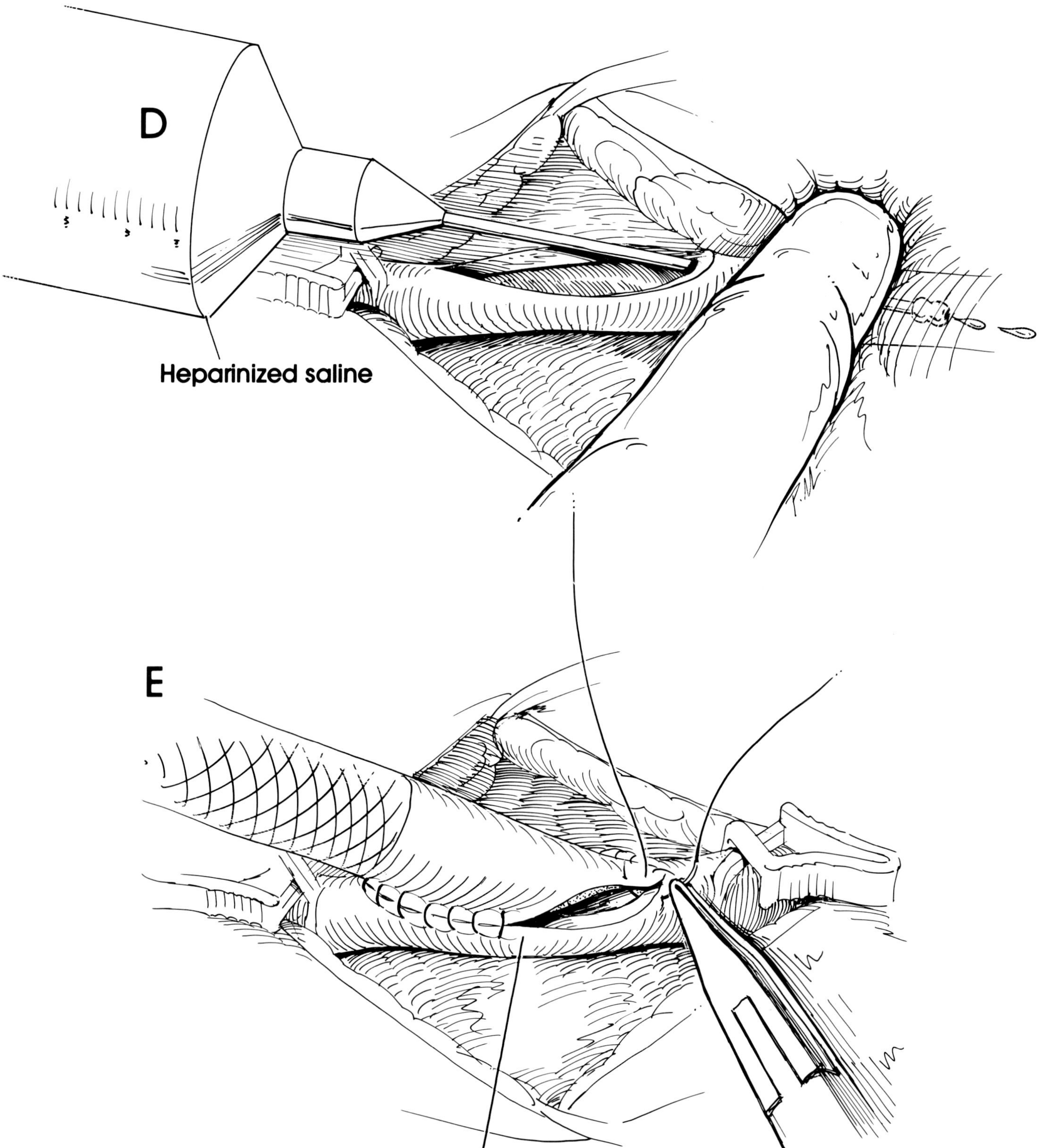
D
Heparinized saline
E

F After the anastomosis is completed, the proximal clamp is removed, allowing the graft to flush. The distal radial artery clamp is removed, and the graft is heparinized and clamped.

G A spongestick is used to construct a subcutaneous tunnel linking the two incisions.

H The graft is clamped immediately distal to the arterial anastomosis and then decompressed.

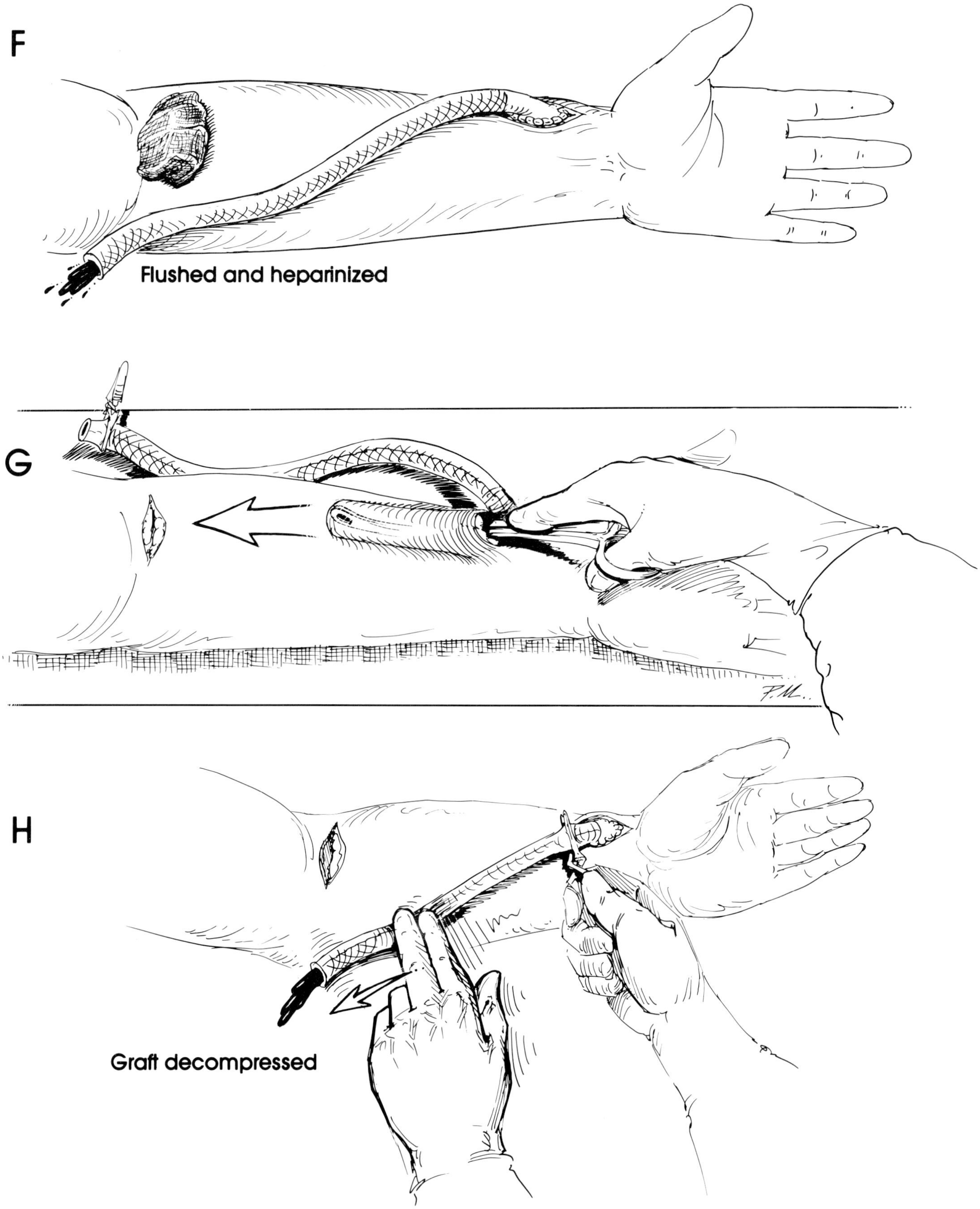
F
Flushed and heparinized
G
H
Graft decompressed

I–K With care to avoid twisting, the decompressed graft is brought through the subcutaneous tunnel and out through the antecubital incision. The graft is unclamped, and its proper position in the tunnel is confirmed. The free end of the graft is clamped following adequate heparinization. The cephalic vein is clamped, and a venotomy incision measuring one and one-half times the graft diameter is made.

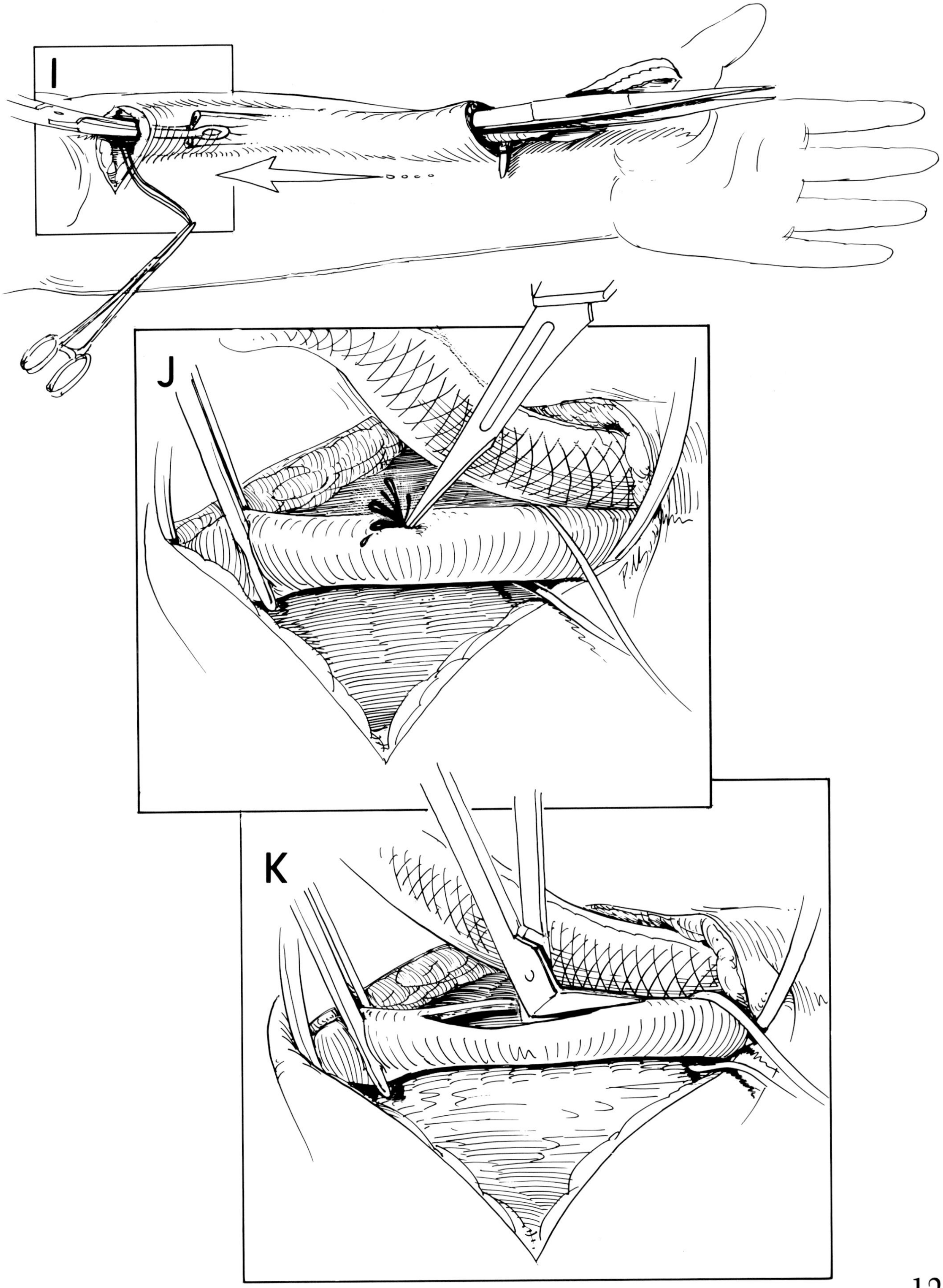
I
J
K

L–M The graft is tapered for the end-to-side anastomosis, which is constructed with 6-0 polypropylene suture. The subcutaneous tissue is closed with 3-0 absorbable suture, and the skin is reapproximated with staples.

N A palpable pulse and thrill confirm adequate flow.

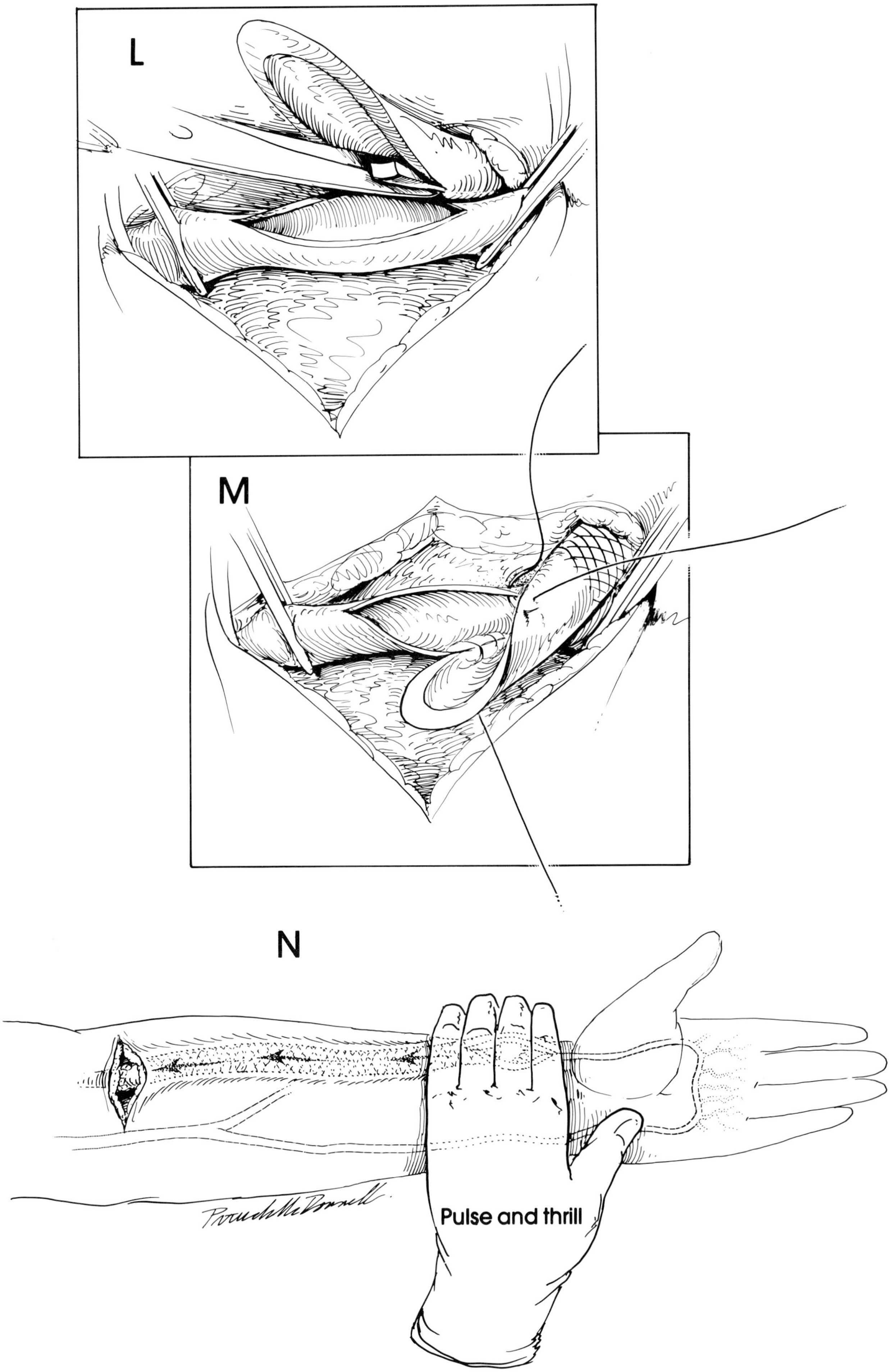
L
M
N
Pulse and thrill

Straight Arm Graft Fistula

A–C Approximately 5 cm distal to the axillary skin crease, a 4-cm transverse incision is made along the medial aspect of the arm overlying the brachial artery. The axillary vein, which is superficial and medial to the artery, is identified and mobilized. Should the axillary vein be unsatisfactory, the corresponding brachial vein may serve as an alternative site for the venous anastomosis. This incision is covered with moist sponges, and a transverse anterolateral incision of equal length is made approximately 3 cm proximal to the antecubital skin crease and overlying the brachial pulse. Dissection is performed, and the artery is mobilized from the surrounding tissue. Bulldog clamps are placed proximal and distal to the intended site of the arteriotomy. The arteriotomy is made with a no. 11 blade and Potts scissors. It should measure one and one-half times the graft diameter.

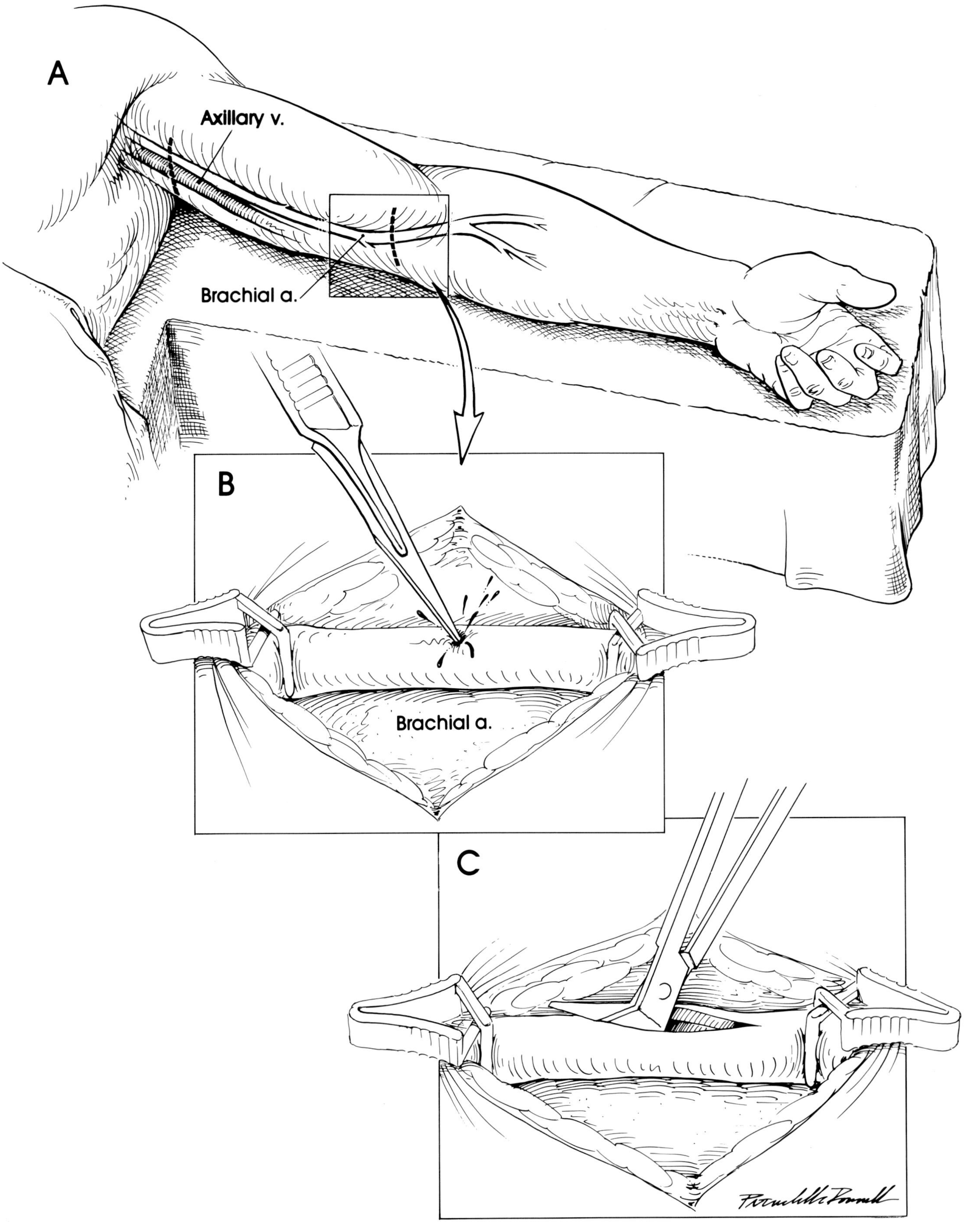
A
Axillary v.
Brachial a.
B
Brachial a.
C

D The vessels are irrigated with heparinized saline, and the clamps are replaced.

E The graft is tapered appropriately for the low-profile end-to-side anastomosis, which is constructed with running 6-0 polypropylene sutures.

F When the anastomosis has been completed, the proximal clamp is removed, allowing the graft to flush. The distal brachial artery is unclamped, and the graft is heparinized.

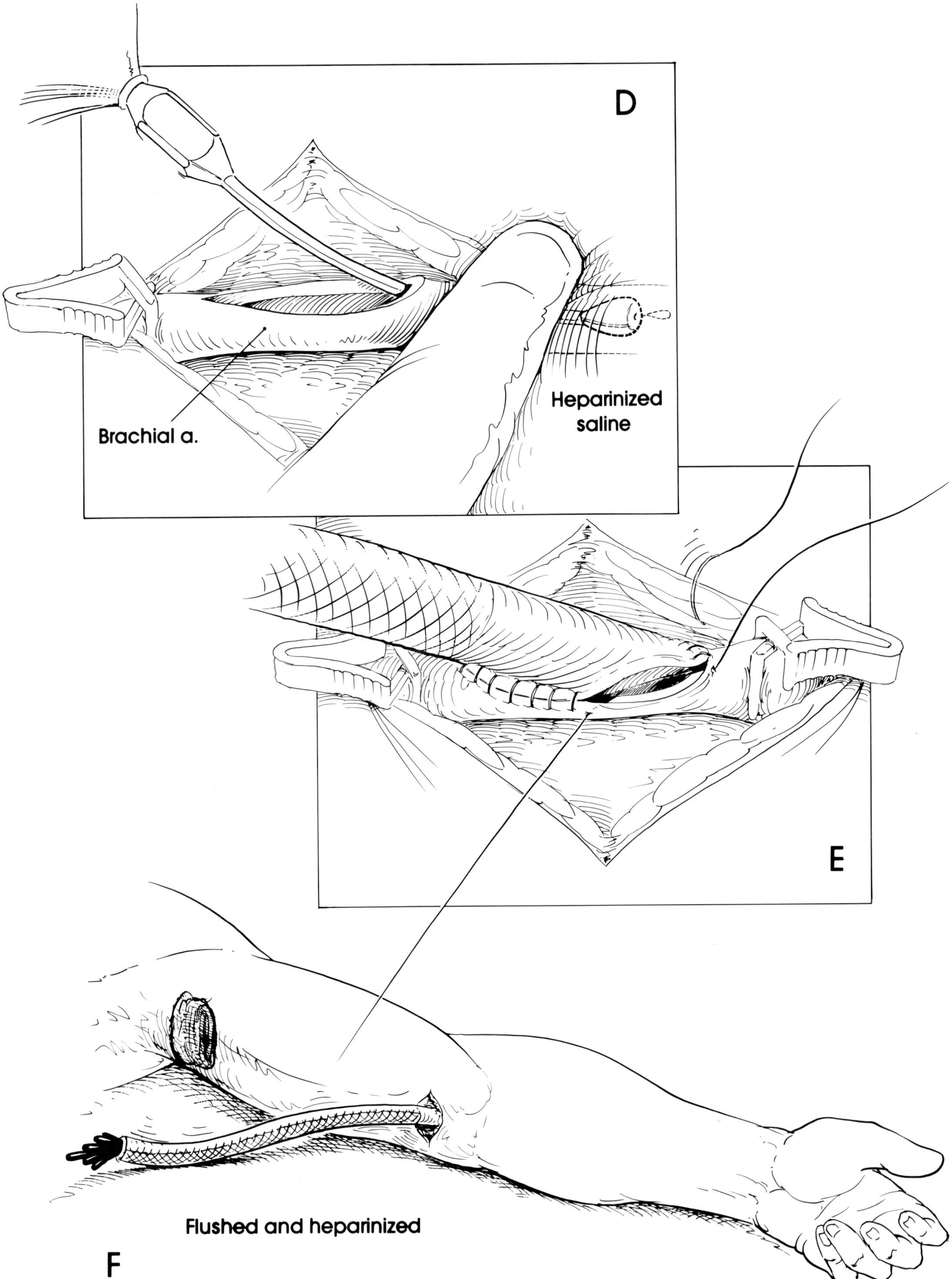

D
Brachial a.
Heparinized
saline
E
Flushed and heparinized
F

G The graft is placed on the skin in the configuration it will occupy in the subcutaneous tunnel. The graft should lie smoothly and without twisting.

H The graft is then clamped at the level of the distal incision and decompressed.

I A tunnel is constructed through the subcutaneous tissue between the two incisions. The depth of the tunnel should facilitate cannulation of the graft without devascularization of the overlying skin.

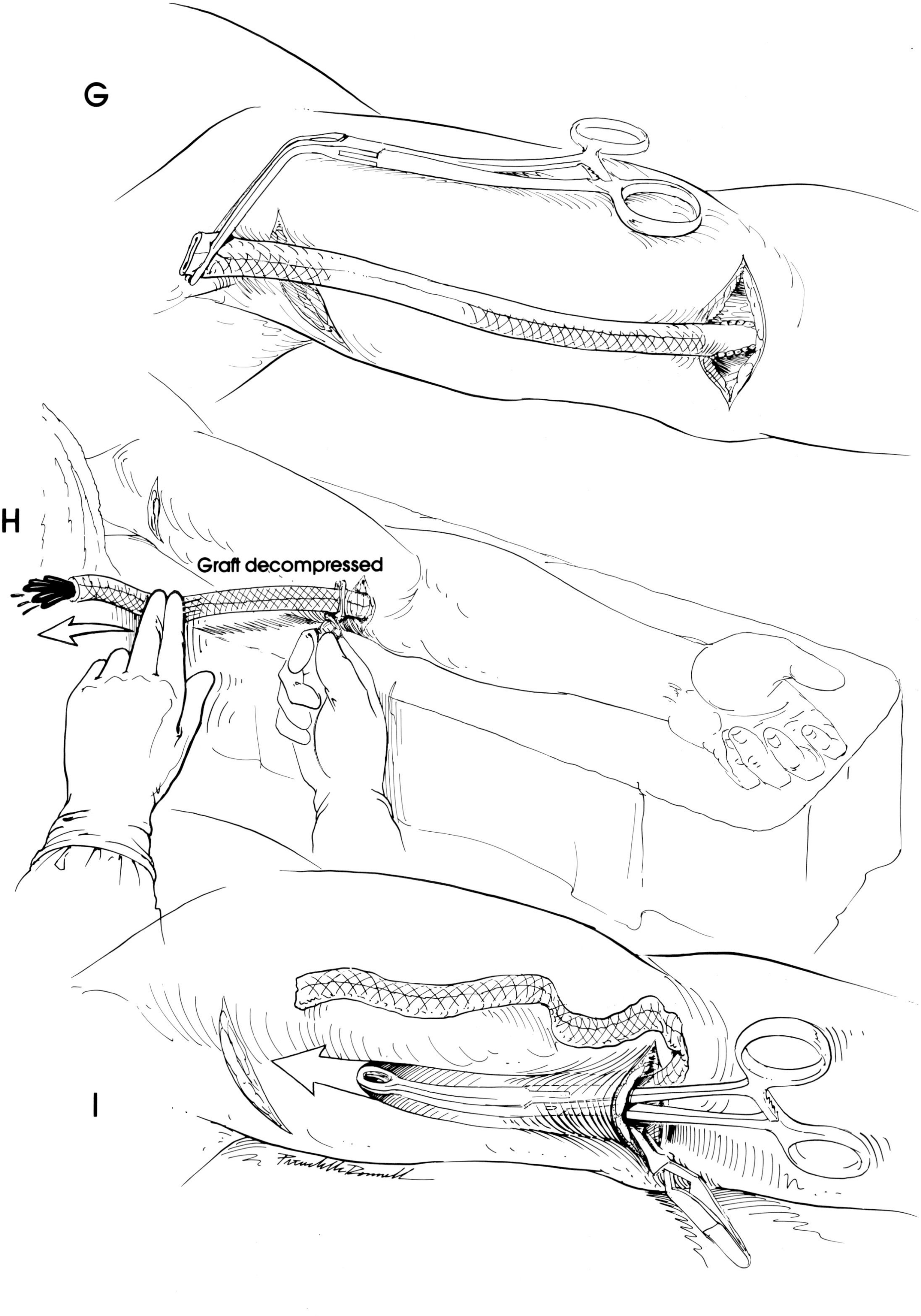
G
H
Graft decompressed
I

J The decompressed graft is delivered through the subcutaneous tissue, with care taken to maintain proper orientation of the graft.

K The graft is unclamped and allowed to flush. It is then heparinized and clamped.

L The vein is clamped, and a venotomy measuring one and one-half times the graft diameter is made.

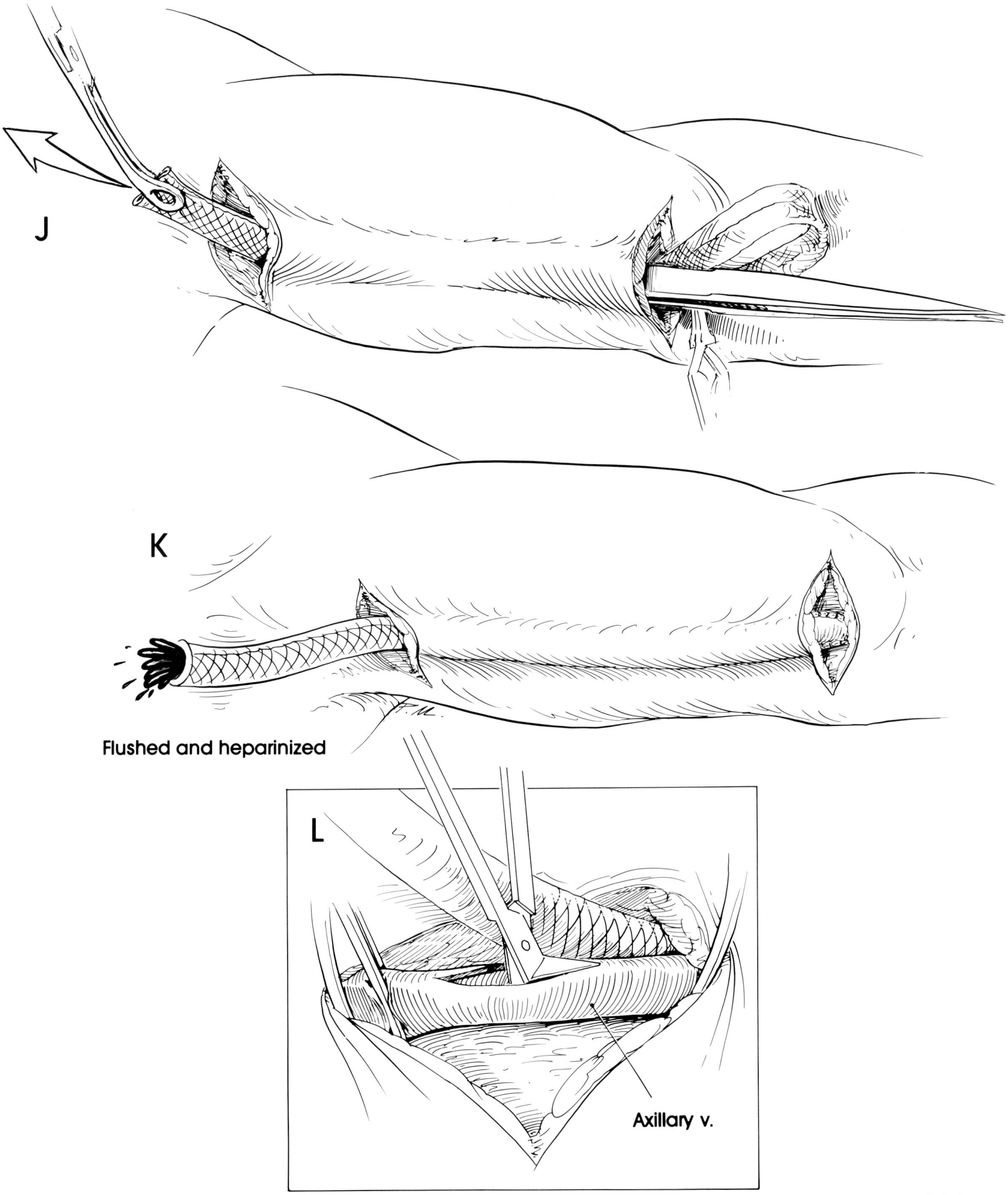
J
K
Flushed and heparinized
L
Axillary v.

M The graft is tapered, and the end-to-side venous anastomosis is completed with running 6-0 vascular sutures.

N Clamps are removed, and the straight graft fistula is allowed to fill. A palpable pulse and thrill confirm adequate flow. Incisions are closed with 3-0 absorbable suture for reapproximation of the subcutaneous tissue and staples for the skin.

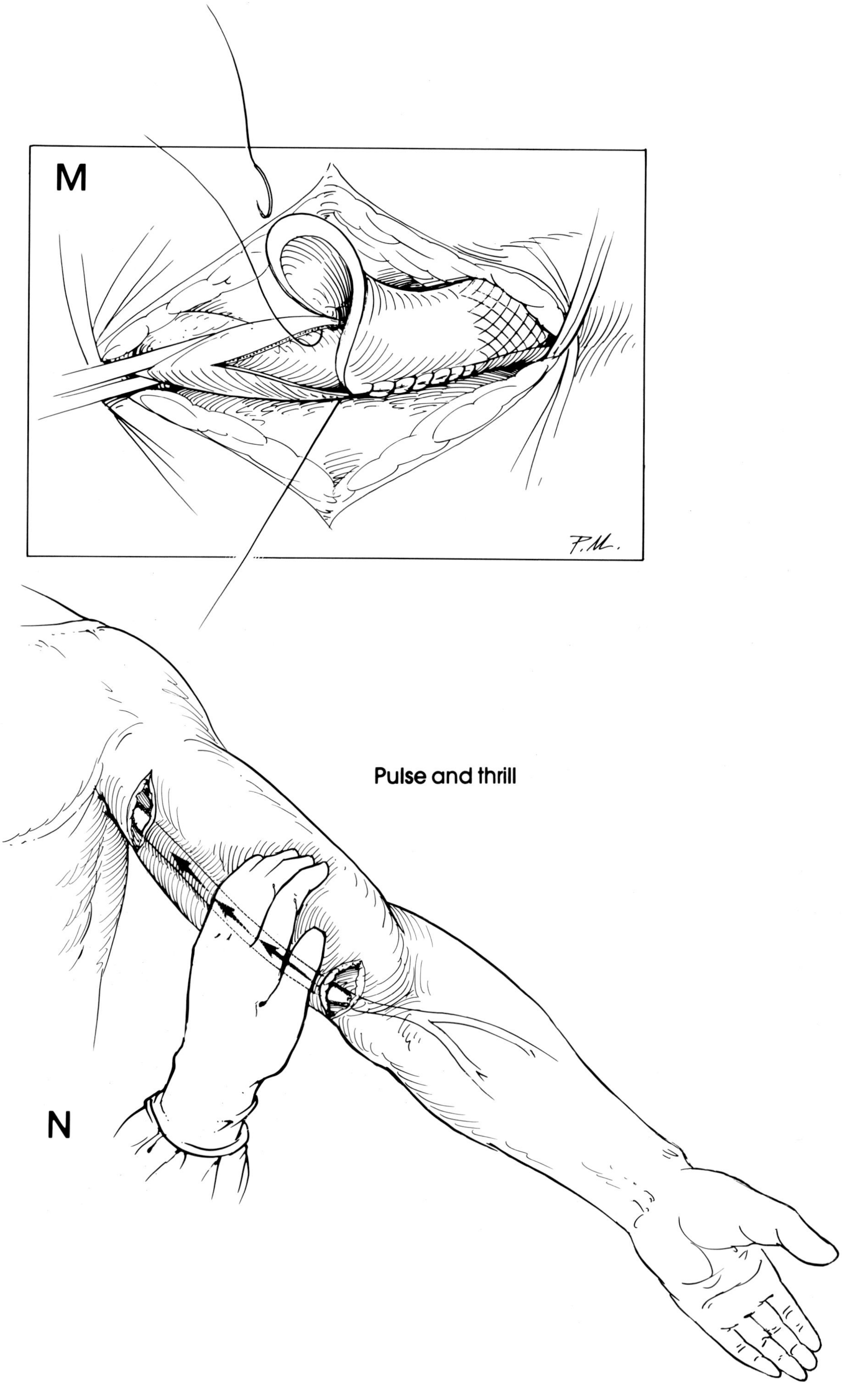
M
N
Pulse and thrill

Looped Thigh Graft Fistula

A A longitudinal incision approximately 8 cm long is made below the inguinal ligament, slightly medial to the femoral pulse.

B The greater saphenous vein and common femoral artery are identified and mobilized.

C A proximal vascular clamp is placed on the common femoral artery, and the vessel is opened with a no. 11 blade.

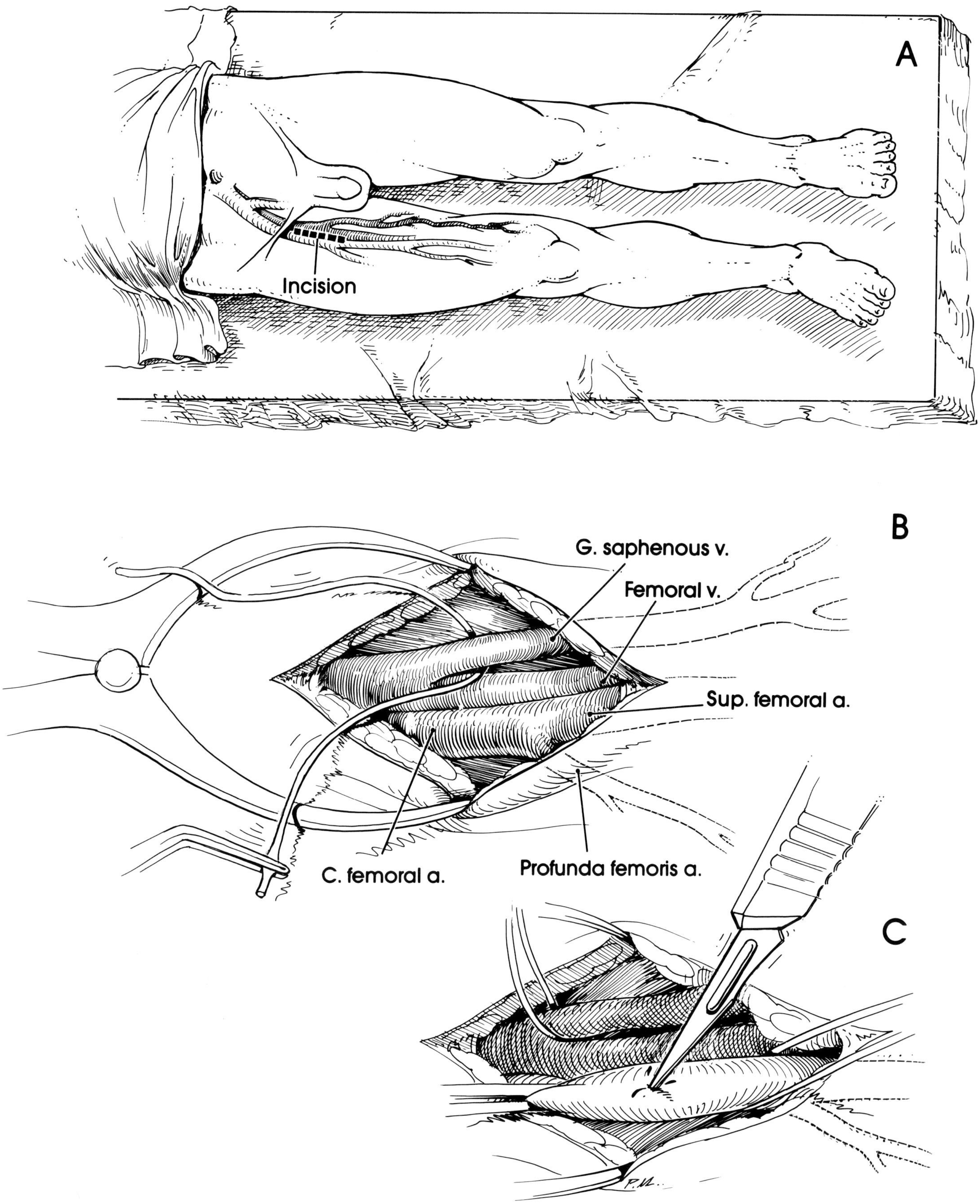
A
Incision
B
G. saphenous v.
Femoral v.
Sup. femoral a.
C. femoral a.
Profunda femoris a.
C

D The length of the arteriotomy is extended to one and one-half times the graft diameter.

E The vessels are heparinized, and a distal clamp is placed on the artery.

F The graft is tapered appropriately, and the end-to-side anastomosis is constructed with 6-0 vascular sutures.

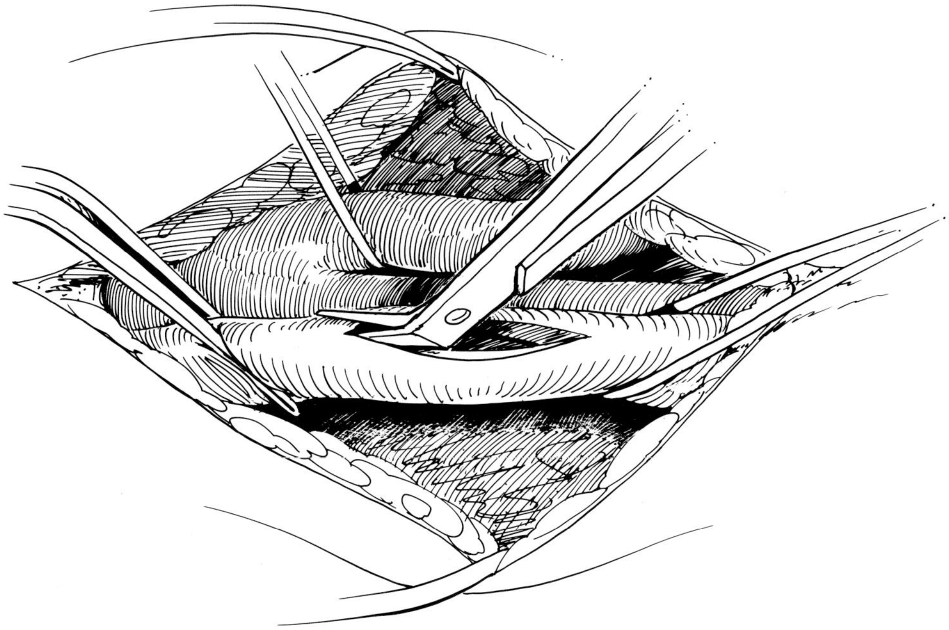

D

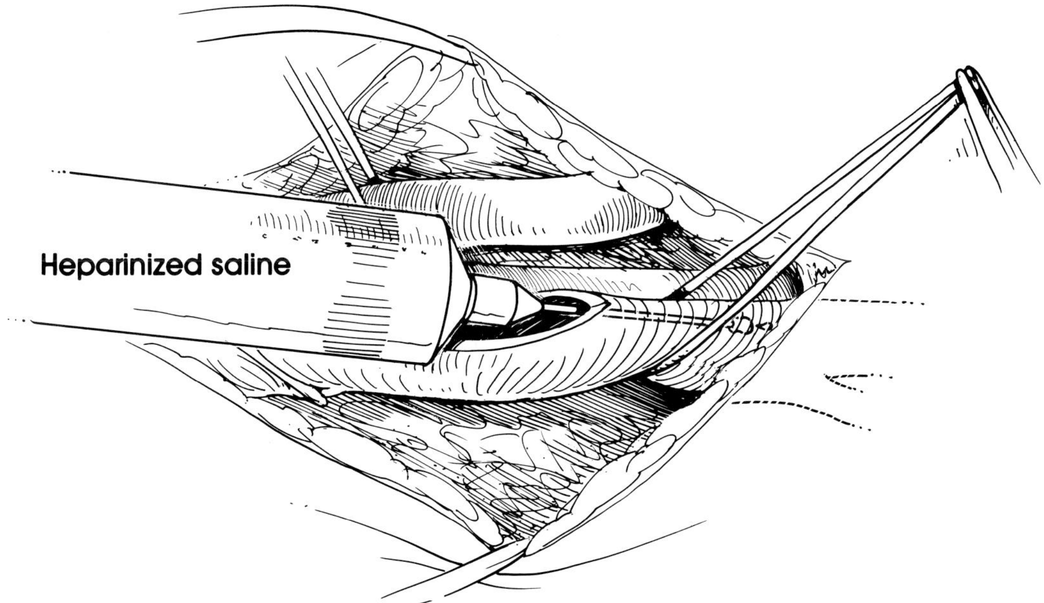

E

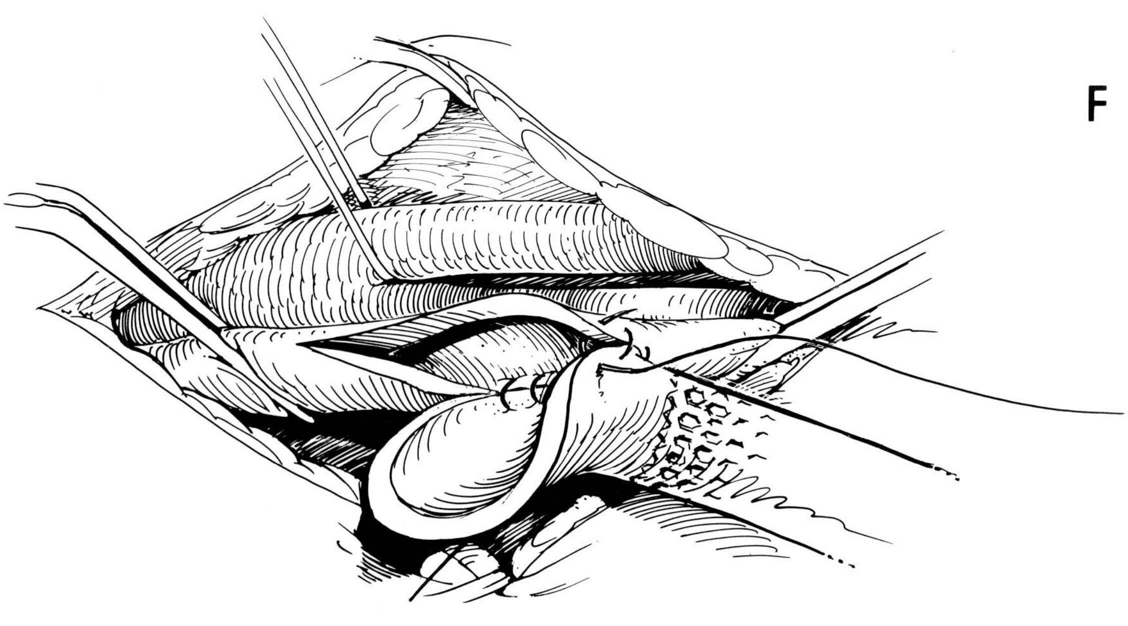

F

G After completion of the arterial anastomosis, the proximal clamp is removed, allowing the graft to flush. The remaining clamp is removed, and the graft is heparinized.

H The graft is placed in the looped configuration that it will assume in the subcutaneous tissue tunnel. A transverse counterincision is made 2 cm below the apex of the graft.

I A curved spongestick is used to form the lateral subcutaneous tunnel. As in the forearm, the tunnel must be deep enough to prevent erosion of the overlying skin without being so deep that cannulation is impeded.

G

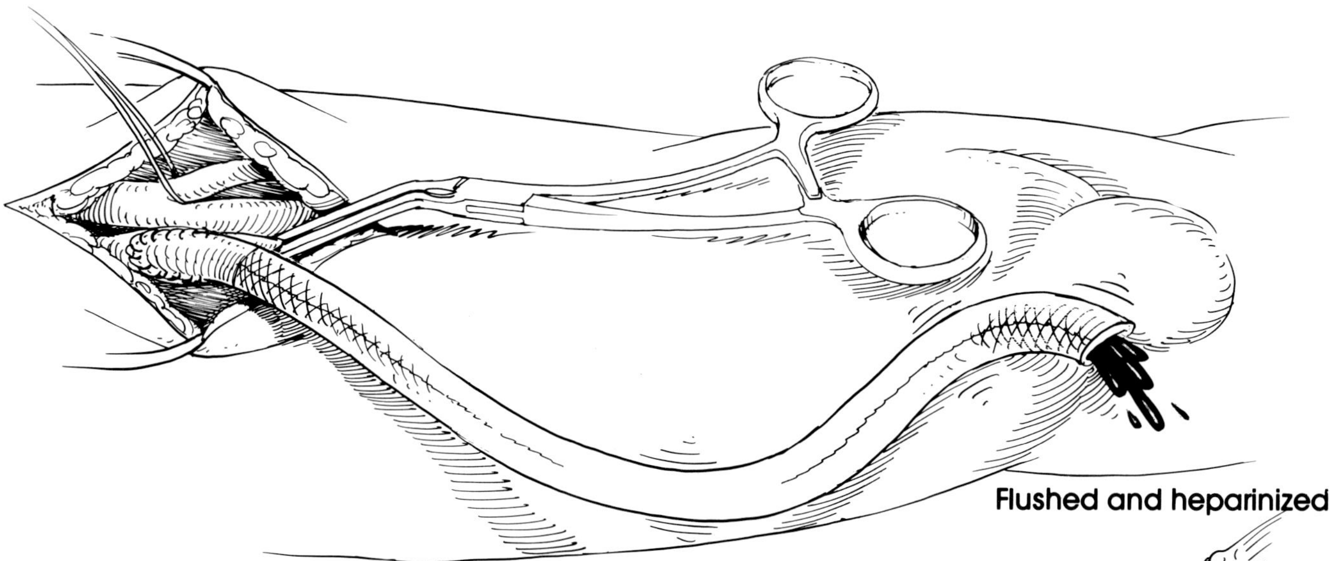

H

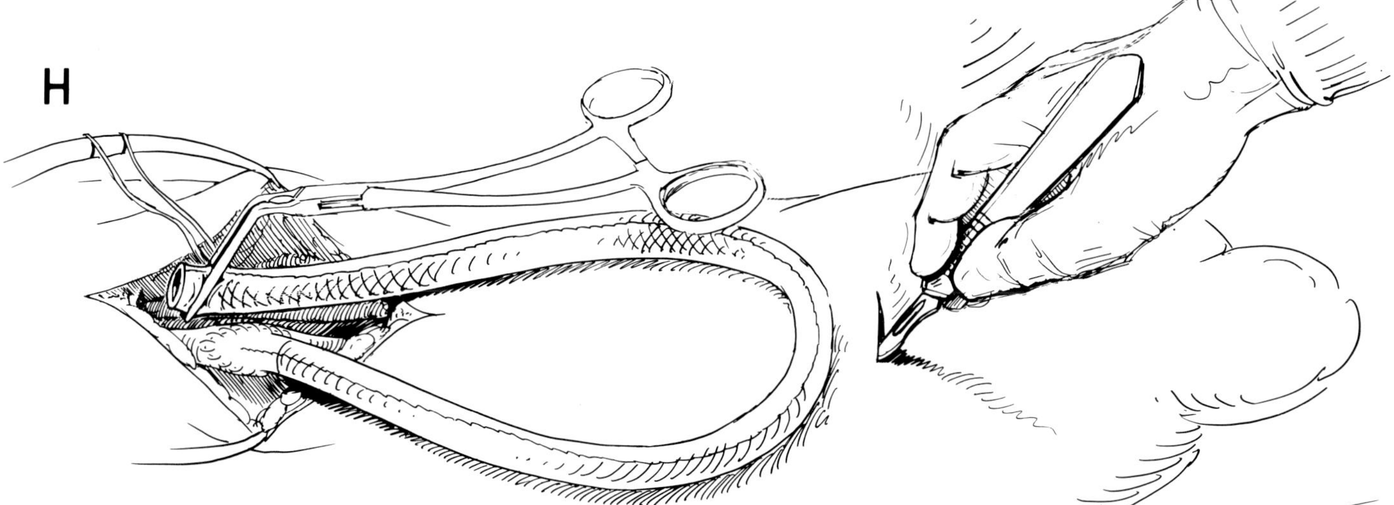

I

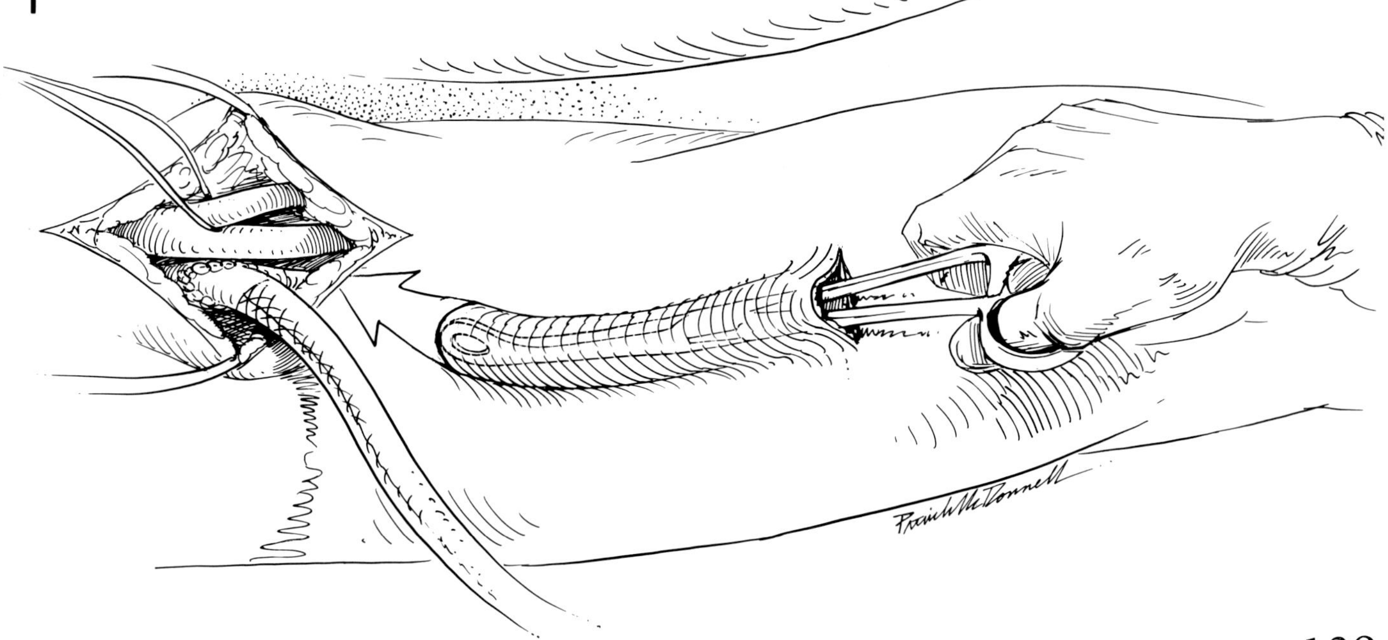

J The graft is clamped immediately distal to the arterial anastomosis and decompressed.

K The graft is brought through the descending tunnel, with care to maintain its orientation.

L The graft is allowed to flush, and proper position is confirmed. Heparinization of the graft is then performed and the free end clamped.

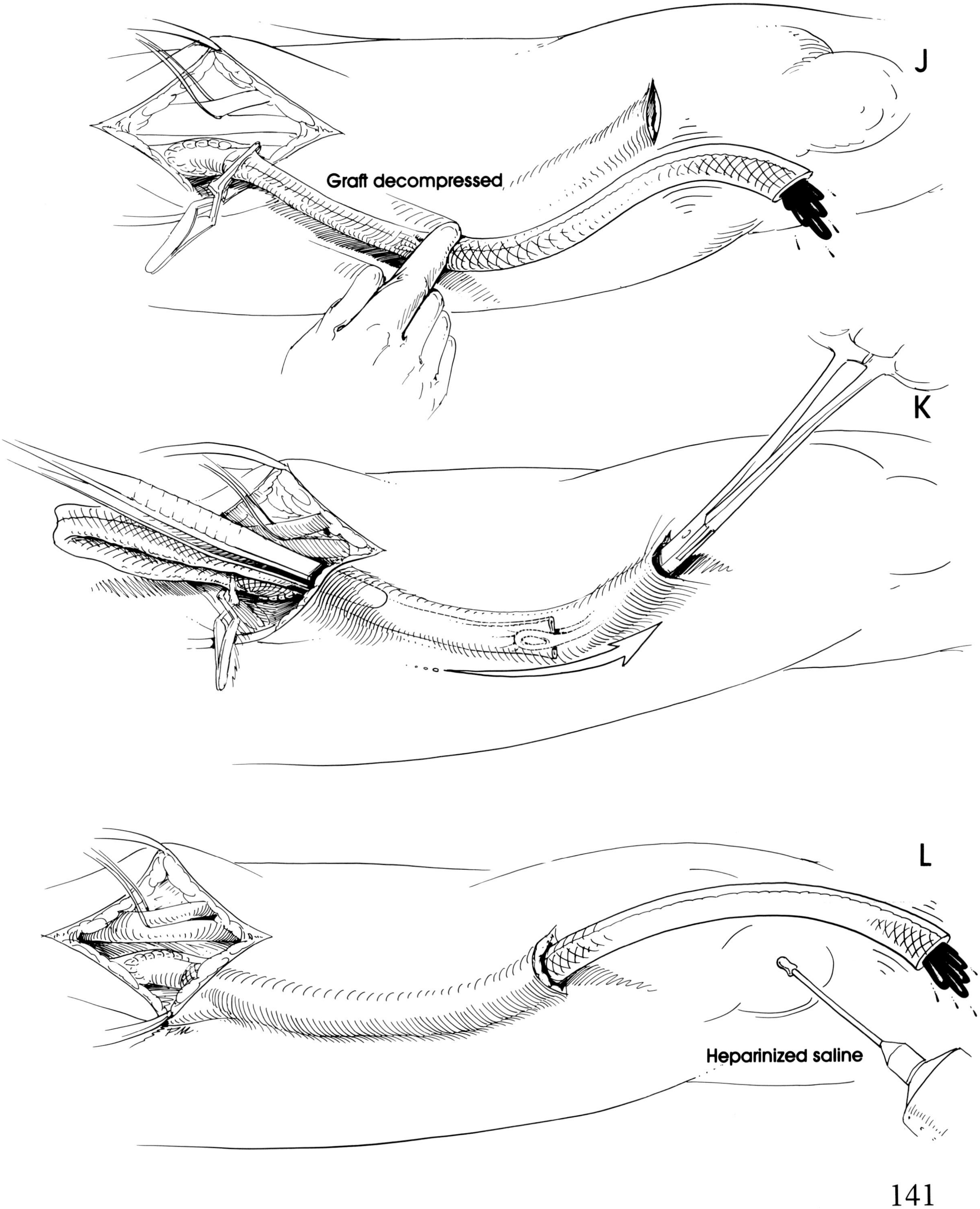
J
Graft decompressed
K
L
Heparinized saline

M A return tunnel is made between the incisions. Following clamping at the level of the counterincision, the distal portion of the graft is decompressed.

N The graft is delivered through the antecubital incision, with care taken to avoid twisting it within the tunnel. A forceps handle is used to prevent rolling of the skin margin of the counterincision.

O The graft is flushed and irrigated with heparinized saline solution, and a clamp is placed on the free end.

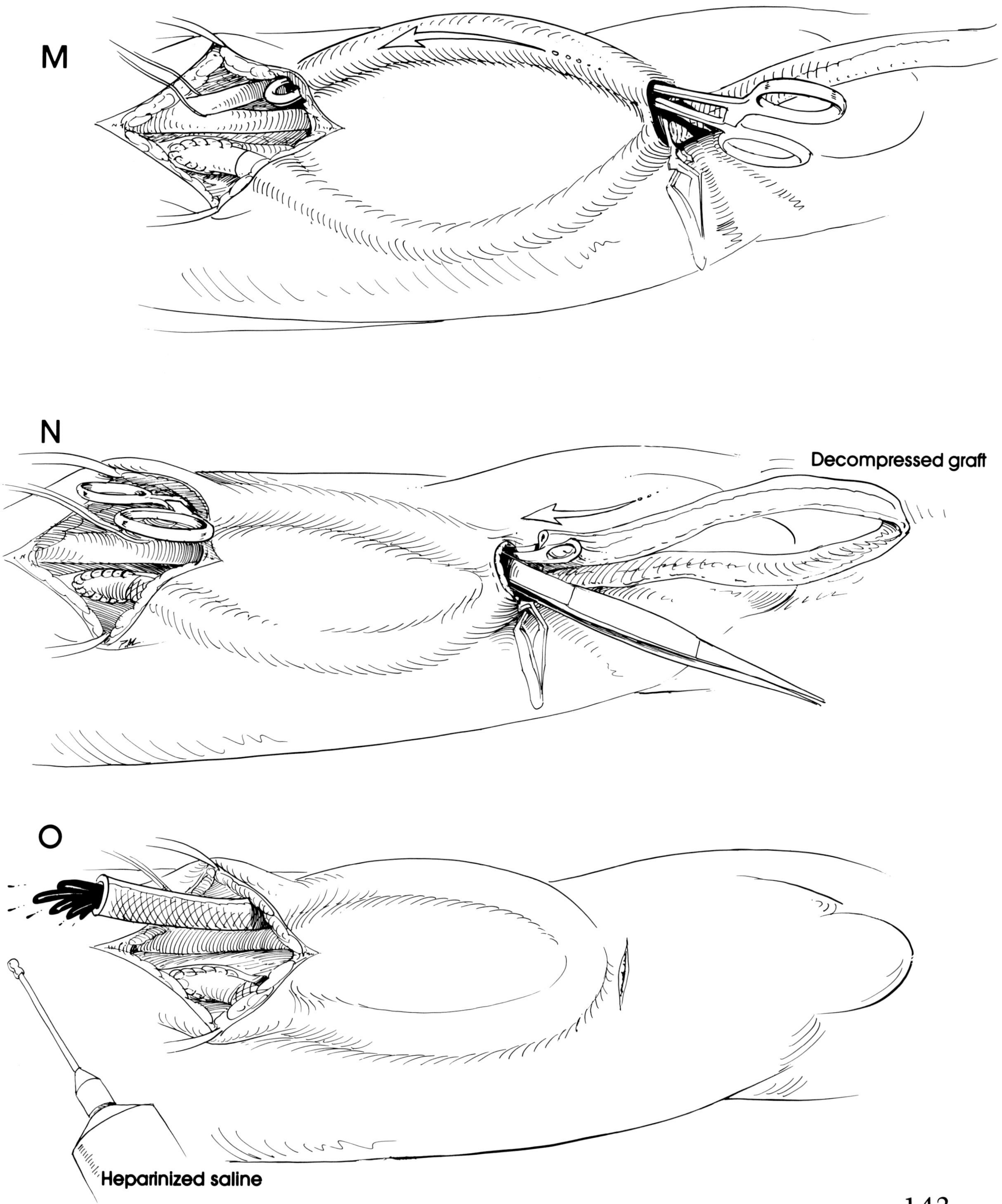
M
N
Decompressed graft
O
Heparinized saline

P The saphenous vein is clamped distally, and the venotomy is extended to a length one and one-half times the graft diameter.

Q Following heparinization of the vein, the graft is tapered and the venous anastomosis is constructed with 6-0 sutures.

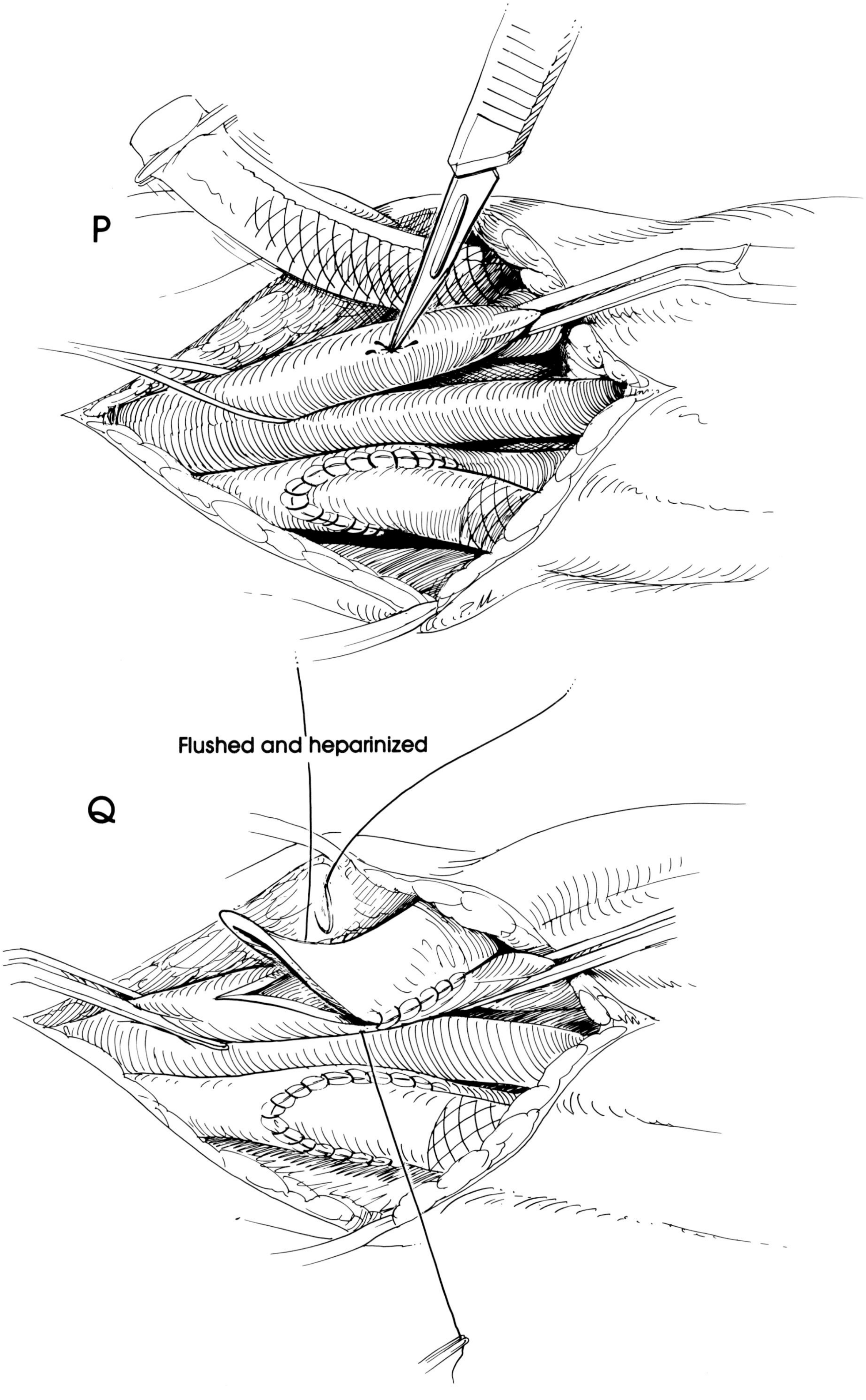
P
Flushed and heparinized
Q

R The clamp on the graft is removed, and the anastomoses are inspected.

S If the greater saphenous vein is too small or absent, the femoral vein may be used as an alternative source of venous runoff.

R

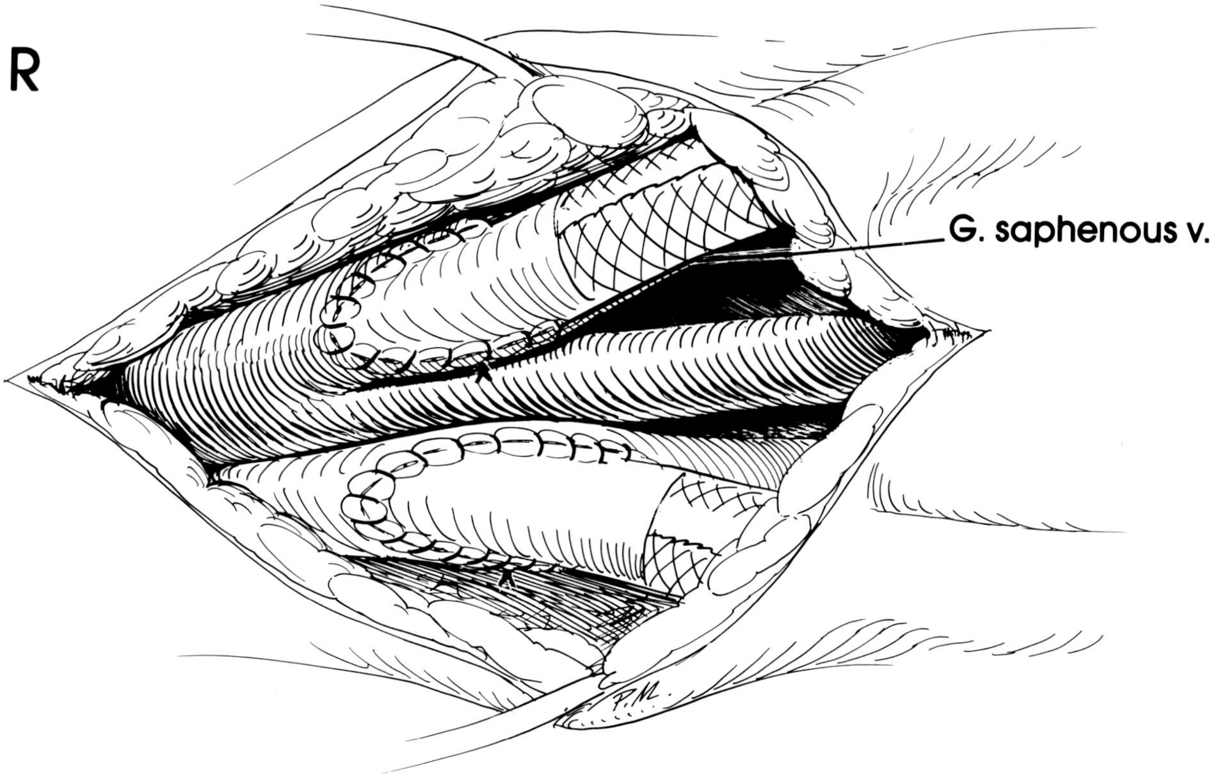

S

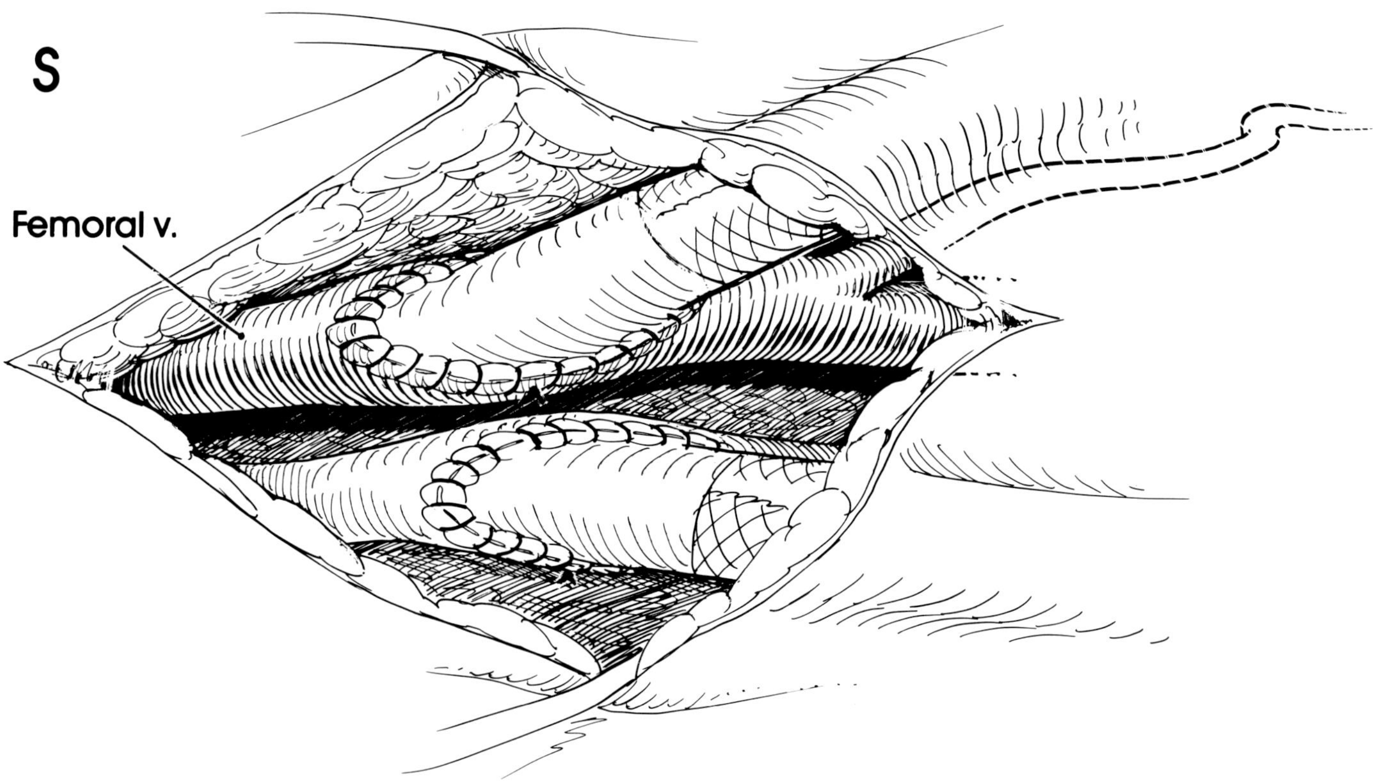

T The position of the graft along the anterolateral aspect of the thigh makes it more accessible, thereby facilitating cannulation.

U A palpable pulse and thrill confirm appropriate function of the fistula. Incisions are closed with 3-0 absorbable suture for the subcutaneous tissue and staples for the skin.

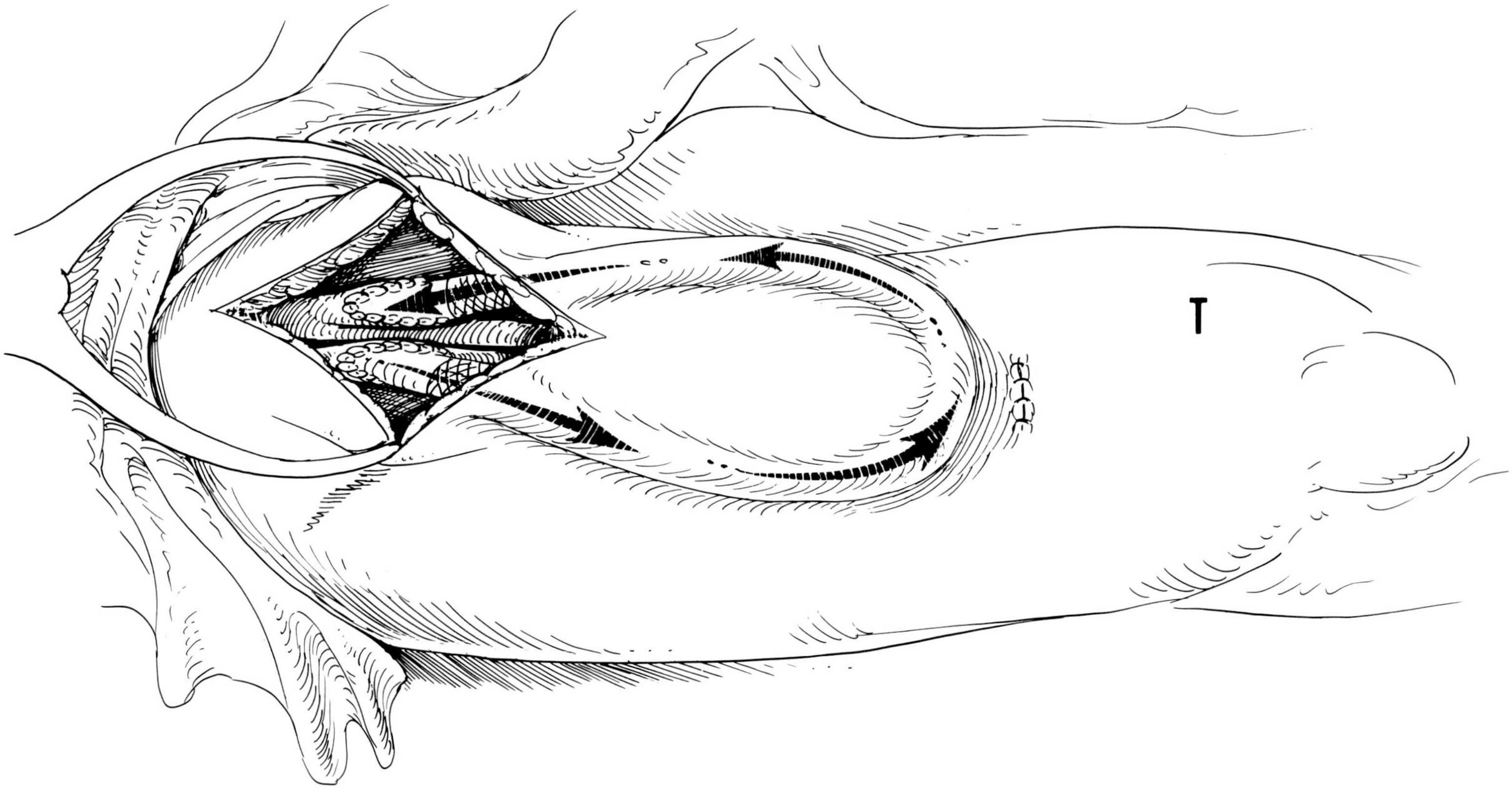

T

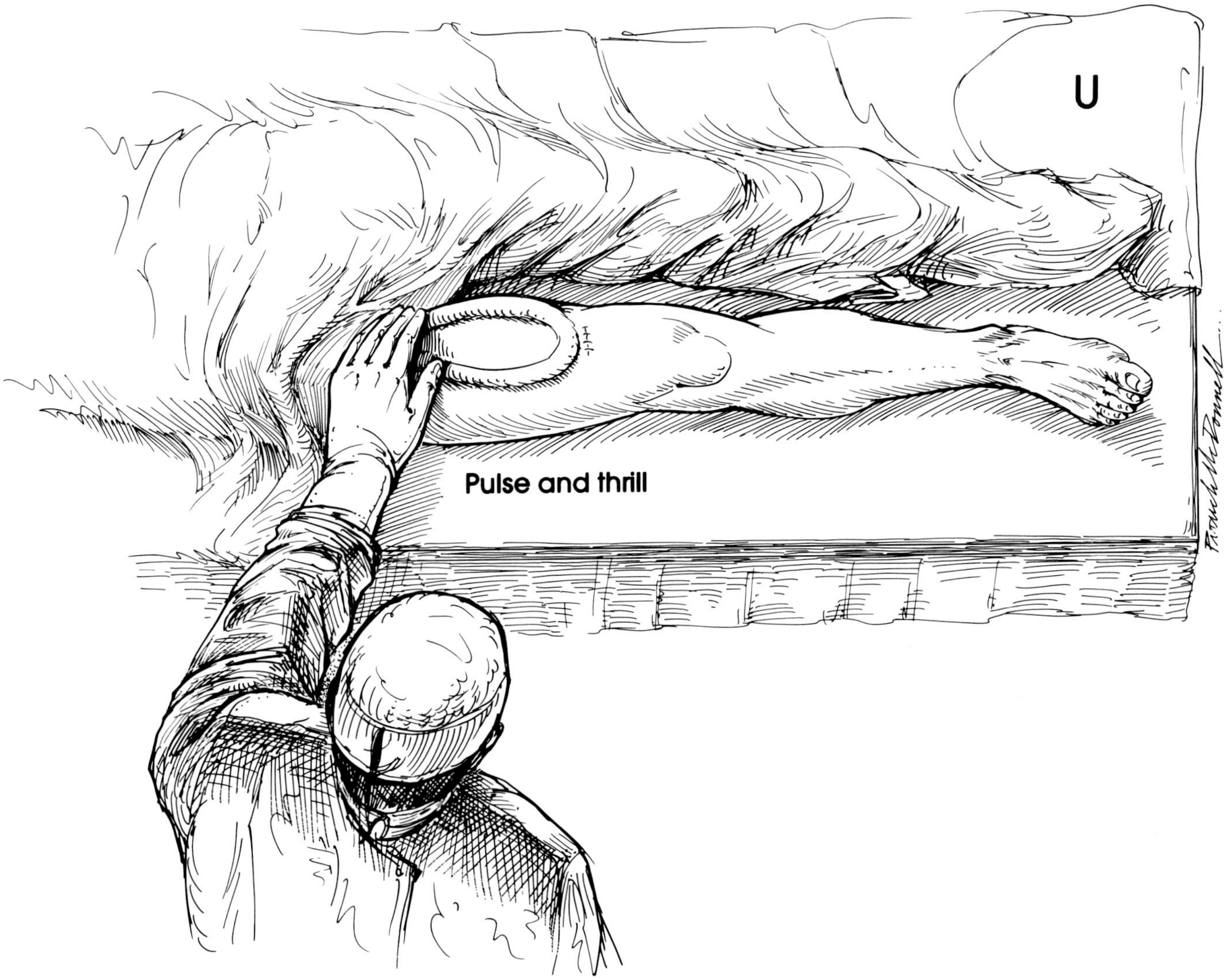

U

Axillary-Axillary Graft Fistula

A Bilateral transverse incisions approximately 6 cm long are made 2 cm below the midportion of the clavicles.

B The axillary vessels are exposed through both incisions and are mobilized to permit construction of the anastomoses. The incision through which the venous anastomosis will be made is packed with moist sponges, and attention is directed to the arterial incision.

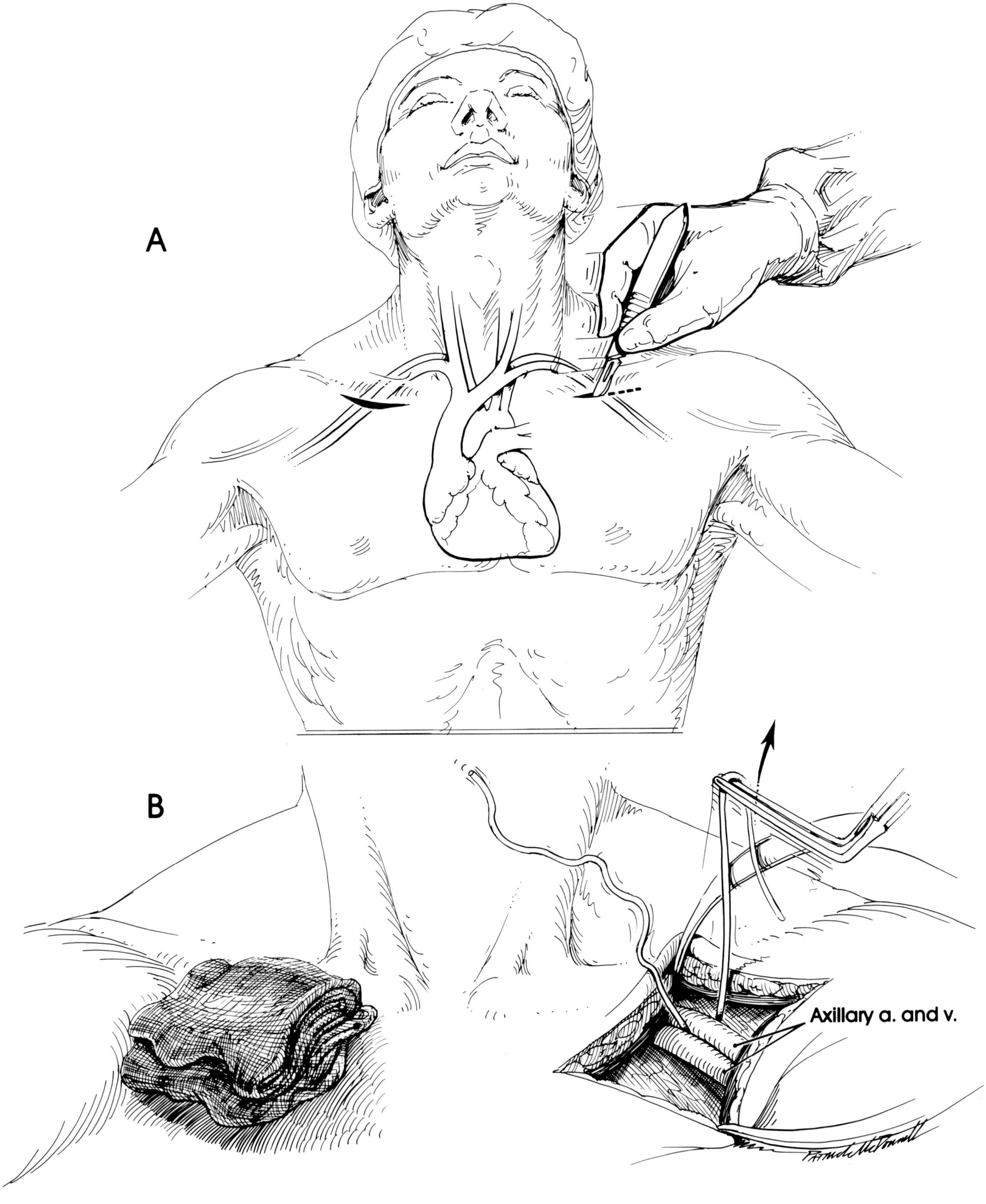
A
B
Axillary a. and v.

C The axillary artery is clamped proximally, and the arteriotomy is begun.

D The arteriotomy is extended to a length approximately one and one-half times the diameter of the graft to be used.

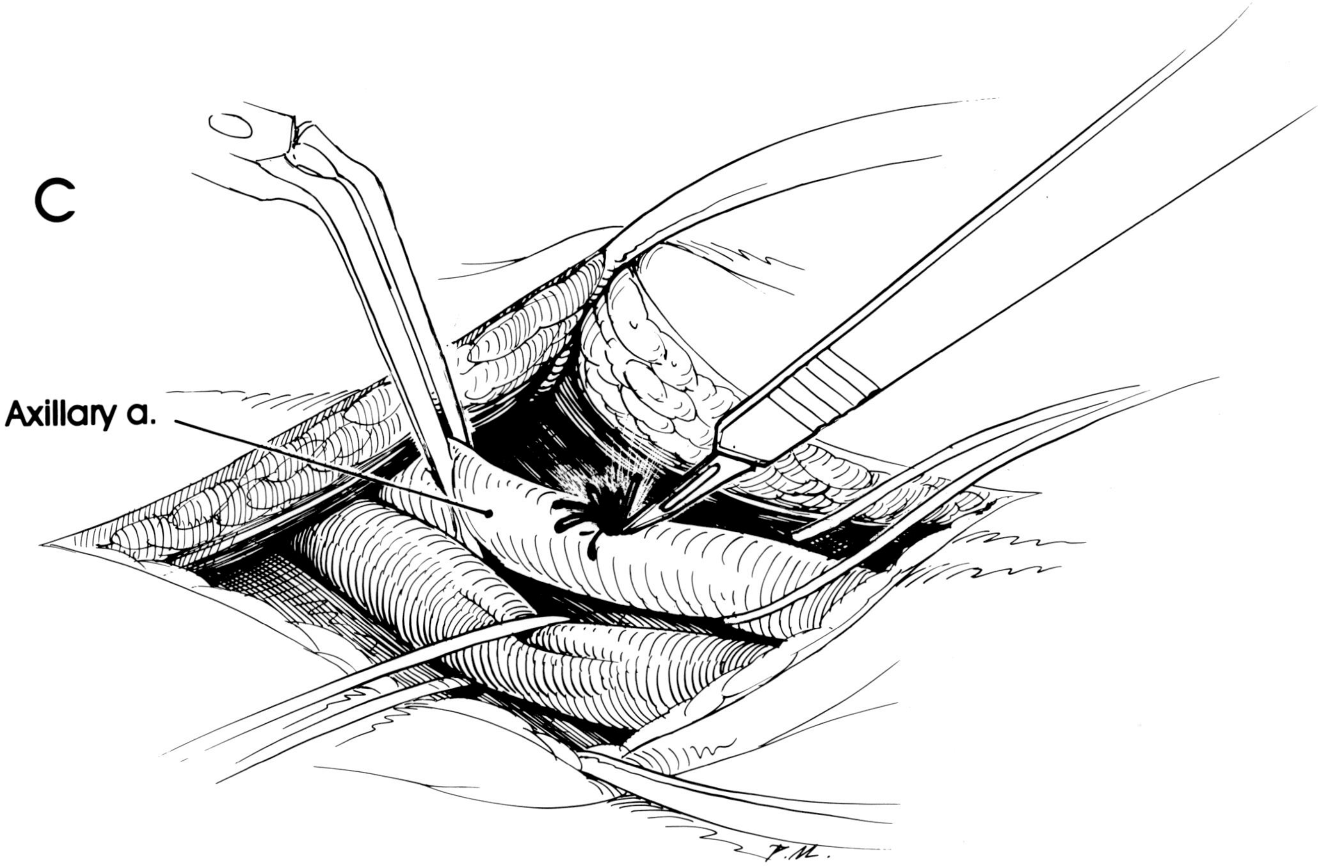
C
Axillary a.

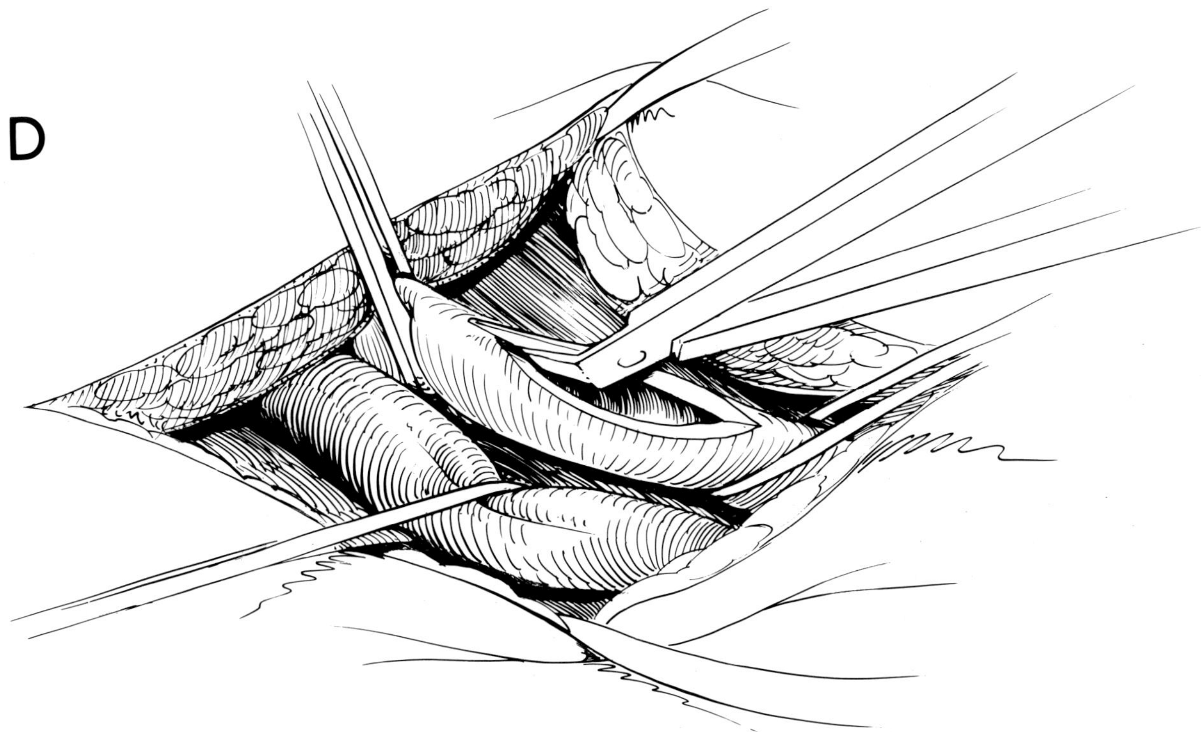
D

E Vessels are heparinized, and a vascular clamp is placed distal to the arteriotomy.

F The graft is tapered for the low-profile, flared end-to-side anastomosis, which is then constructed with running 6-0 polypropylene sutures.

G As always, the graft is flushed before removal of the distal arterial clamp to prevent the possible entry of debris into the distal circulation. The graft is then filled with heparinized saline and clamped.

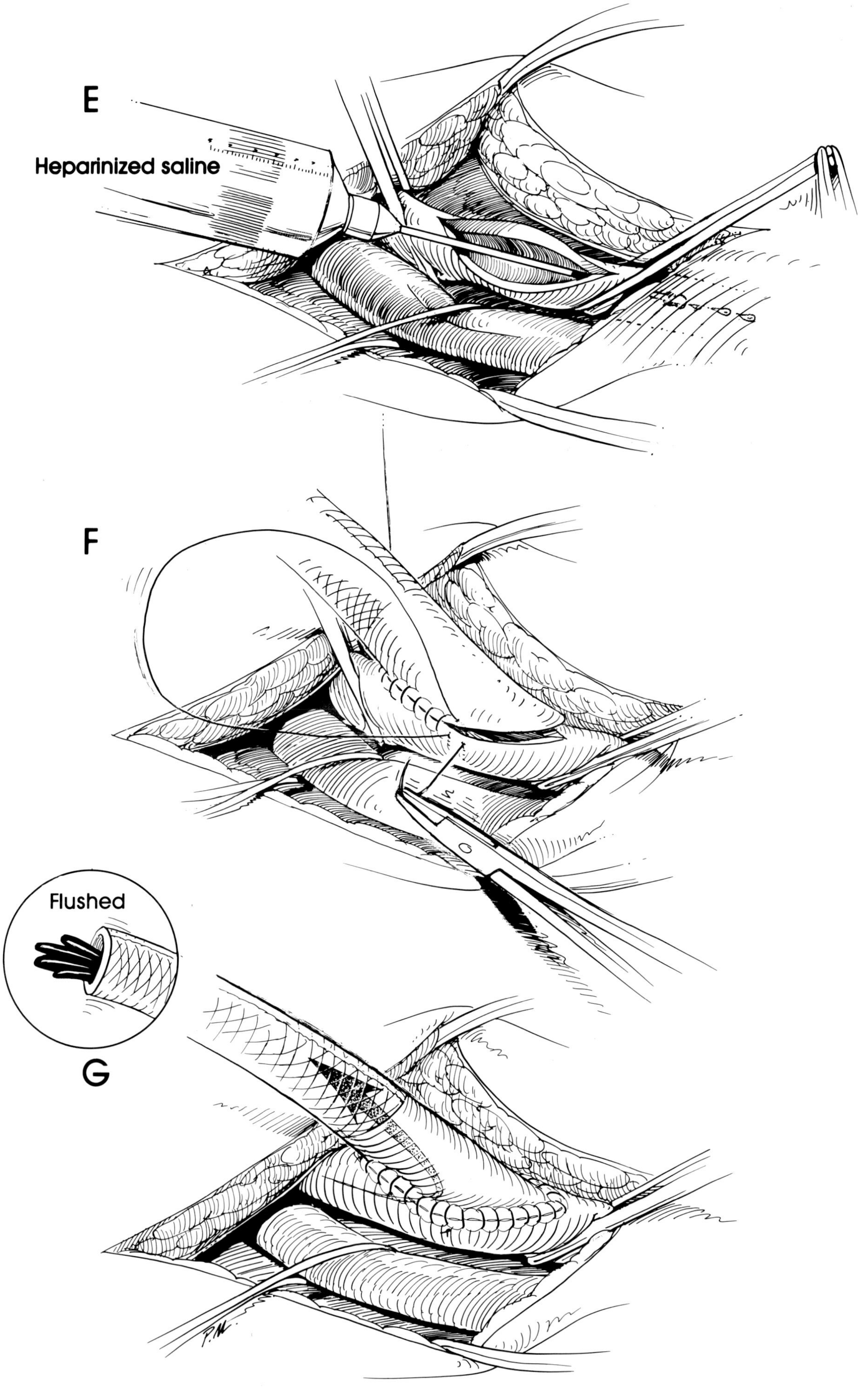
E
Heparinized saline
F
Flushed
G

H A subcutaneous tissue tunnel of appropriate depth is made with a curved spongestick. The inferior aspect of the tunnel should be slightly convex so that the graft will have a smooth course without tension on the anastomosis.

I A clamp is placed immediately distal to the arterial anastomosis, and the graft is decompressed. The spongestick is used to draw the graft through the tunnel without tension.

J The graft is allowed to fill, and proper position within the tunnel is confirmed.

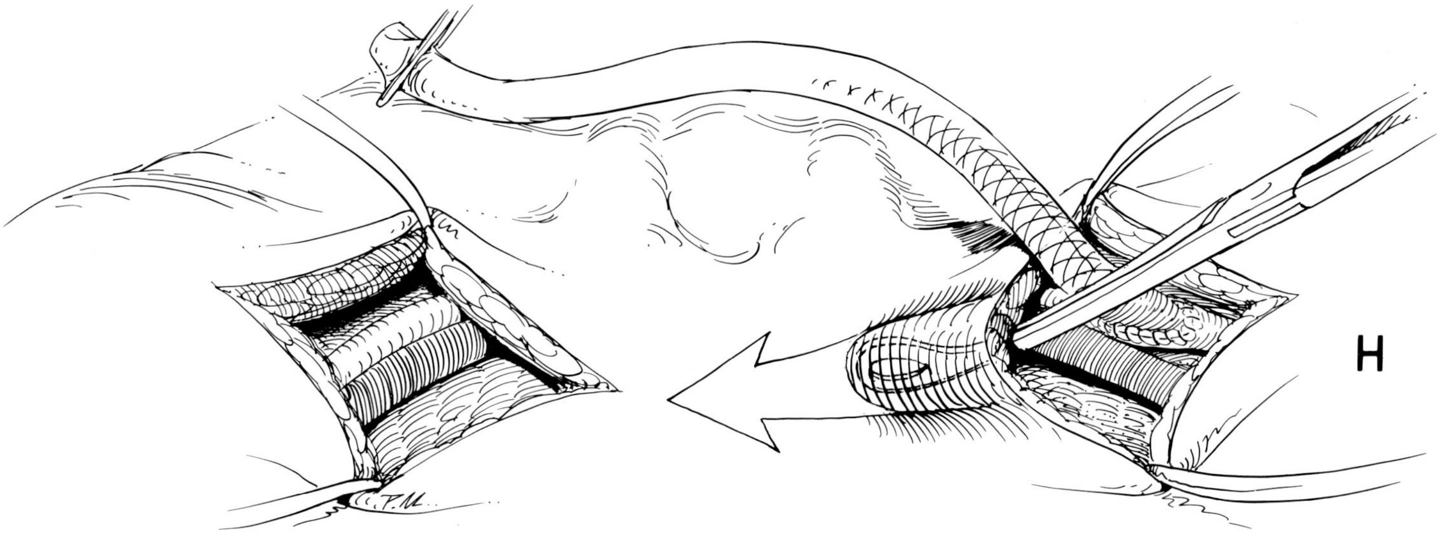

H

I

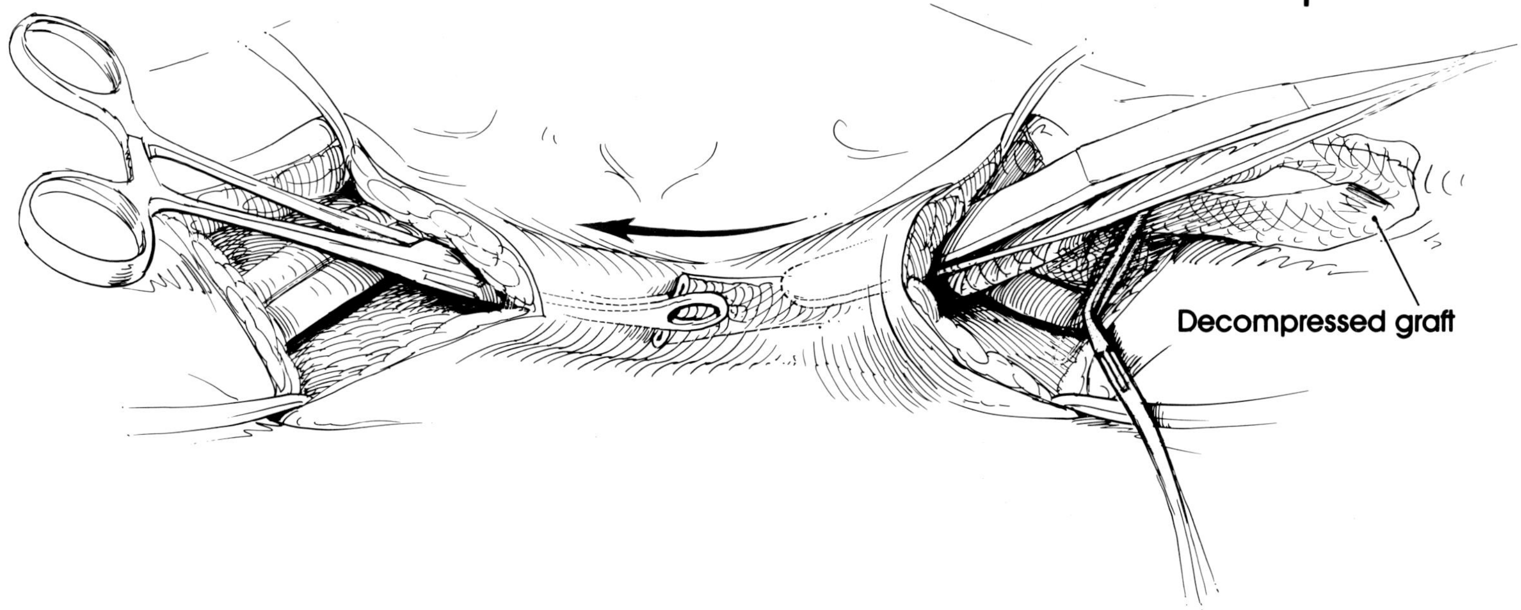

J

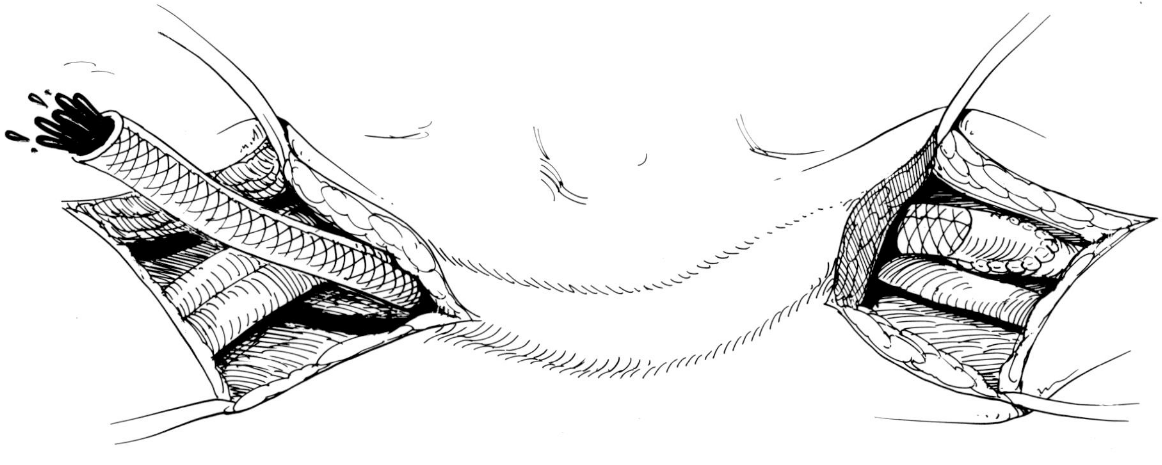

K–N The graft is again heparinized, and attention is directed to the venous incision. The axillary vein is clamped distally, and the venotomy is begun. As before, the venotomy length should be one and one-half times the graft diameter. The axillary vein is irrigated proximally, and the graft is tapered appropriately. The end-to-side venous anastomosis is completed with 6-0 vascular sutures.

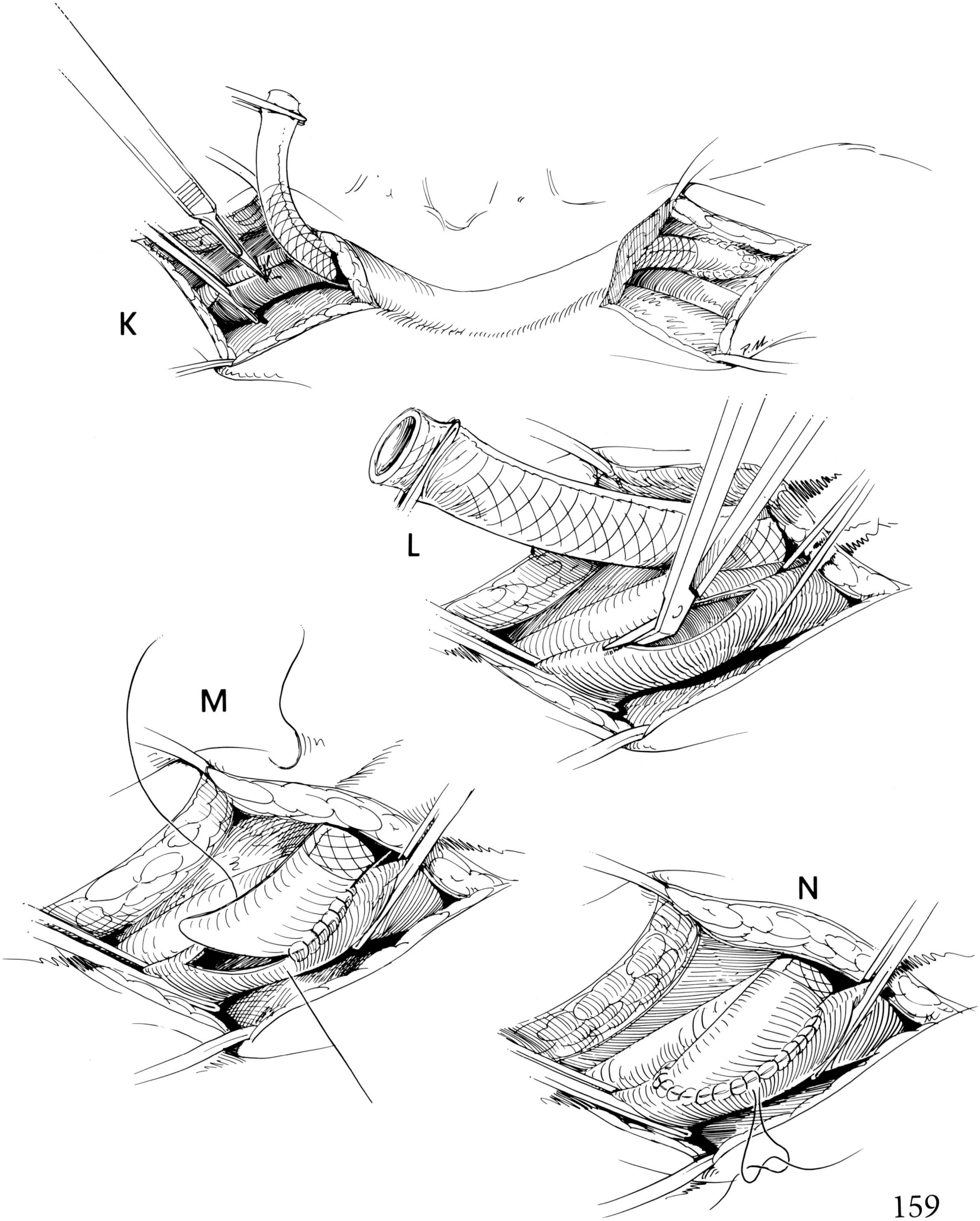
K
L
M
N

O After the anastomosis has been completed, the clamps are removed and flow through the fistula is assessed. The subcutaneous tissue is closed with 3-0 absorbable suture, and staples are used to reapproximate the skin.

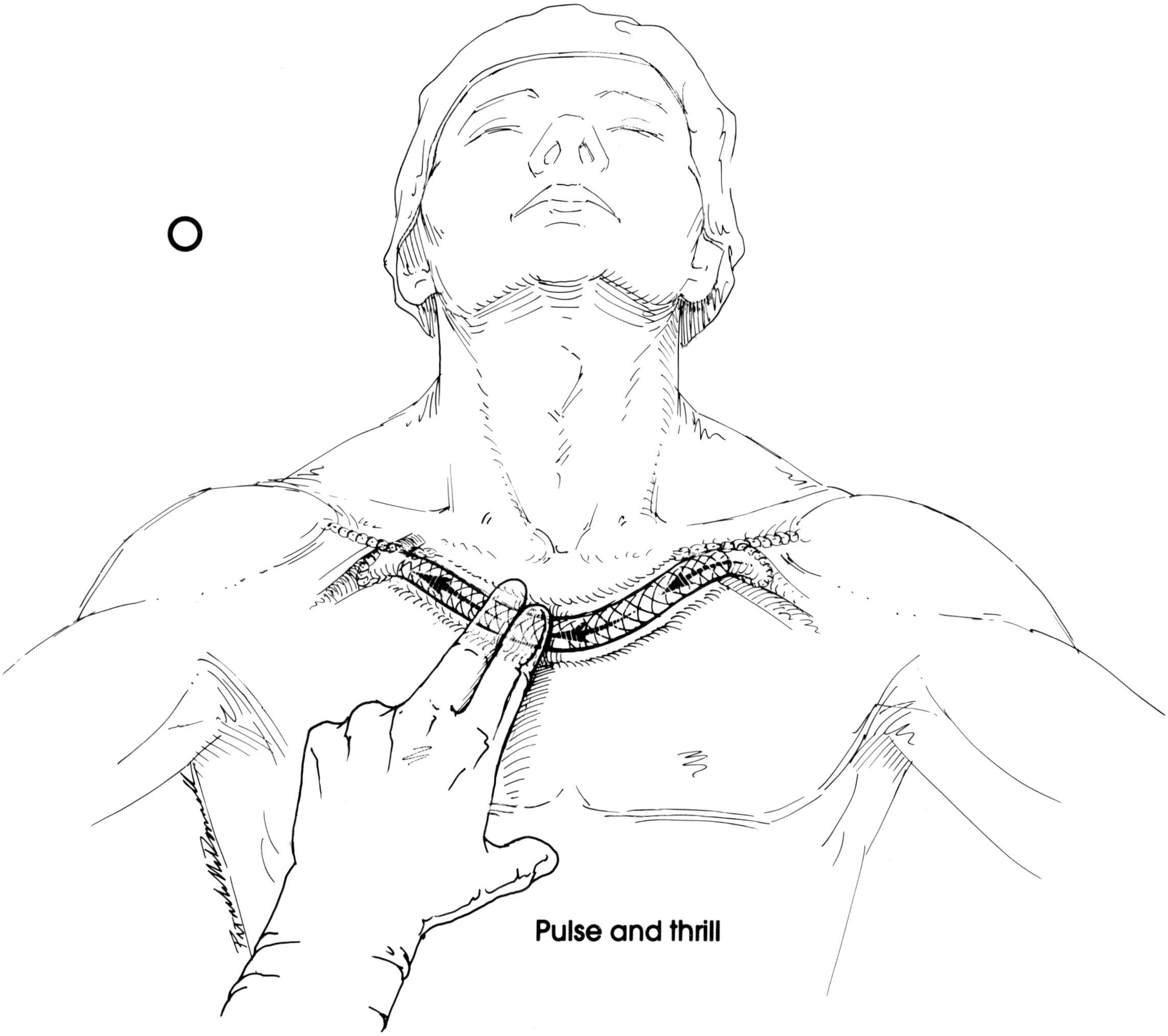
Pulse and thrill

Complications of Graft Arteriovenous Fistulas

6

THE MOST COMMON COMPLICATION associated with graft arteriovenous fistulas is thrombosis. Thrombosis may be due to extrinsic forces, such as inappropriate pressure following withdrawal of the needles, or it may be secondary to intrinsic abnormalities of the graft. It is for the purpose of making this distinction that angiography is indicated following thrombectomy. The most common long-term complication of graft fistulas is outflow tract obstruction secondary to hyperplastic changes of the vein proximal to the graft anastomosis. Hyperplastic changes are thought to be a reaction of the vessel to the greatly increased flow being diverted into it by the fistula. Arterial hyperplasia also occurs, but much less frequently. Some studies indicate that trauma to the vessel wall at the time of instrumentation with embolectomy catheters is a significant factor in the production of hyperplastic changes. Regardless of etiology, extension grafts are curative in cases of inadequate vessel diameter. Complications that occur less frequently include graft dissection, aneurysm formation, arterial steal, and infection. Dissection of graft fistulas is a result of inappropriate cannulation technique, and treatment requires partial resection of the graft. Aneurysms are treated according to their size, with the larger ones requiring resection rather than plication. The treatment of arterial steal is based on reduction of flow through the graft with a concomitant increase in brachial artery flow. If this is not possible, graft closure is indicated. Limited resection of infected grafts is not usually successful; however, reconstruction of the vessels may be avoided by leaving the graft stumps in place as long as there is no evidence of infection in that area.

All efforts must be expended to salvage graft arteriovenous fistulas, as the vessels available for their construction are limited.

Graft Thrombosis

Fogarty Thrombectomy

A A transverse incision approximately 3 cm long is made overlying the most inferior edge of the looped graft arteriovenous fistula.

B–C Vessels are mobilized sufficiently to allow clamp placement, and the graft is opened with a transverse incision.

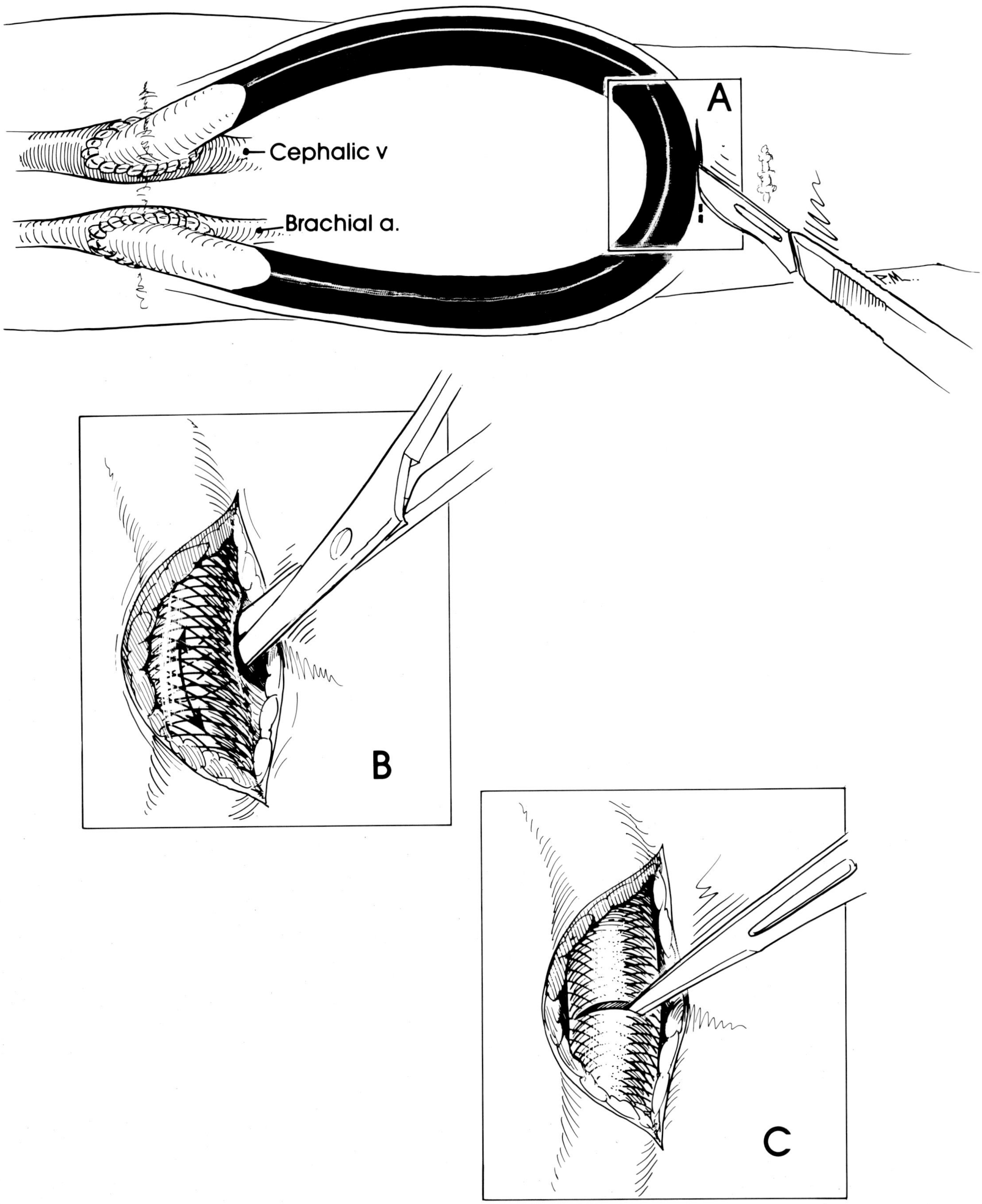
A
Cephalic v
Brachial a.
B
C

D–E A 5 F thrombectomy catheter is inserted into the venous limb of the graft and advanced until the balloon is beyond the anastomosis. The balloon is then inflated and the catheter withdrawn. Successive passes of the catheter are made until no additional thrombus is retrieved.

F–G The venous limb of the graft is then heparinized and clamped.

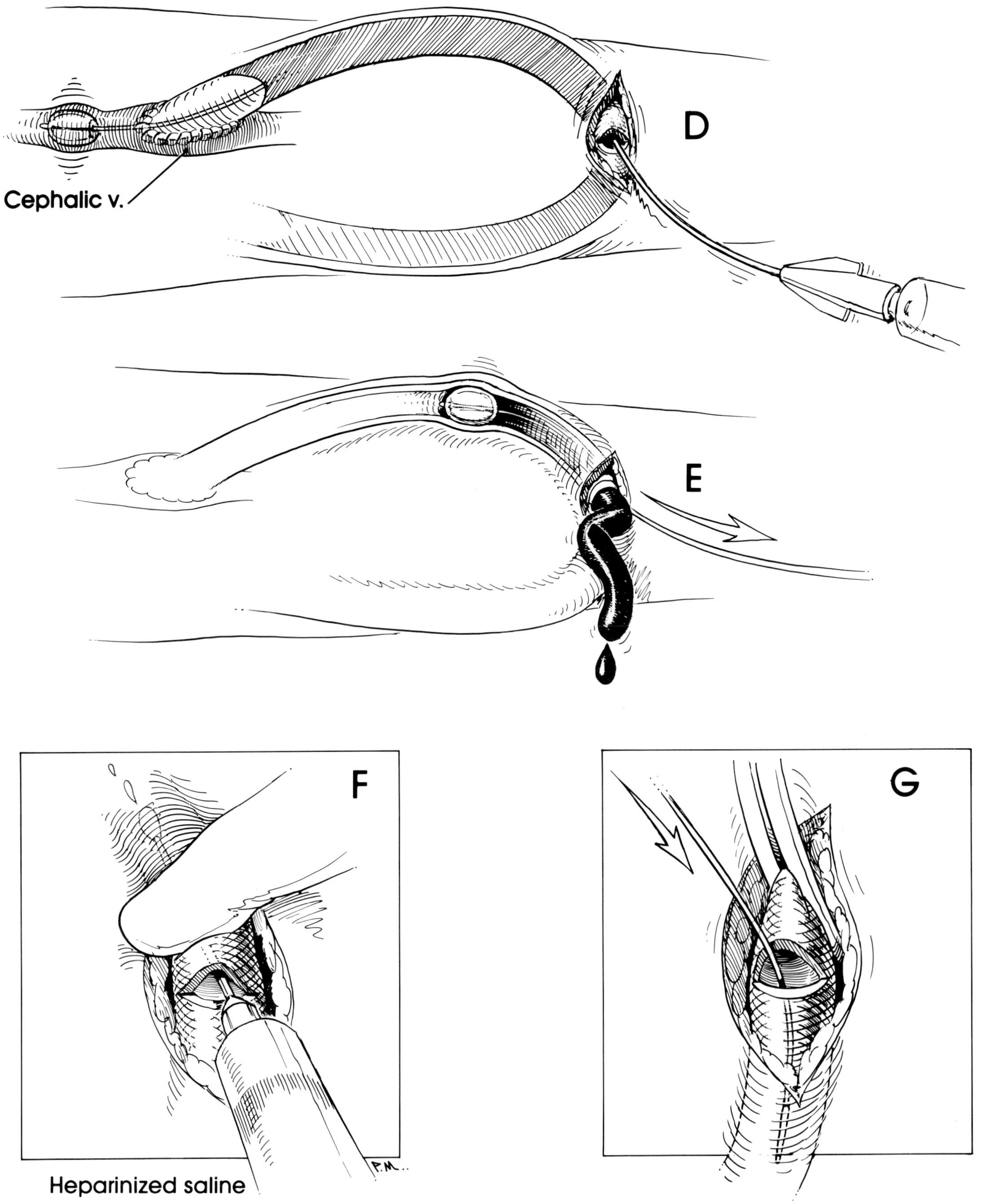
D
Cephalic v.
E
F
G
Heparinized saline
P.M.

H The thrombectomy catheter is inserted into the arterial limb of the fistula and advanced into the brachial artery.

I–J The clot is removed, and the graft is heparinized and clamped.

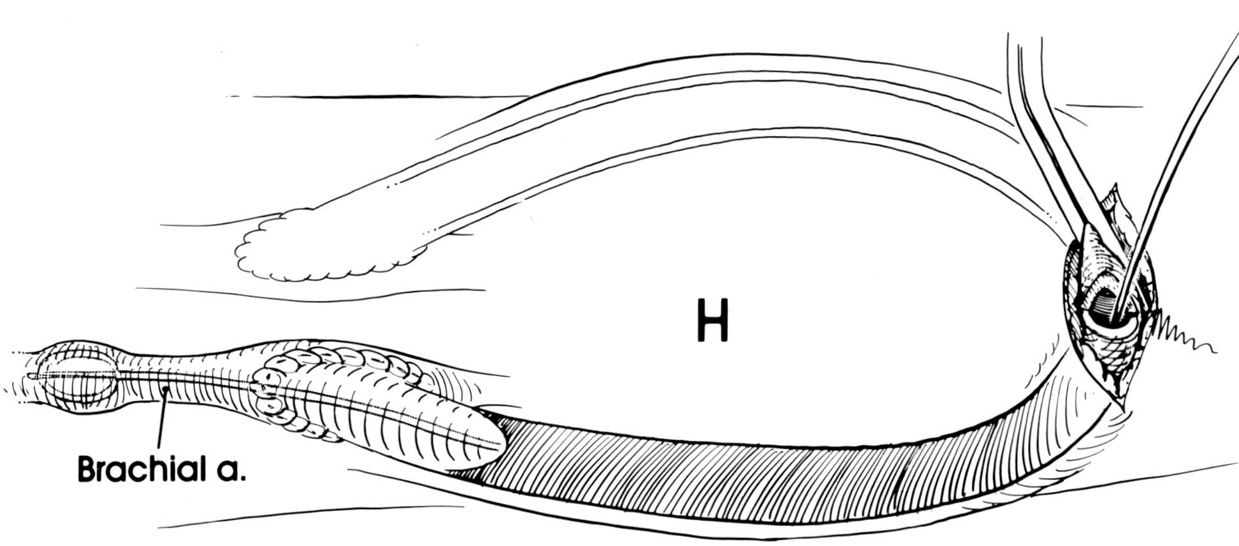
H
Brachial a.

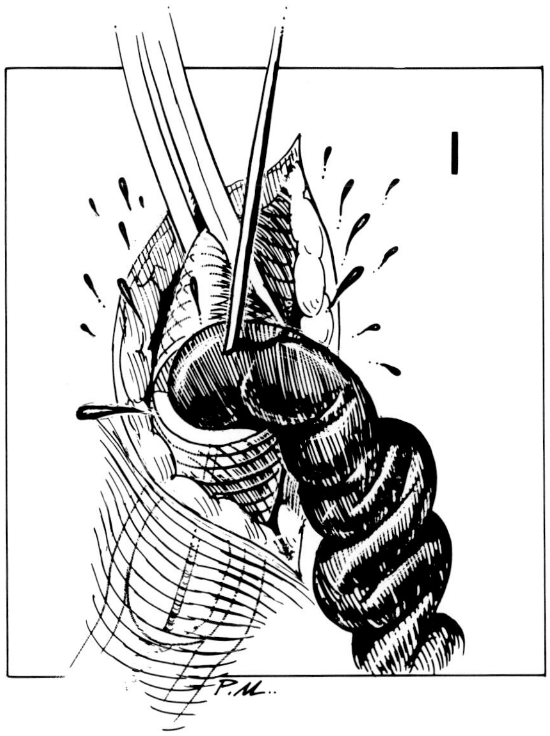
I

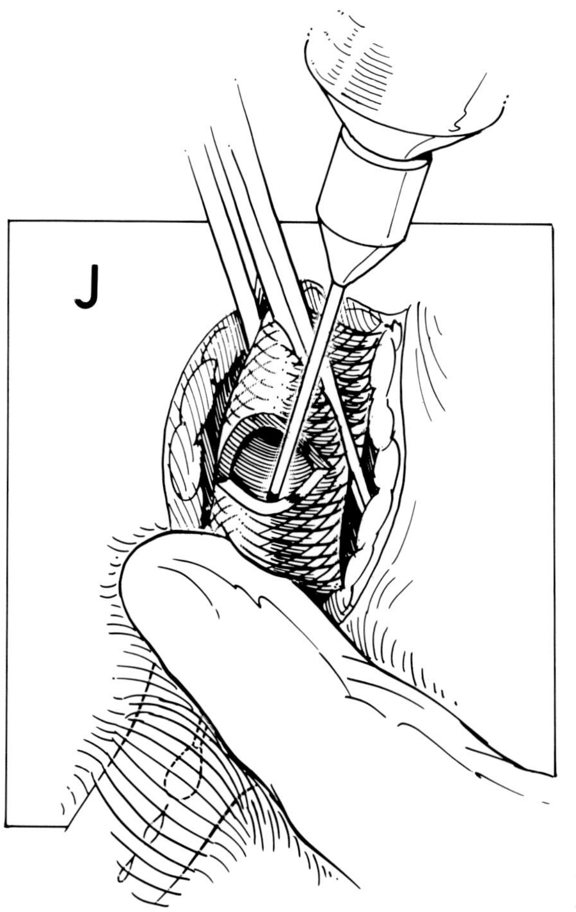
J

K–M The two edges of the graft incision are approximated and joined with running 6-0 polypropylene sutures.

K

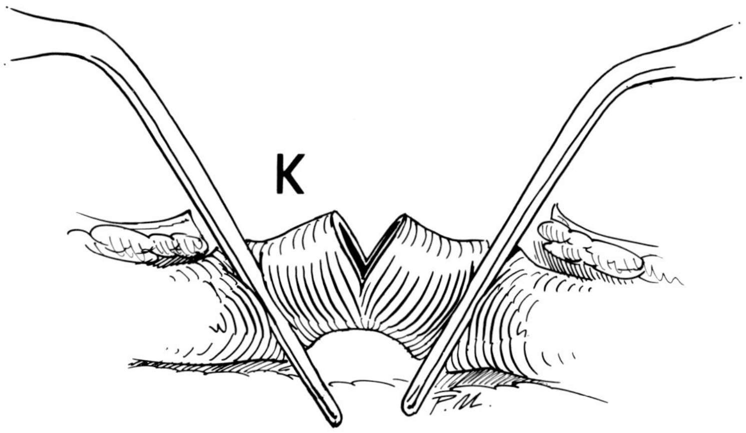

L

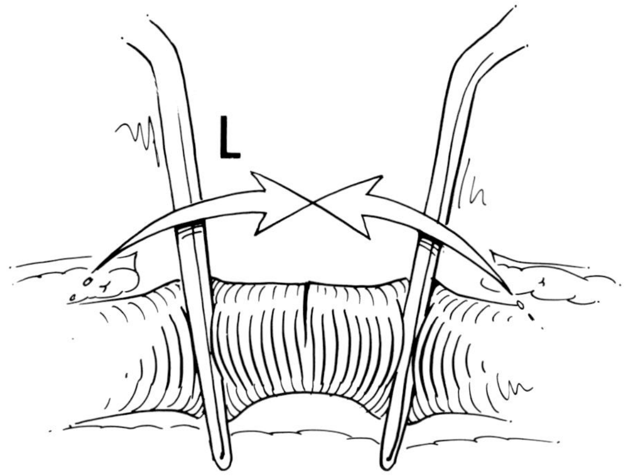

M

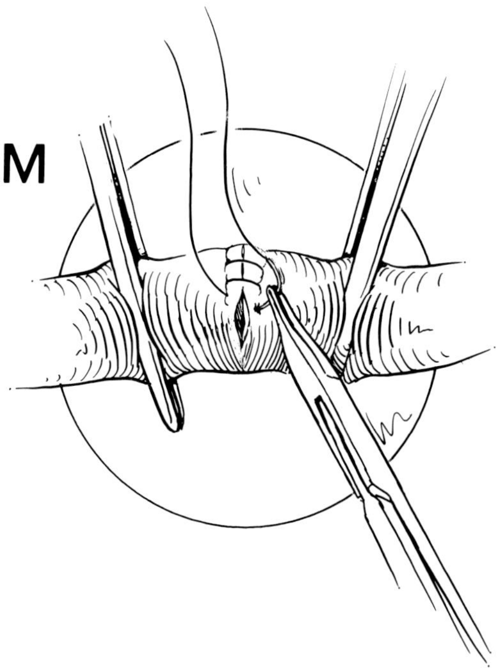

N A palpable pulse and thrill confirm adequate flow.

Angiography should be performed if a pulse and thrill are not present or if there is reason to suspect that the thrombosis could have been secondary to an intrinsic abnormality of the graft.

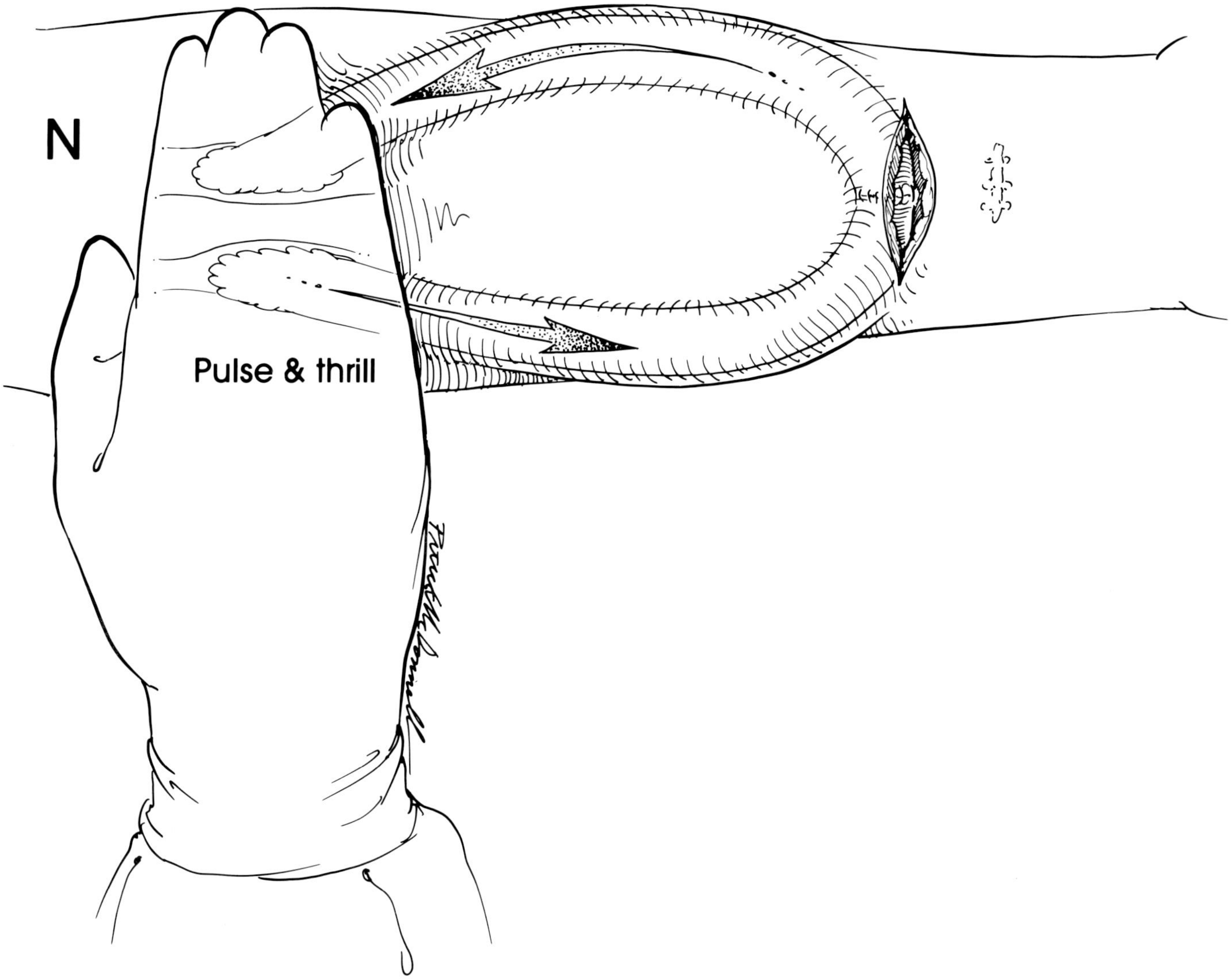
N
Pulse & thrill

Angiography

The arterial limb of the graft fistula is cannulated in a central direction with a 19-gauge butterfly needle. The angiography tubing is filled with heparinized saline and clamped. A syringe containing the radiopaque dye is connected, and the tubing clamp is removed. Positive pressure is then applied on the syringe, forcing dyc retrograde beyond the arterial anastomosis and filling the graft and cephalic vein distally. The radiographic plate is exposed immediately before the syringe empties.

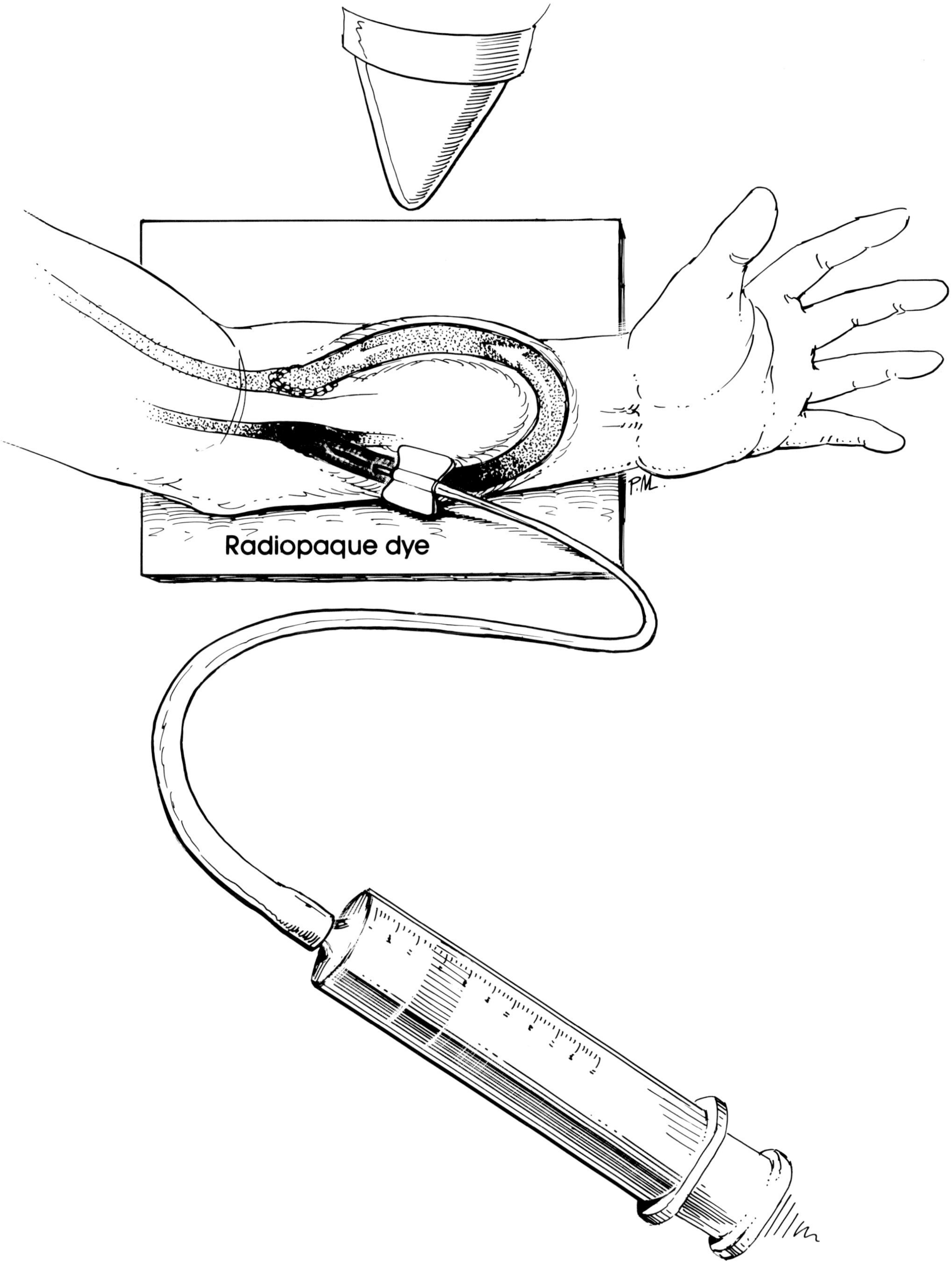
Radiopaque dye
P.M.

Outflow Tract Obstruction

Venous Limb Extension

A–C A longitudinal incision approximately 5 cm long is made overlying the distal portion of the venous limb of the graft. This segment of the fistula is identified and mobilized.

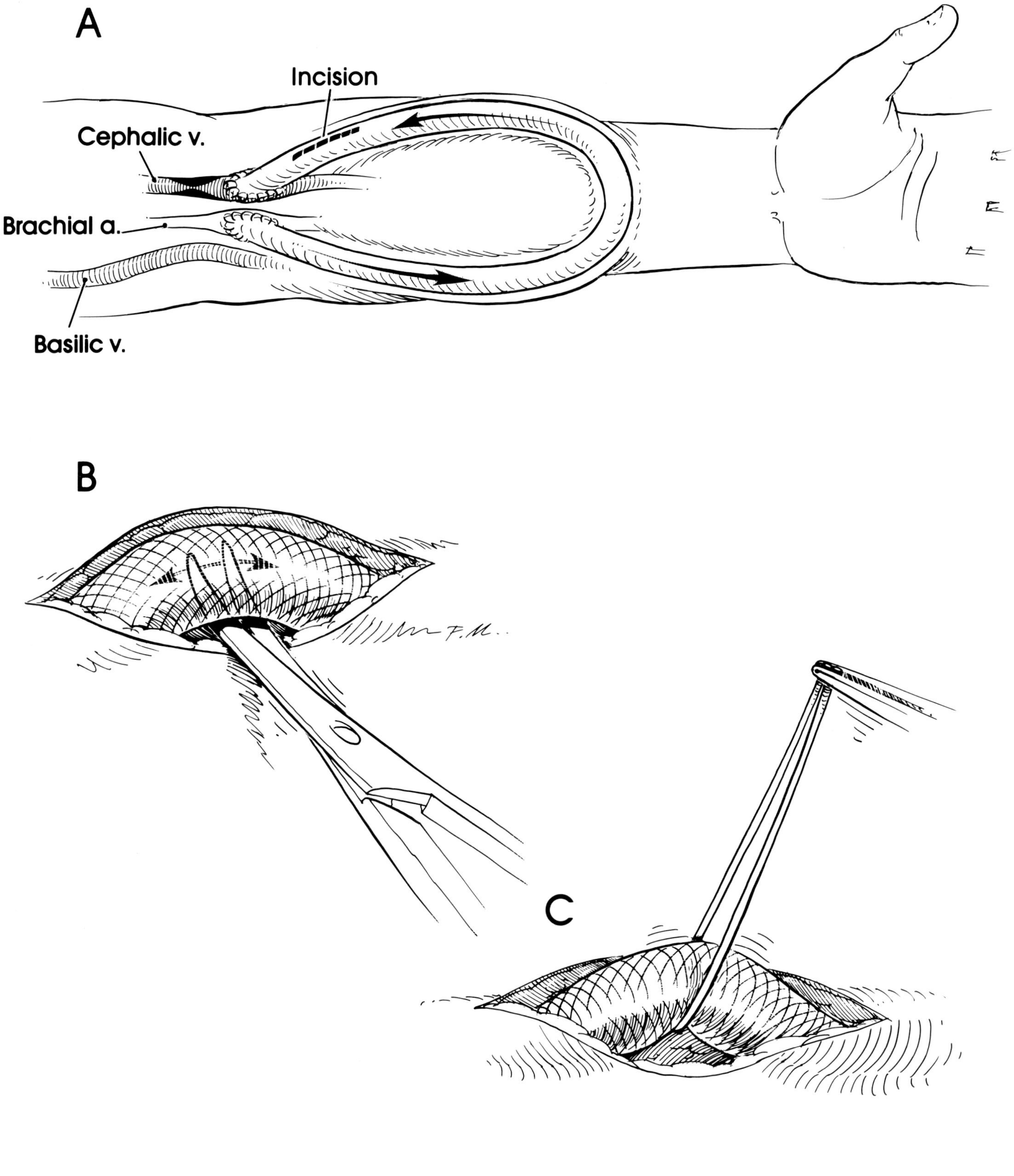
A
Incision
Cephalic v.
Brachial a.
Basilic v.
B
C

D–F The incision is packed with moist sponges, and a 5-cm longitudinal incision is made along the medial aspect of the arm. The basilic vein is identified and mobilized.

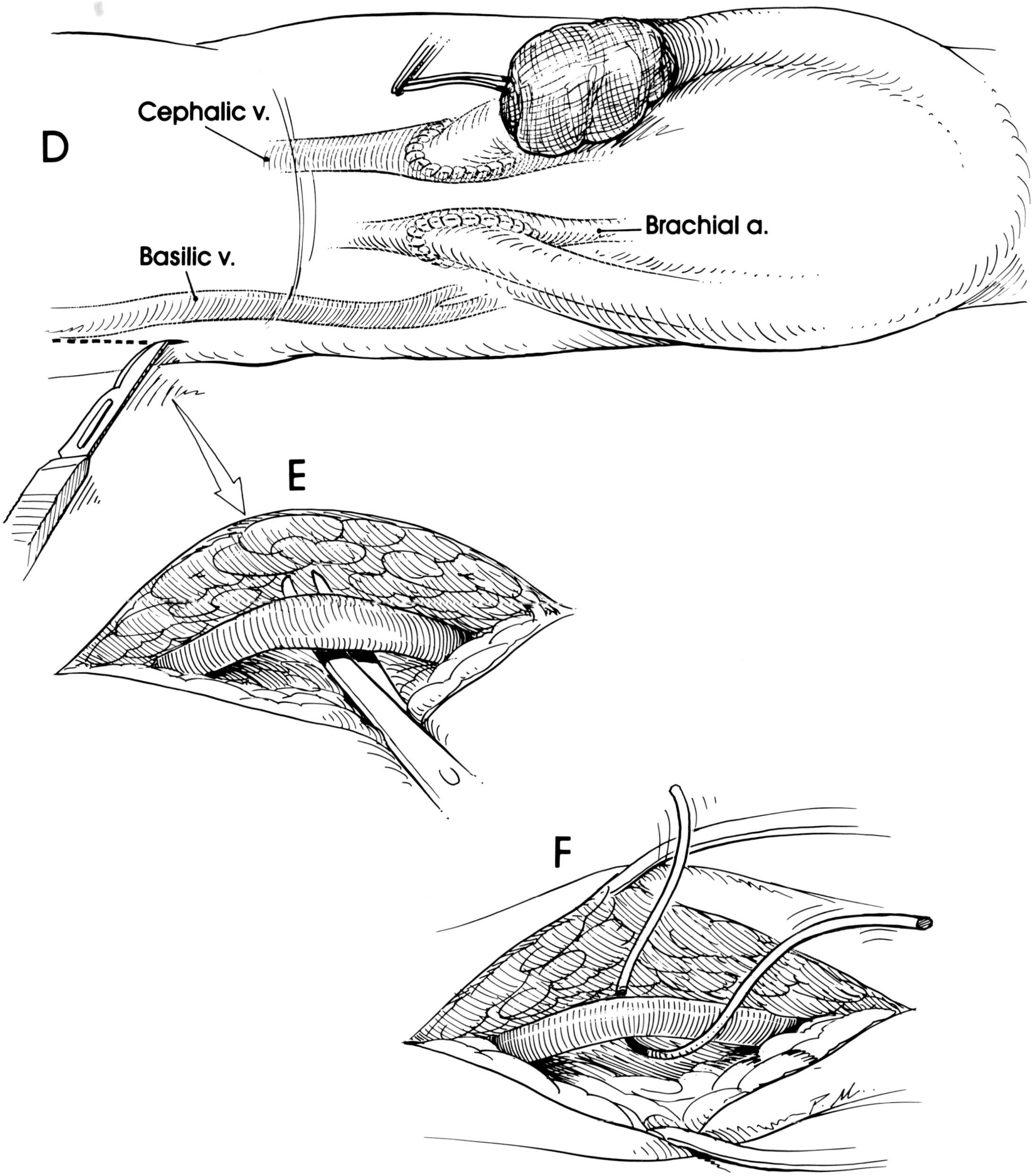
D
Cephalic v.
Brachial a.
Basilic v.
E
F

G–H A vascular clamp is placed on the graft, and the graft is opened with a no. 11 blade.

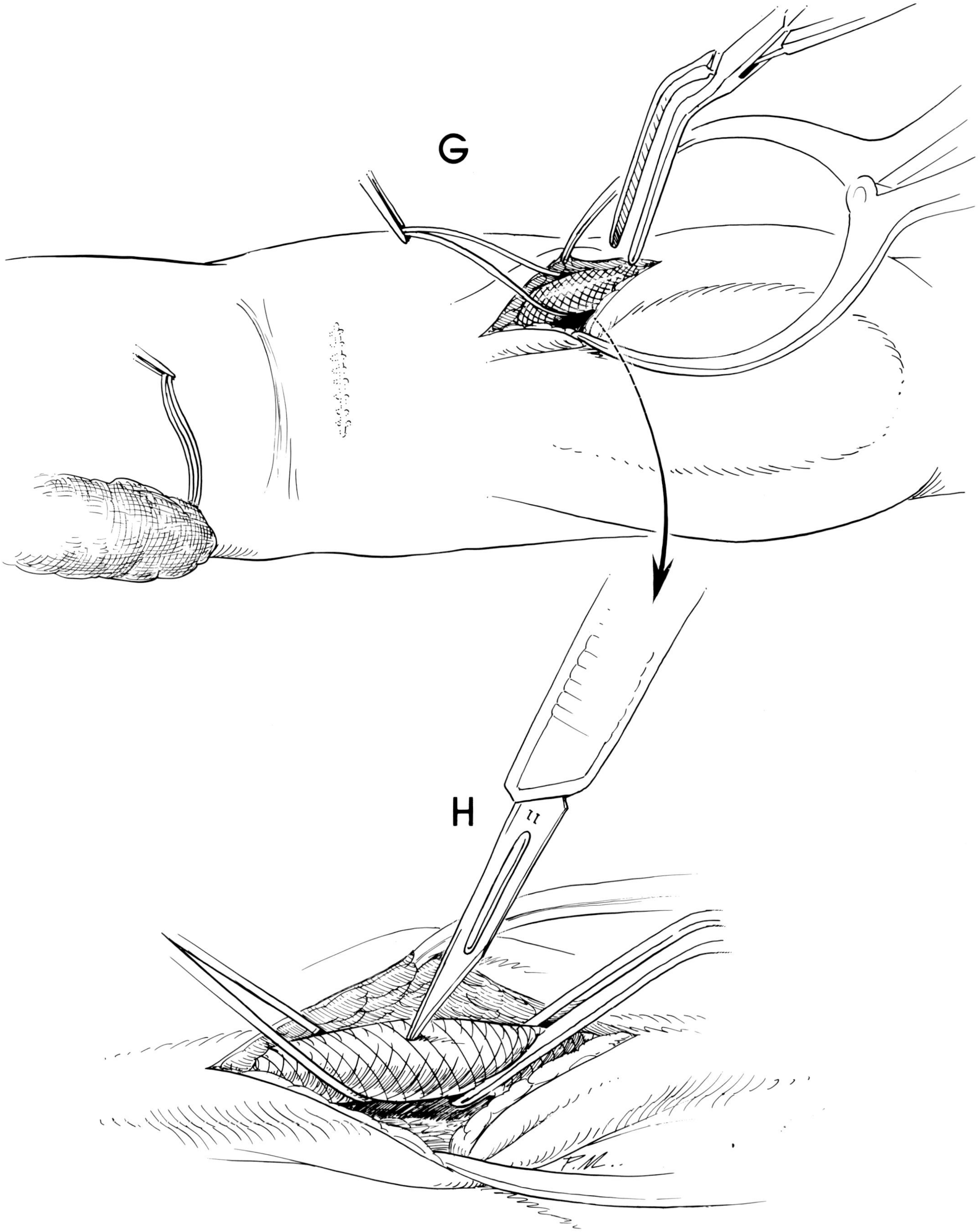
G
H

I The incision is extended to a length one and one-half times the graft diameter.

J The graft is heparinized, and a proximal clamp is placed.

K The interposition graft is tapered appropriately for the flared end-to-side anastomosis, which is constructed with running 6-0 polypropylene sutures.

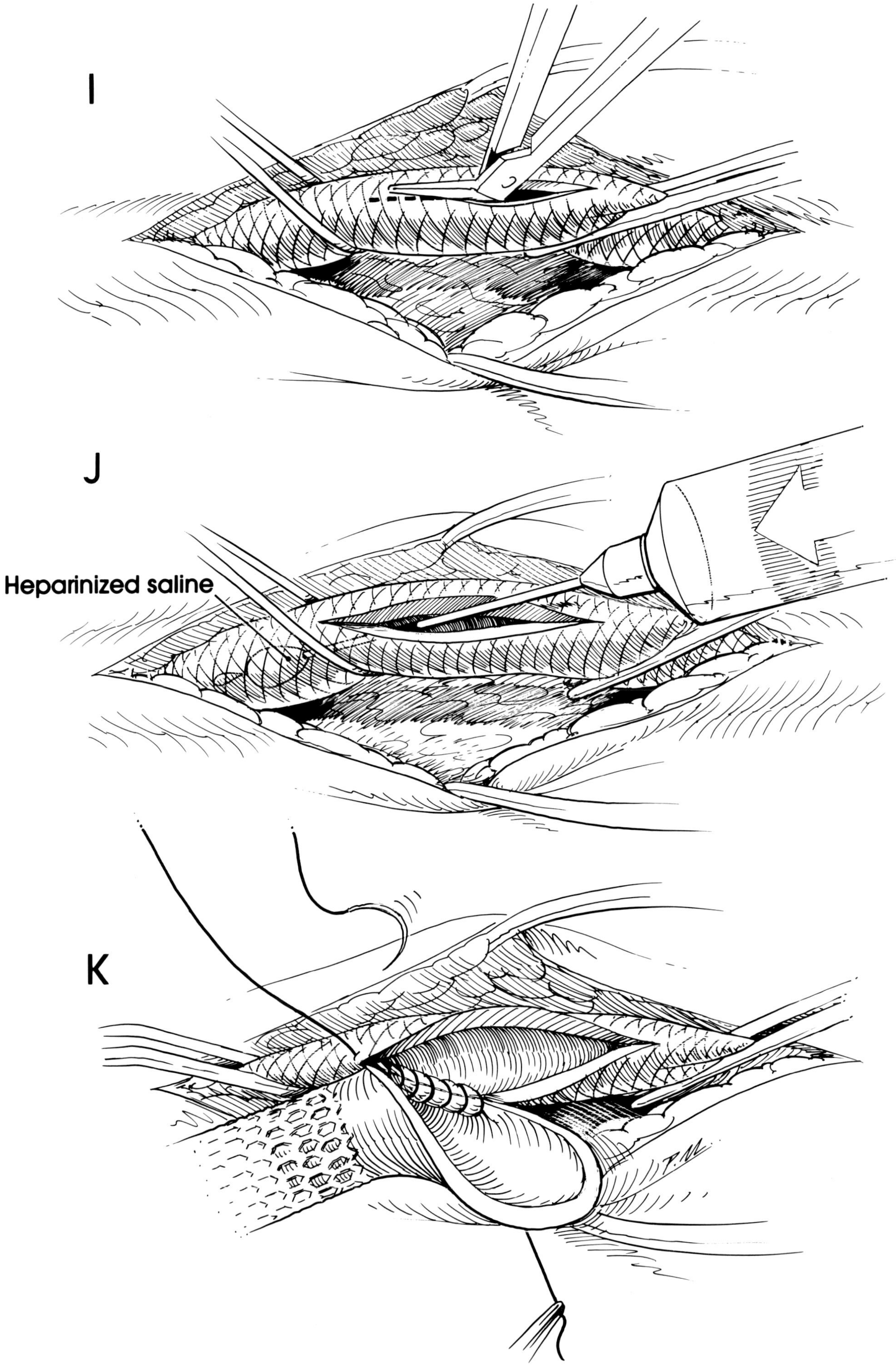
I
J
Heparinized saline
K

L When the anastomosis has been completed, the clamps are removed and the graft is flushed.

M The interposition graft is then filled with heparinized saline and clamped.

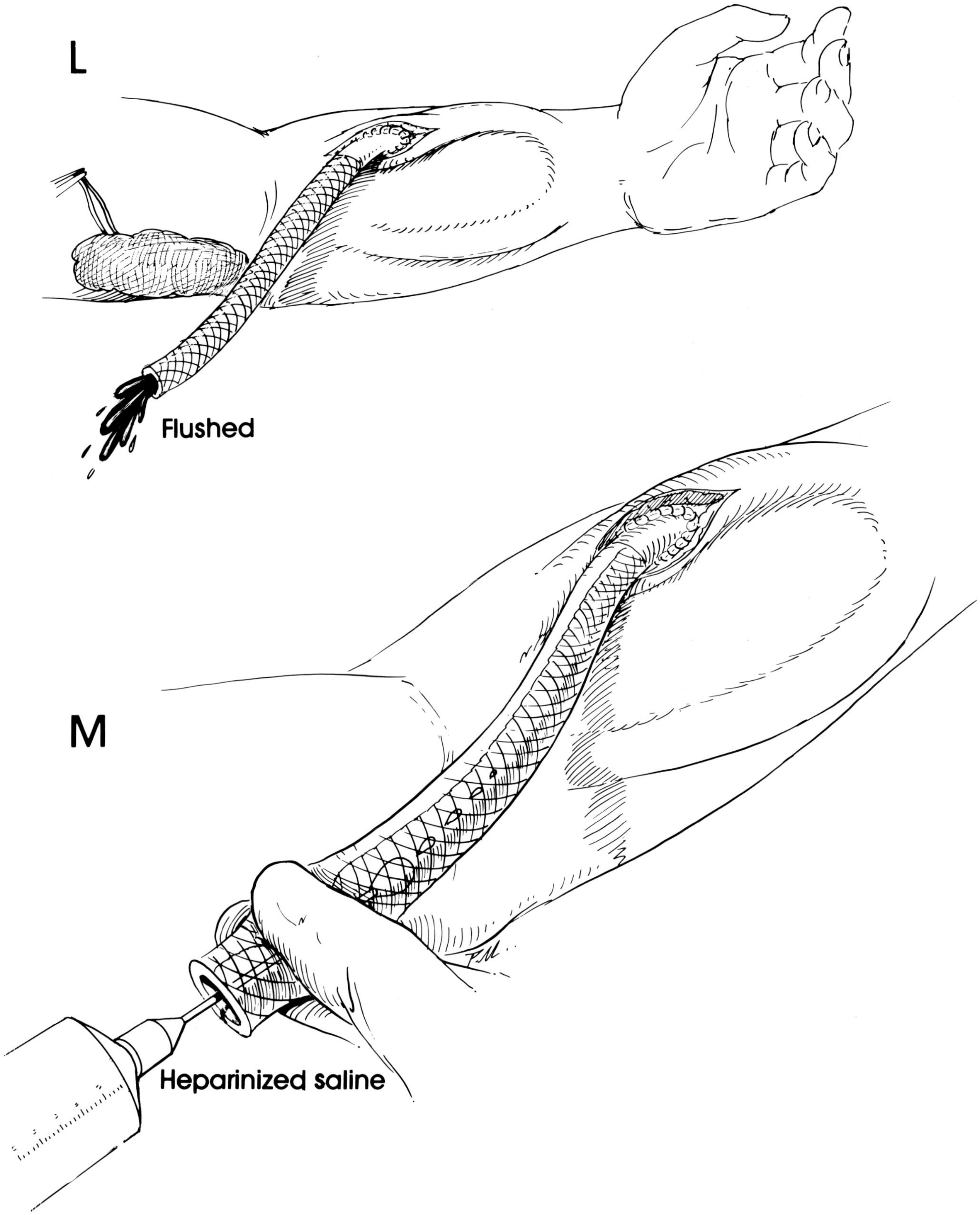
L
Flushed
M
Heparinized saline

N The graft is placed on the skin in the position that it will occupy in the subcutaneous tissue. There should be no twists in the graft.

O The curved spongestick is used to create a tunnel between the two incisions.

P The graft is clamped immediately proximal to the anastomosis and decompressed.

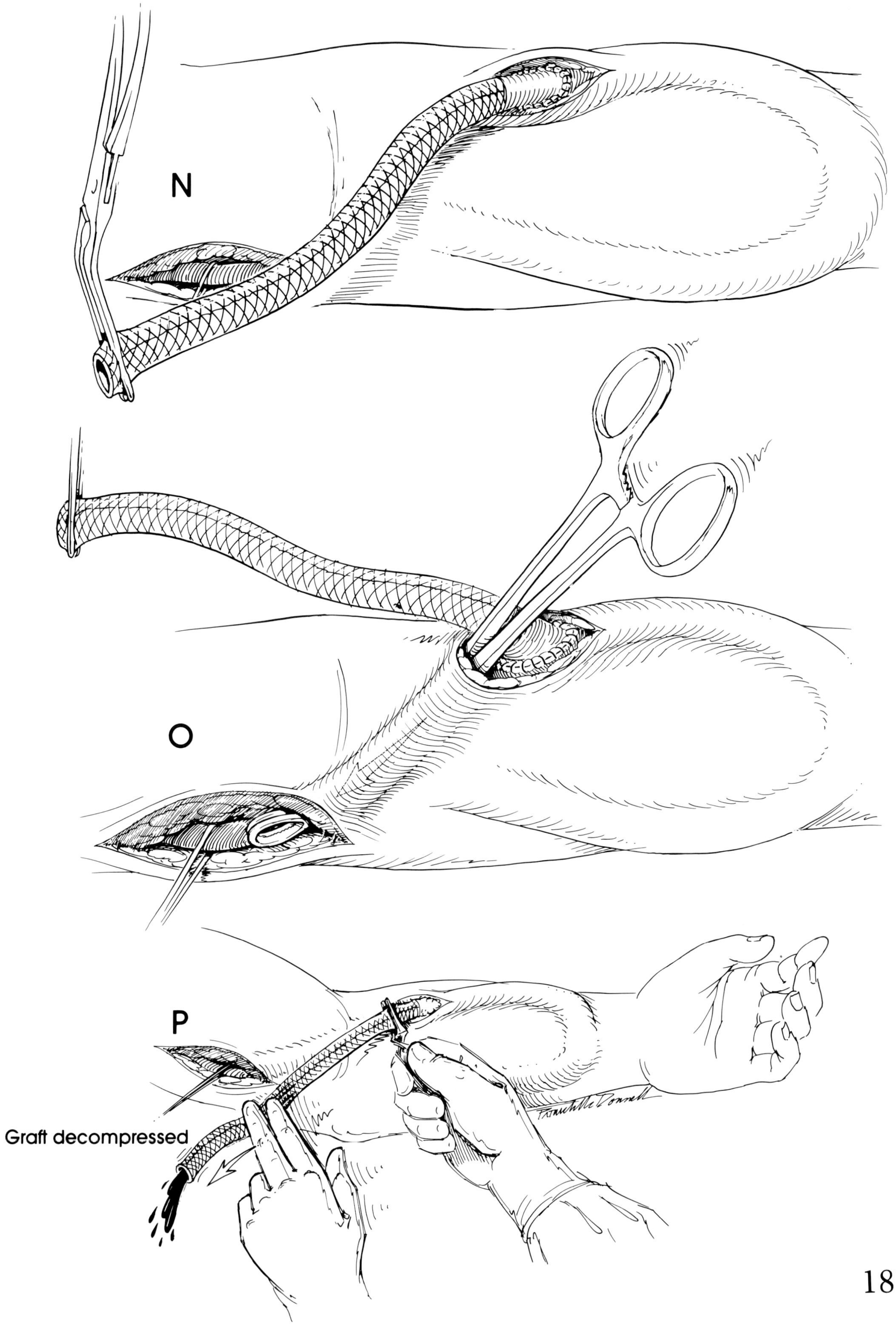
N
O
P
Graft decompressed

Q With care taken to maintain proper orientation, the free end of the graft is inserted into the jaws of the spongestick.

R The graft is gently drawn through the tunnel and out the proximal incision.

S The position of the graft is confirmed, and the graft is flushed and heparinized.

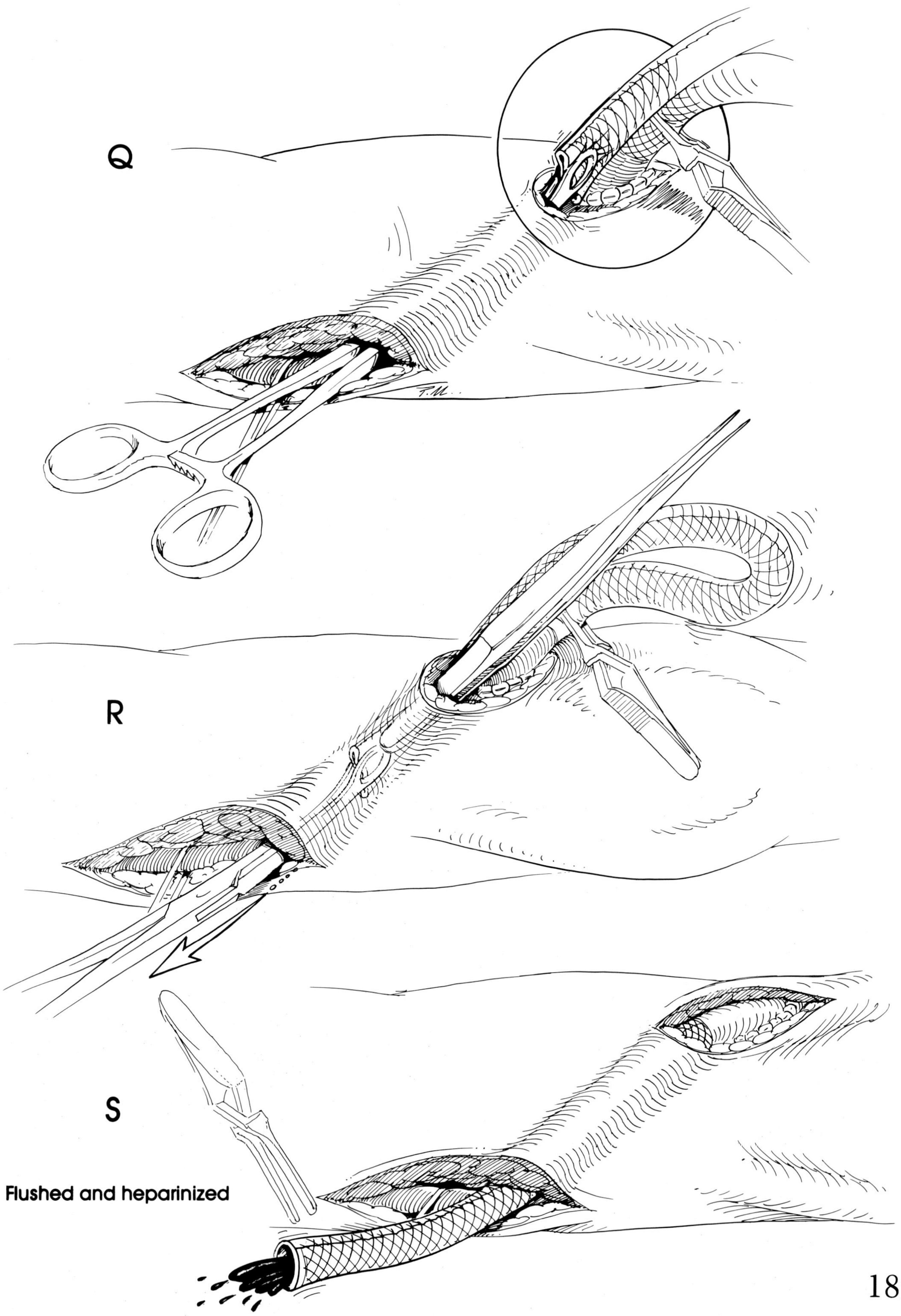
Q
R
S
Flushed and heparinized

T The basilic vein is clamped proximally and distally, and a venotomy one and one-half times the graft diameter is made. The vein is then heparinized.

U Initial tapering of the graft is done with both a proximal and a distal clamp in place. This permits control of bleeding and allows the transected segment to be distended when it is measured and cut. If this technique is used, the length of the graft will not be distorted.

V The graft is further tailored for the flared end-to-side anastomosis.

T

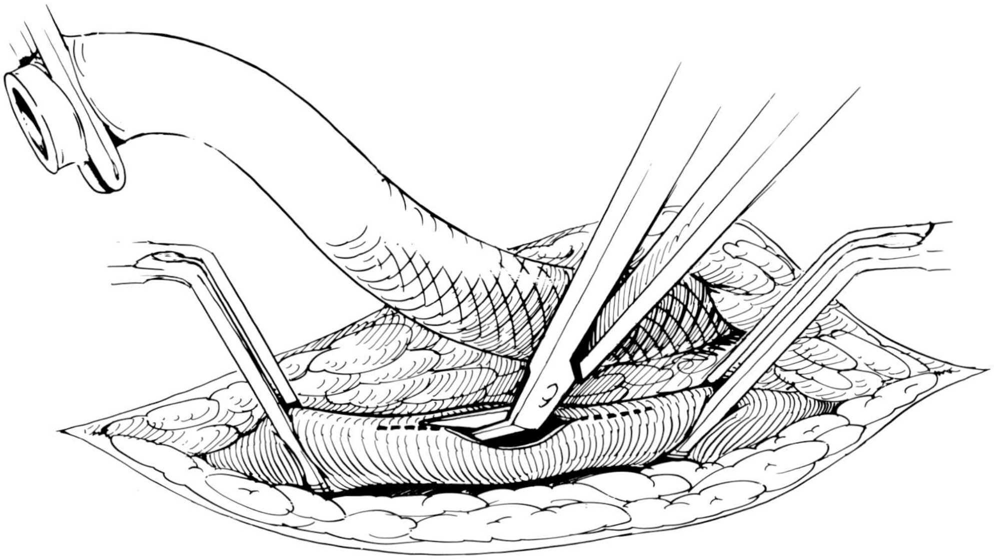

U

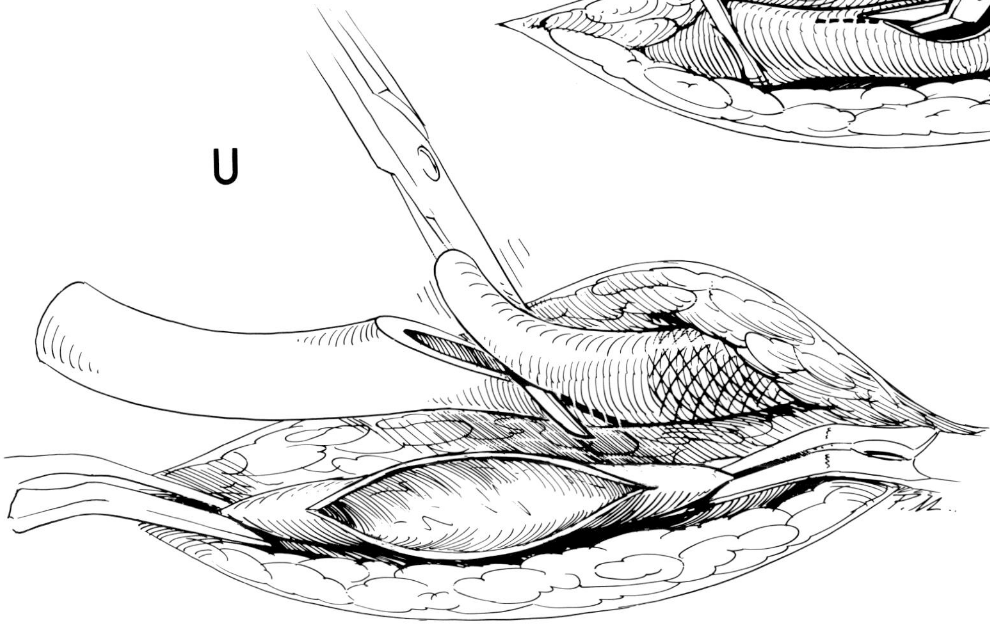

V

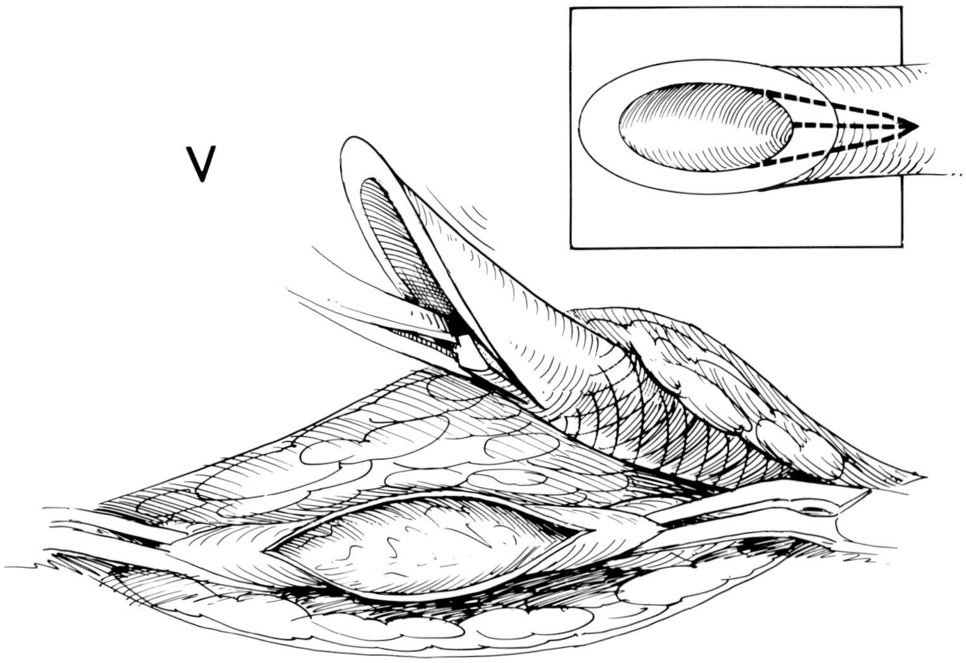

W The anastomosis is completed with running 6-0 vascular sutures.

X Clamps are removed, and the interposition graft is allowed to fill.

Y A palpable pulse and thrill confirm adequate relief of outflow tract obstruction. Lack of a pulse and thrill is an indication for angiography. Incisions are closed with 3-0 absorbable sutures for the subcutaneous layer and with staples to reapproximate the skin.

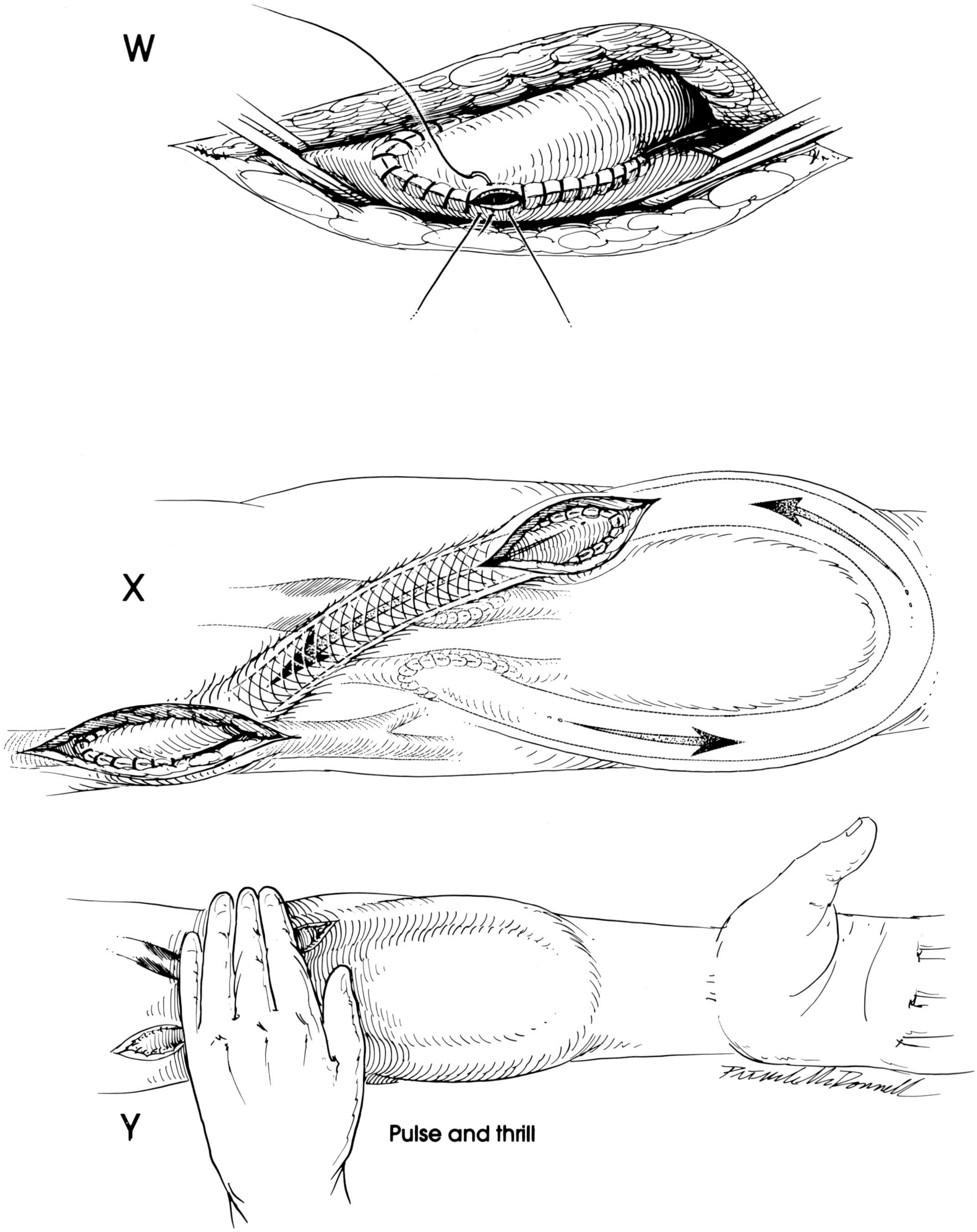
W
X
Y
Pulse and thrill

The hemodynamic alterations that brought about the initial venous hyperplasia are still operative in a graft that has been extended. Consequently, additional hyperplastic changes may occur at the new site of pressure gradient change. Should outflow tract obstruction recur, subsequent venous bypass grafts may be used for correction.

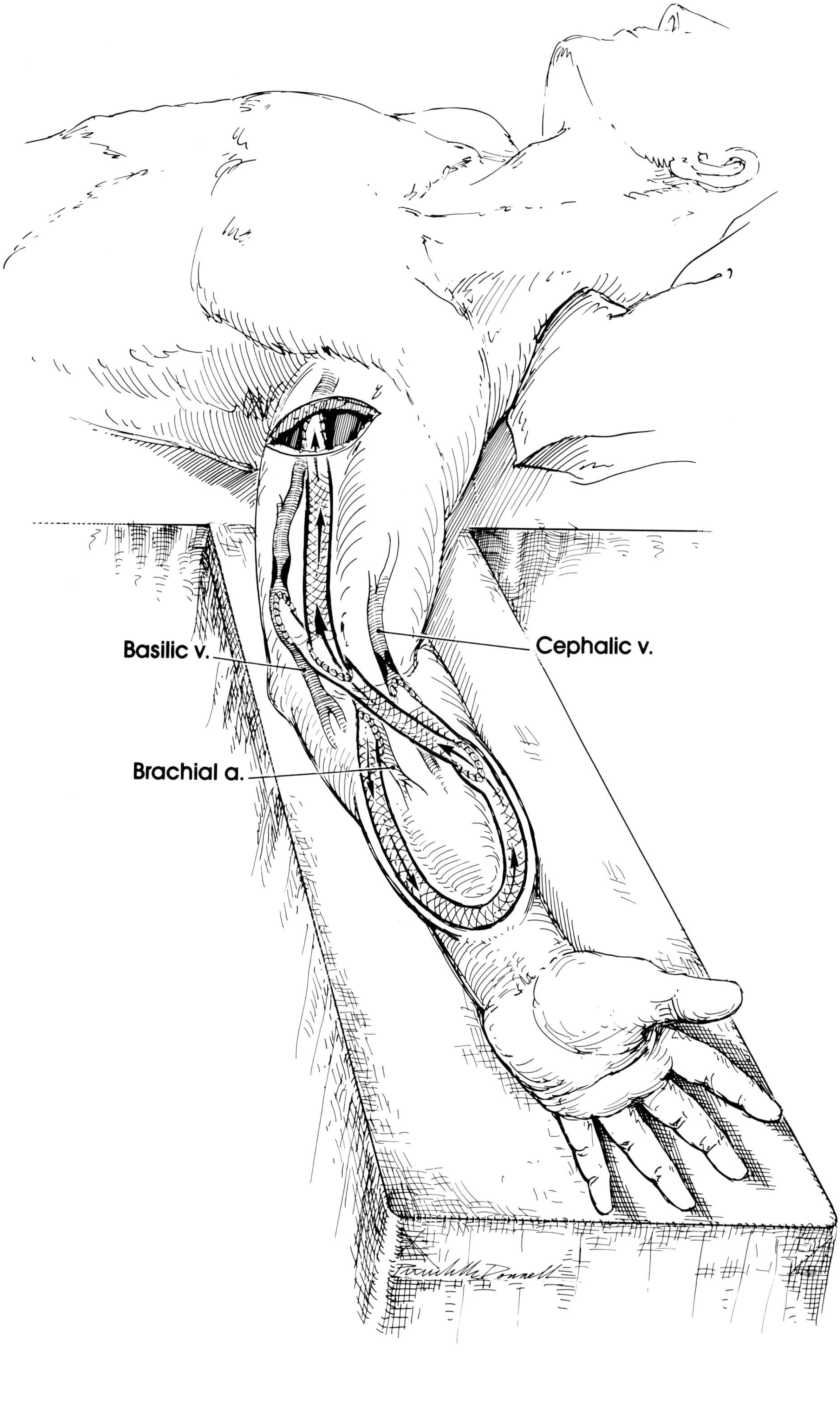
Basilic v.
Cephalic v.
Brachial a.

Outflow Tract Obstruction

Limb Interposition

A A transverse incision approximately 8 cm long is made 4 cm below the antecubital skin crease.

B The basilic vein is identified and mobilized. It should be of adequate caliber to provide sufficient venous runoff. The portions of the graft immediately distal to the anastomoses are likewise identified and mobilized.

C Graft segments at least 5 cm long are mobilized.

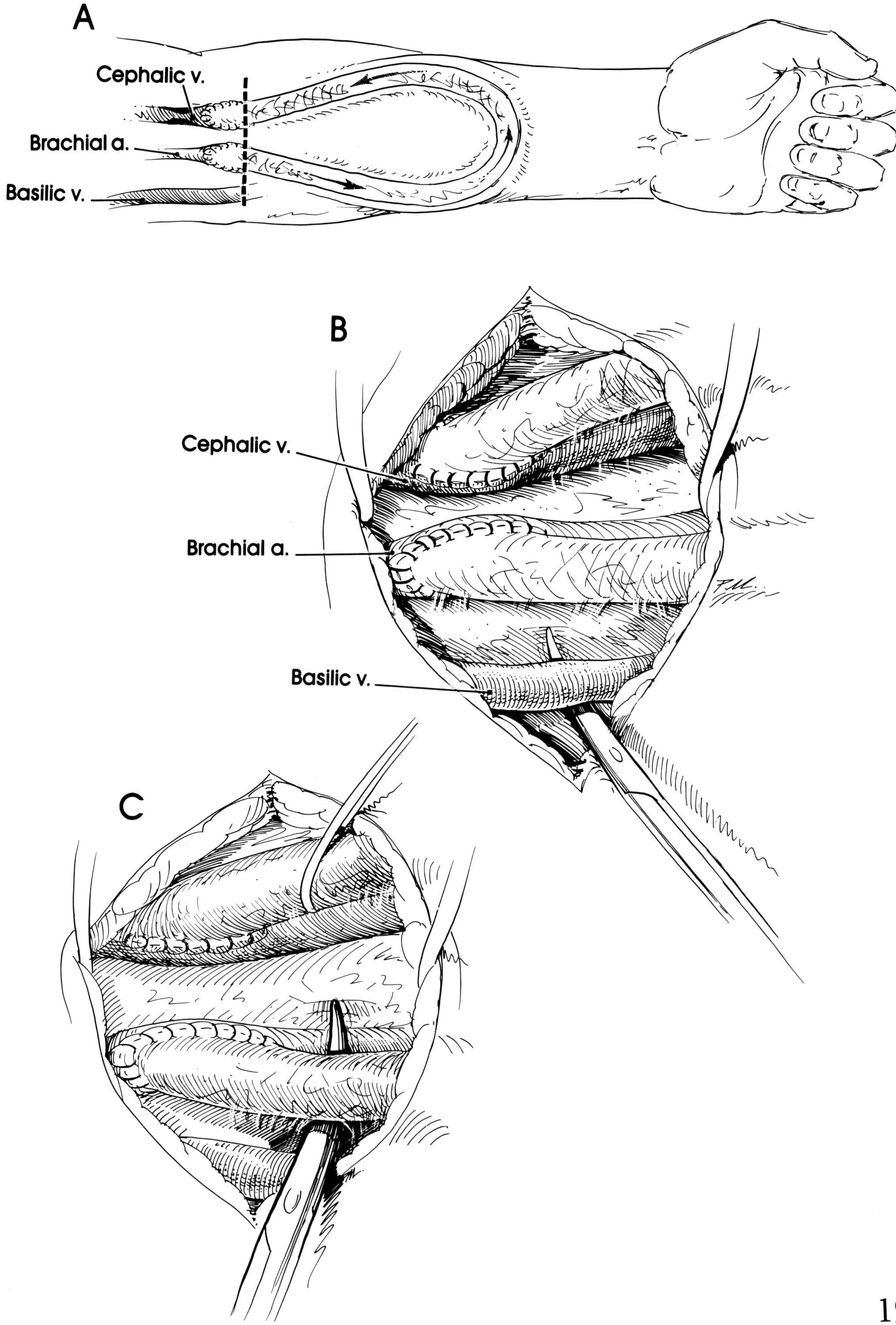
A
Cephalic v.
Brachial a.
Basilic v.
B
Cephalic v.
Brachial a.
Basilic v.
C

D The arterial limb of the graft is clamped immediately distal to the anastomosis, and the graft is transected approximately 3 cm beyond the clamp.

E This proximal graft segment is filled with heparinized saline and again clamped.

D

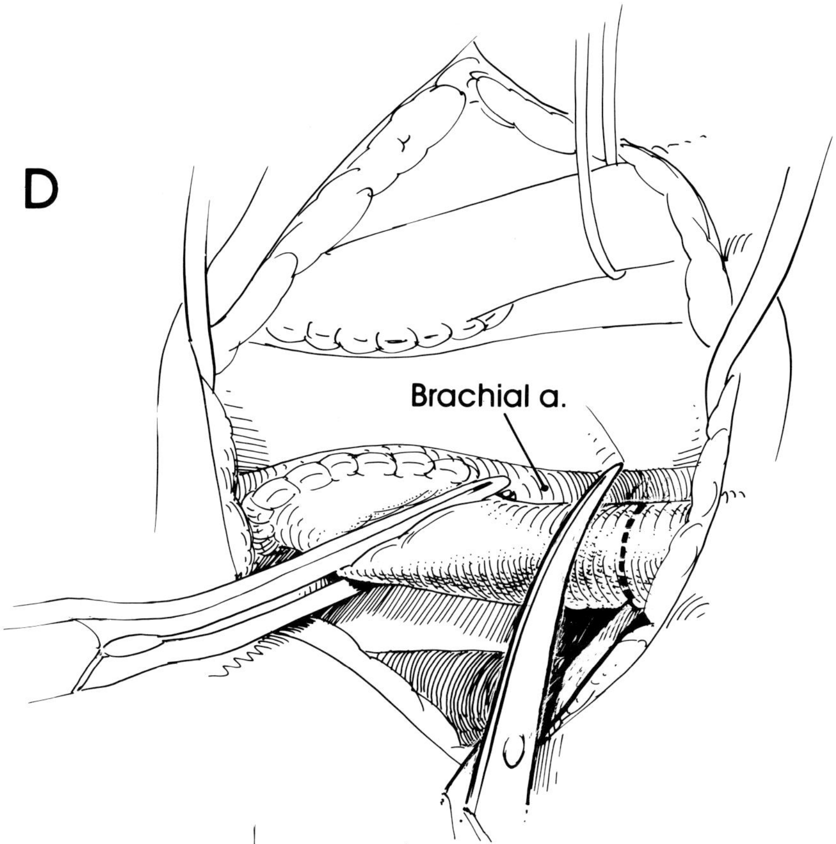

E

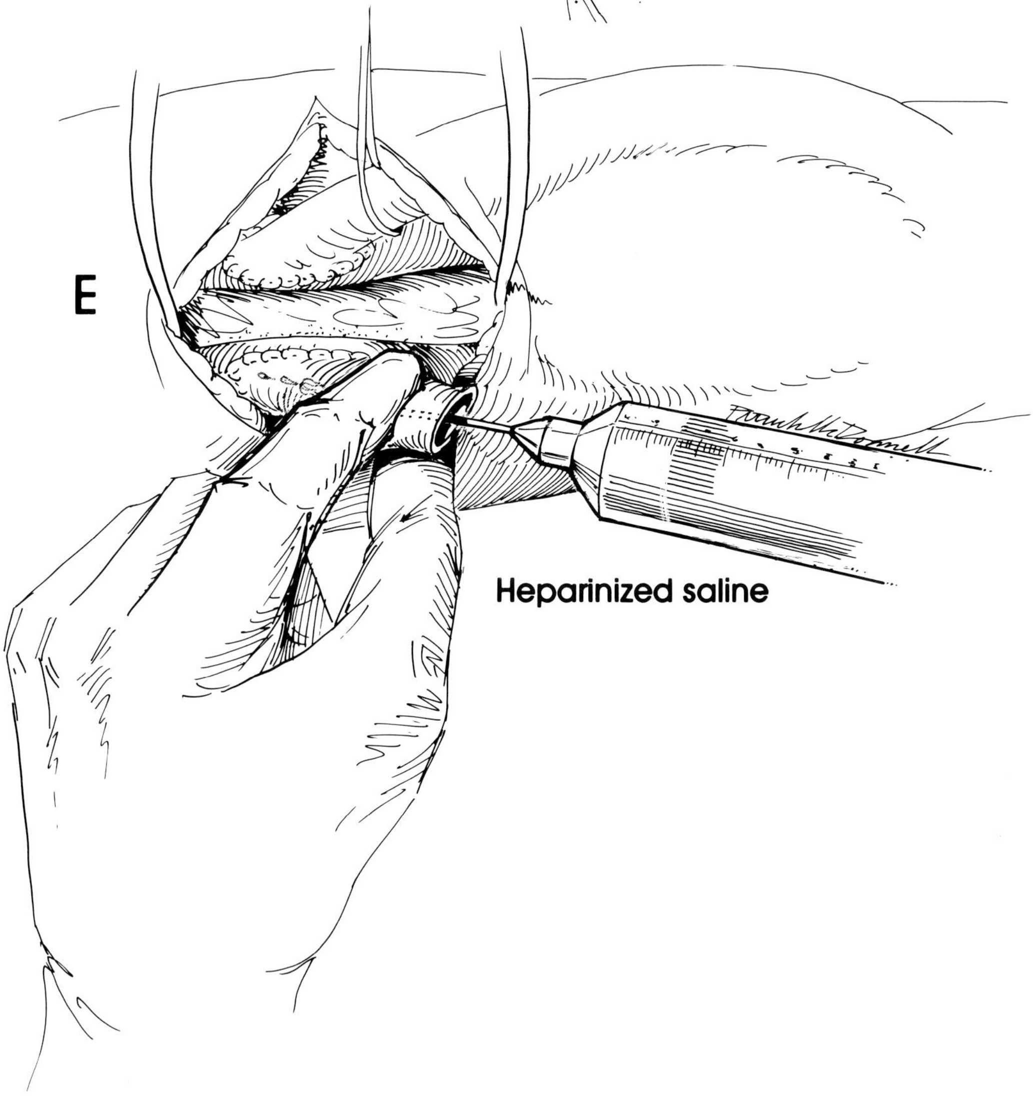

F A vascular clamp is placed immediately below the venous anastomosis, and the graft is divided adjacent to the clamp, leaving enough tissue for adequate closure.

G The distal venous segment is then oversewn with running 4-0 polypropylene sutures. A TA-30 stapler with 3.5-mm staples can also be used for this purpose.

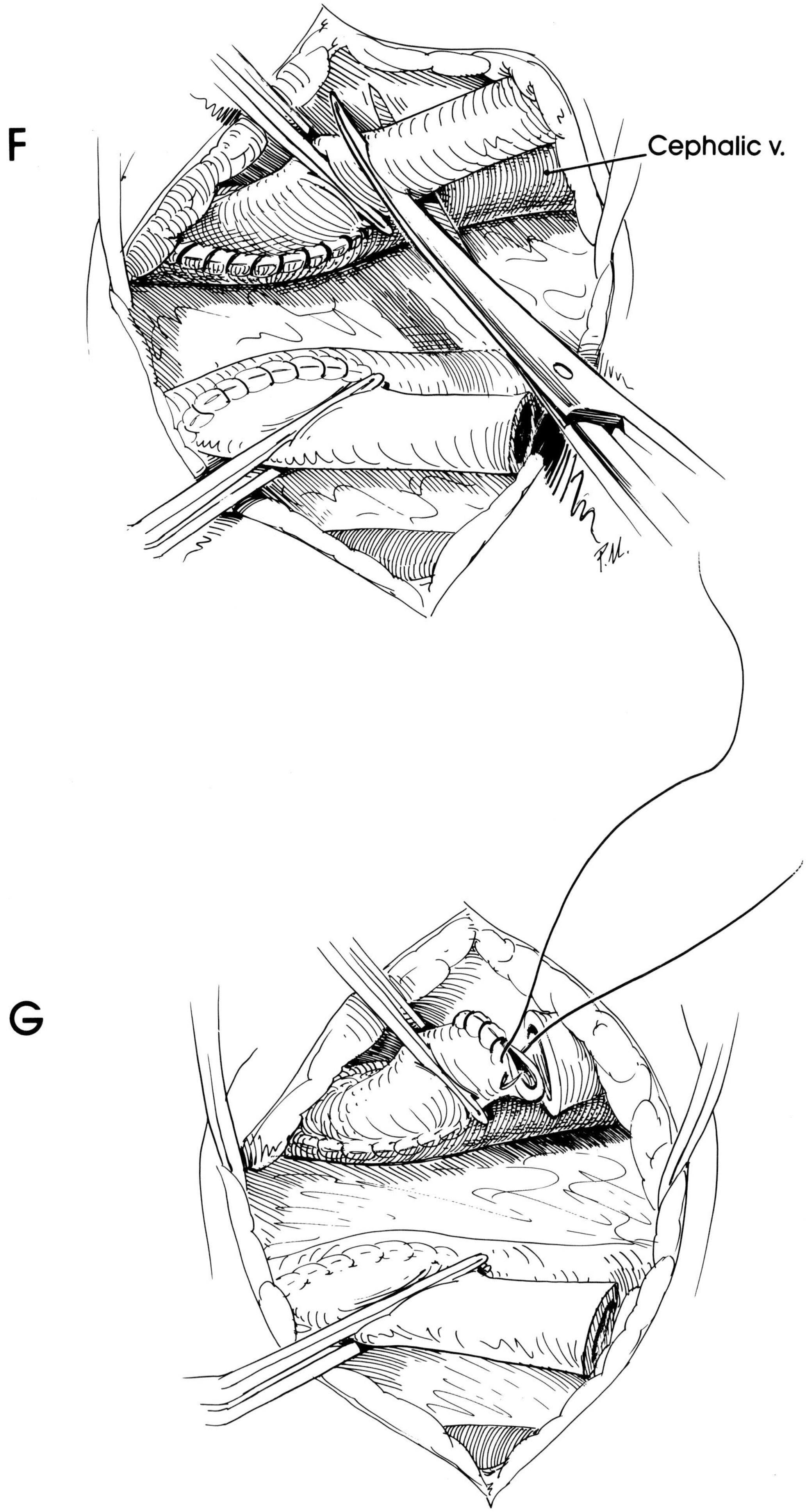
F
Cephalic v.
G

H The end of the proximal arterial segment is placed adjacent to the end of what was previously the venous limb of the graft. An end-to-end anastomosis of the two graft segments is constructed with running 6-0 polypropylene sutures. If primary union is not possible, an interposition graft is used to join these two segments.

I The clamp is removed, and the graft is allowed to flush.

J Vessels are heparinized, and the graft is clamped.

H

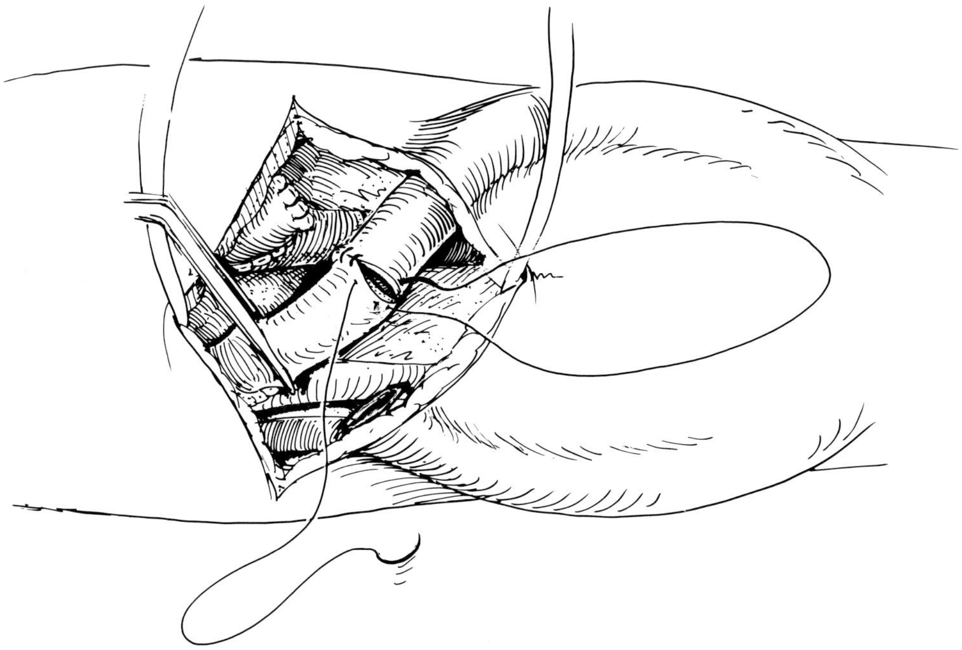

I

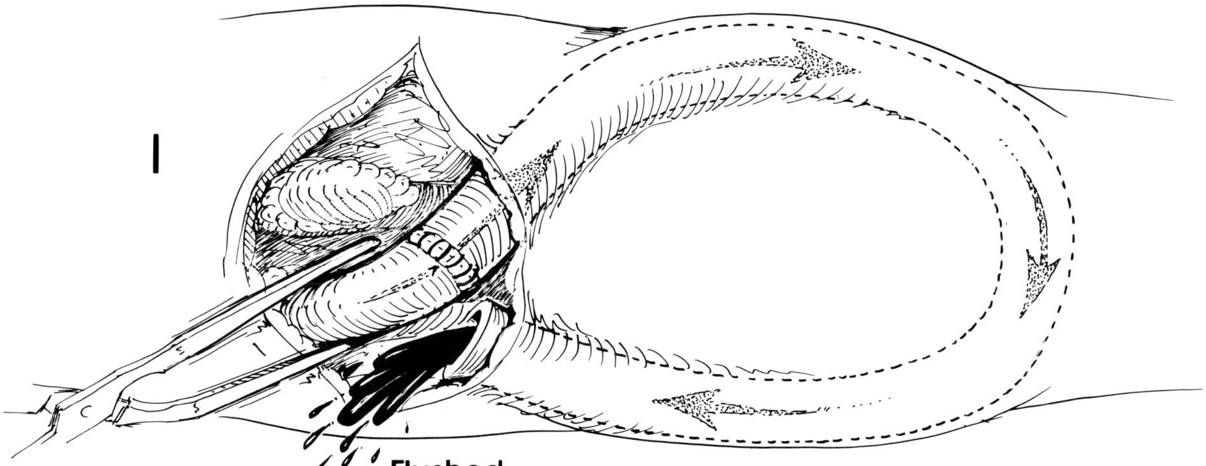

J

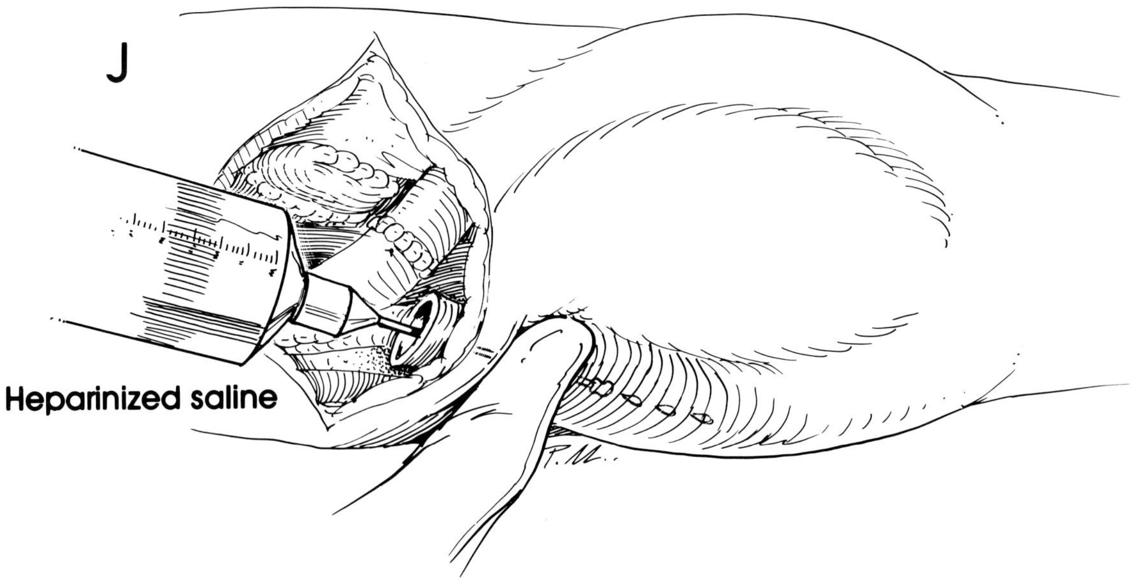

K An end-to-end anastomosis is constructed between the free end of the fistula and the interposition graft with running 6-0 vascular sutures.

L The basilic vein is clamped distally, and the venotomy is extended appropriately for the end-to-side anastomosis. Following adequate heparinization, the basilic vein is clamped proximally. The interposition graft is allowed to fill and is then measured for the anastomosis and tapered appropriately.

K

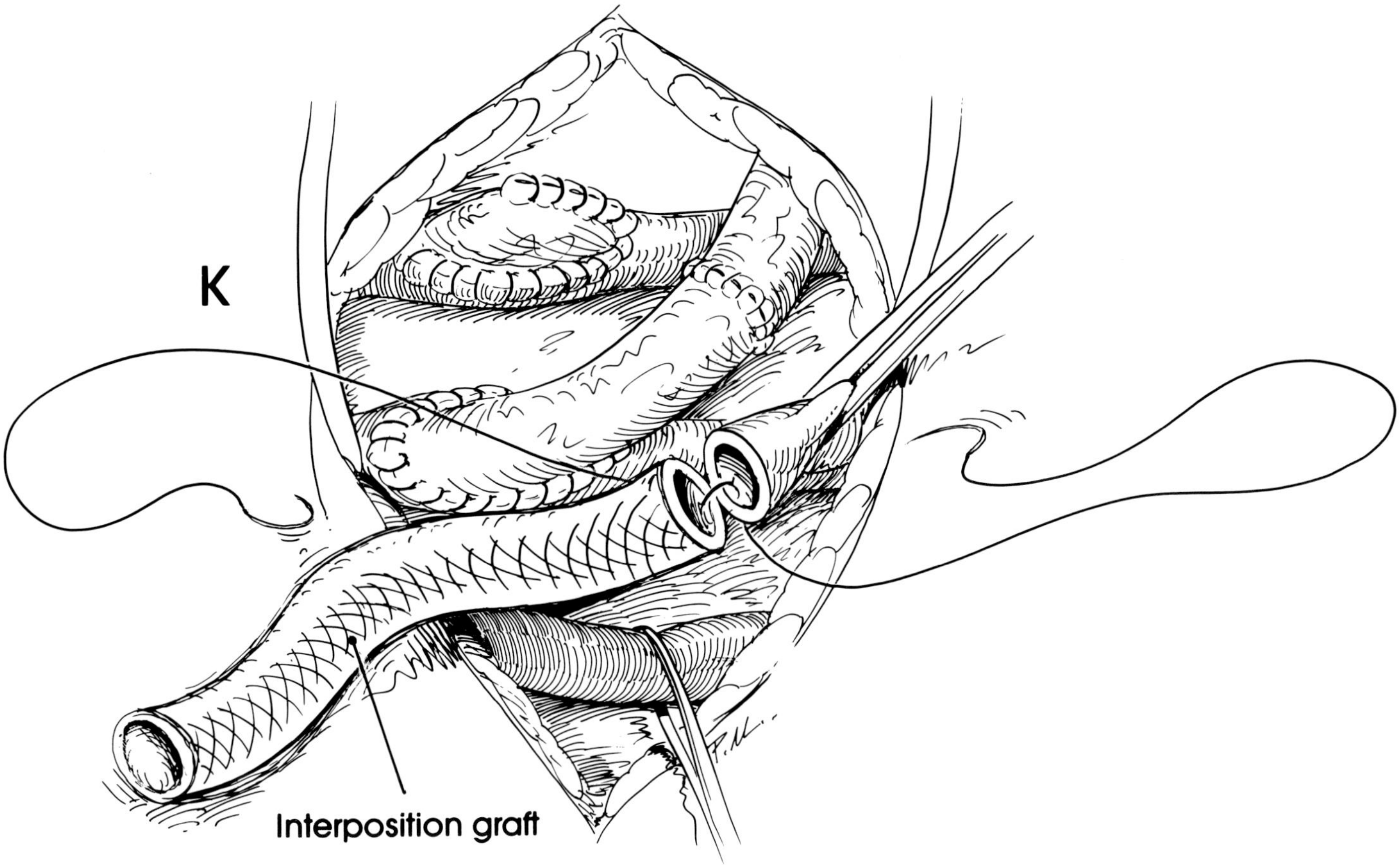

L

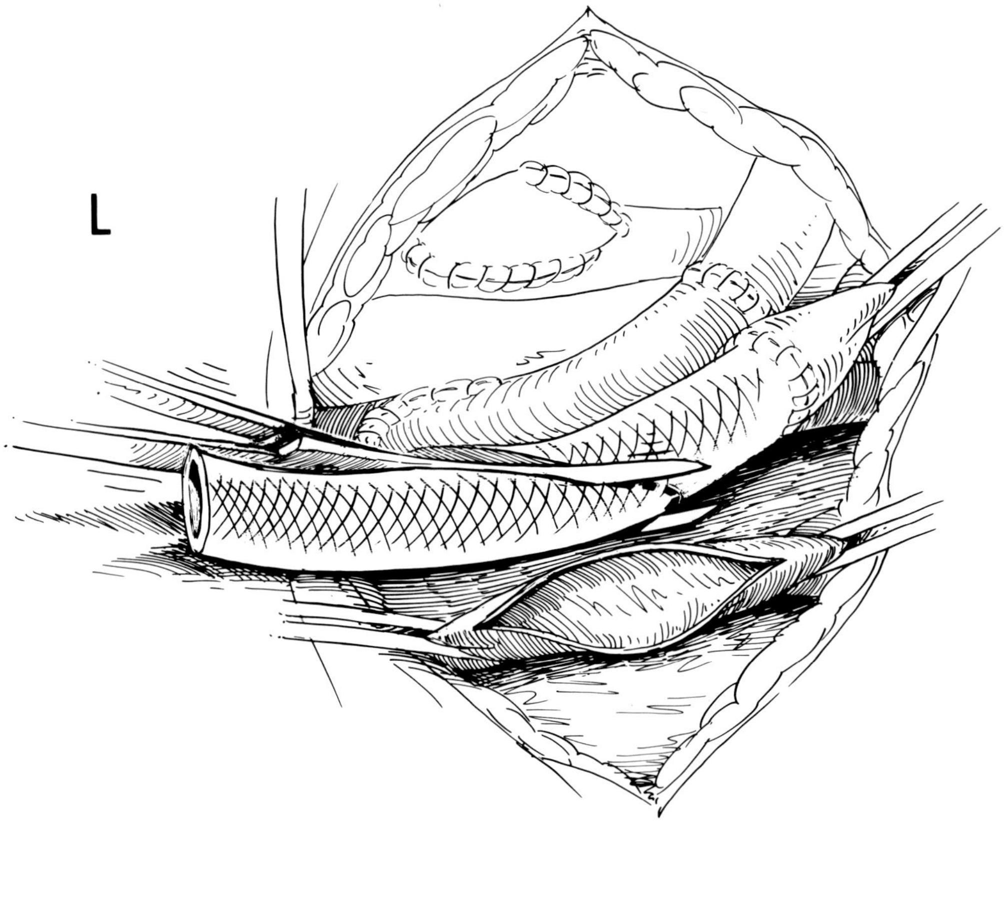

M–N The low-profile, flared end-to-side anastomosis is constructed with running 6-0 polypropylene sutures. The clamps are removed, and flow is established through the graft. The anastomoses and configuration of the fistula are checked.

O A palpable pulse and thrill confirm adequate function of the fistula. The subcutaneous tissue is closed with 3-0 absorbable suture, and staples are used to reapproximate the skin.

This technique allows salvage of the graft and leaves the vasculature of the upper arm available for future procedures, should they become necessary.

M

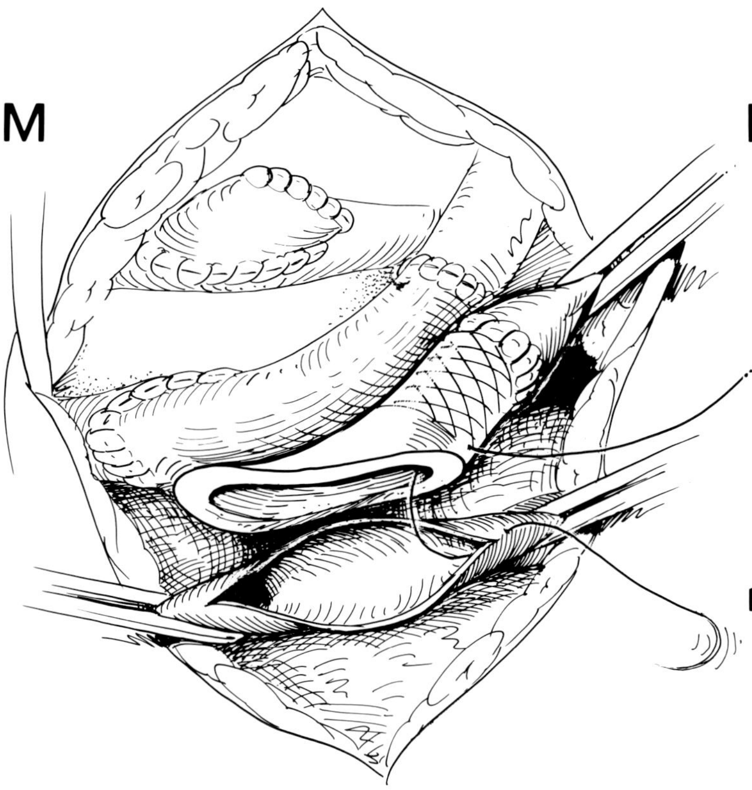

N

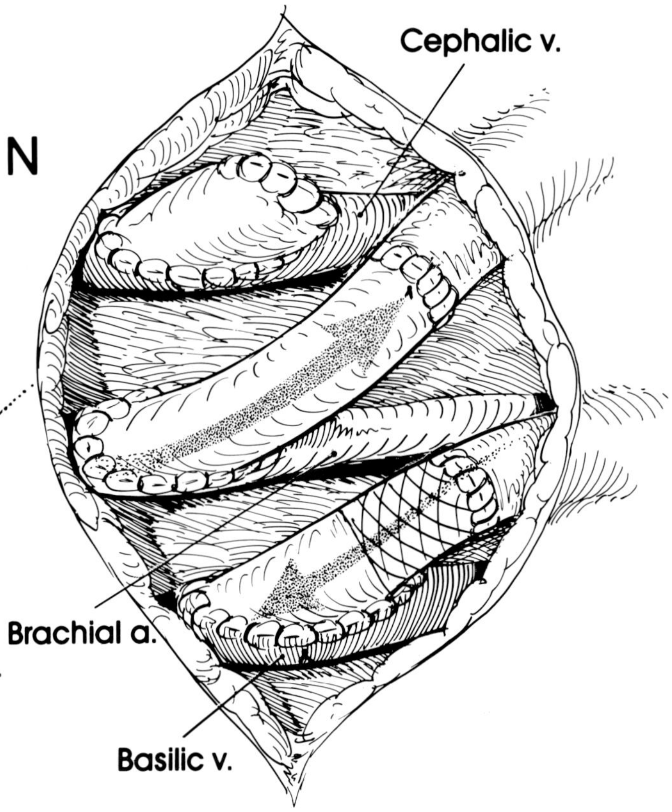

O

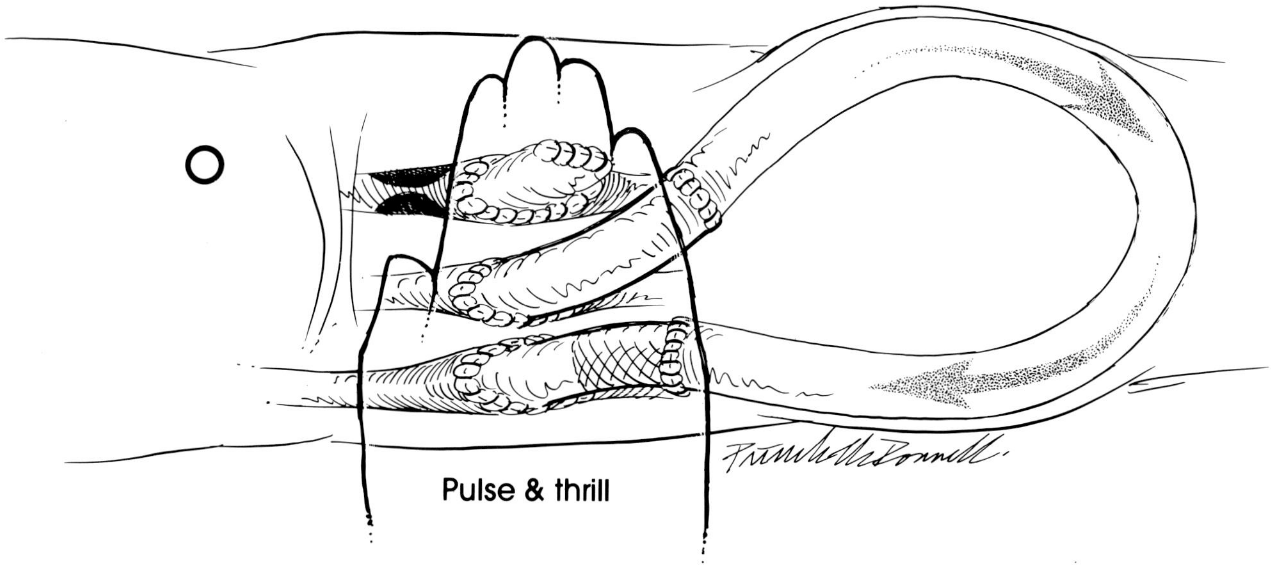

Inflow Tract Obstruction

Arterial Limb Extension

A A longitudinal incision approximately 6 cm long is made overlying the proximal portion of the arterial limb of the graft. The graft is mobilized from the surrounding tissue.

B Moist sponges are placed on the exposed graft, and another 6-cm longitudinal incision is made along the medial aspect of the arm overlying the brachial pulse. Dissection is performed, and the brachial artery is identified and mobilized.

C The brachial artery is clamped proximally.

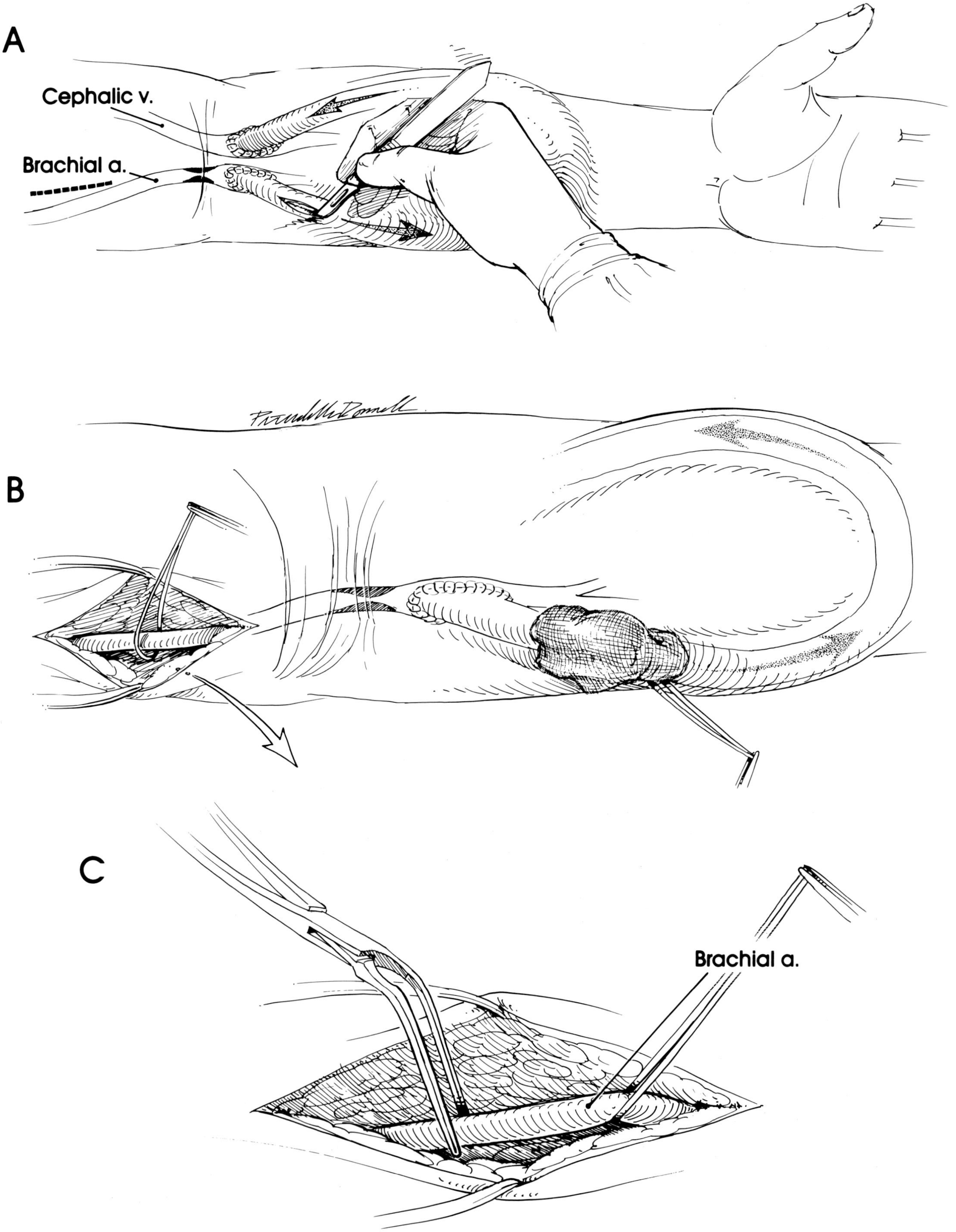
A
Cephalic v.
Brachial a.
B
C
Brachial a.

D A proximal vascular clamp is placed and the arteriotomy is begun with a no. 11 blade.

E The arteriotomy is extended to a length measuring one and one-half times the graft diameter. Heparinization is performed and the artery is clamped distally.

F The graft is tapered, and the end-to-side anastomosis is constructed with running 6-0 polypropylene sutures.

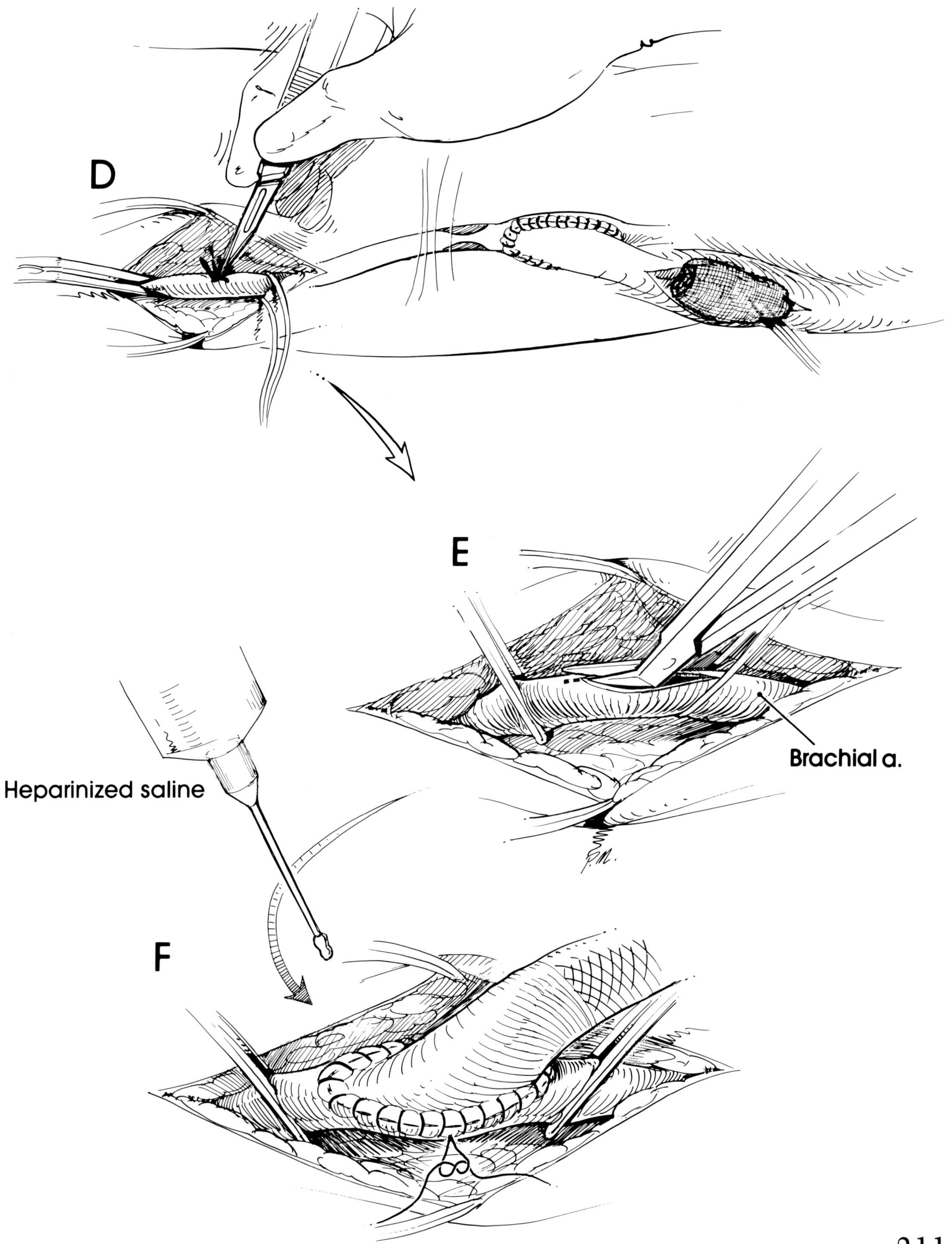
D
E
Brachial a.
Heparinized saline
F

G The graft is allowed to flush, and the distal clamp is removed. The interposition graft is then heparinized.

H A subcutaneous tunnel is created between the two incisions.

I The interposition graft is clamped proximally and decompressed. The graft is gently drawn through the tunnel, with care taken that it is not twisted.

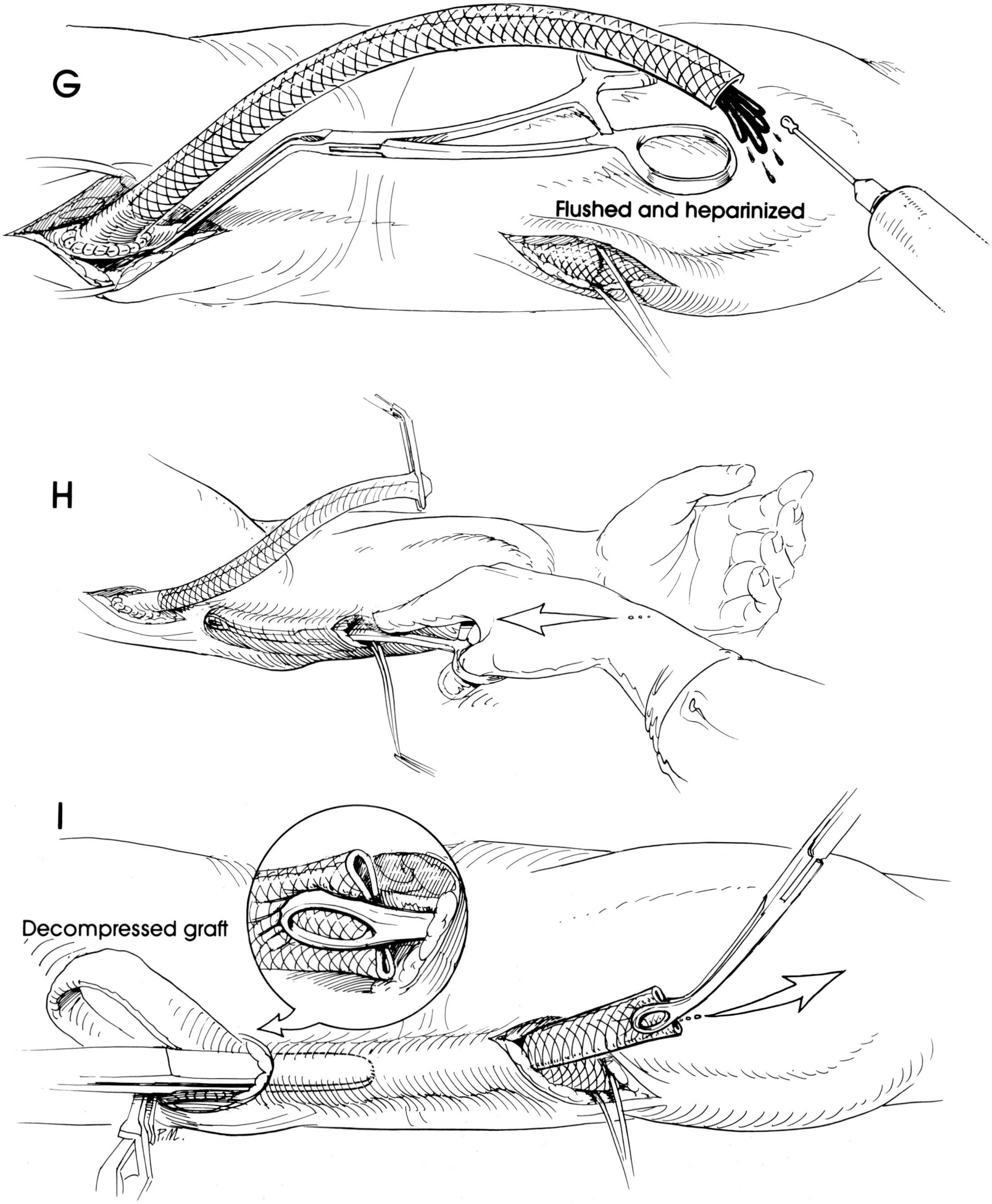
G
Flushed and heparinized
H
I
Decompressed graft

J After proper position of the graft is confirmed, it is filled with heparinized saline and clamped.

K The arterial limb of the previously inserted graft is clamped proximally, and a longitudinal arteriotomy is performed.

L–M The arteriotomy is extended, and distal heparinization is performed.

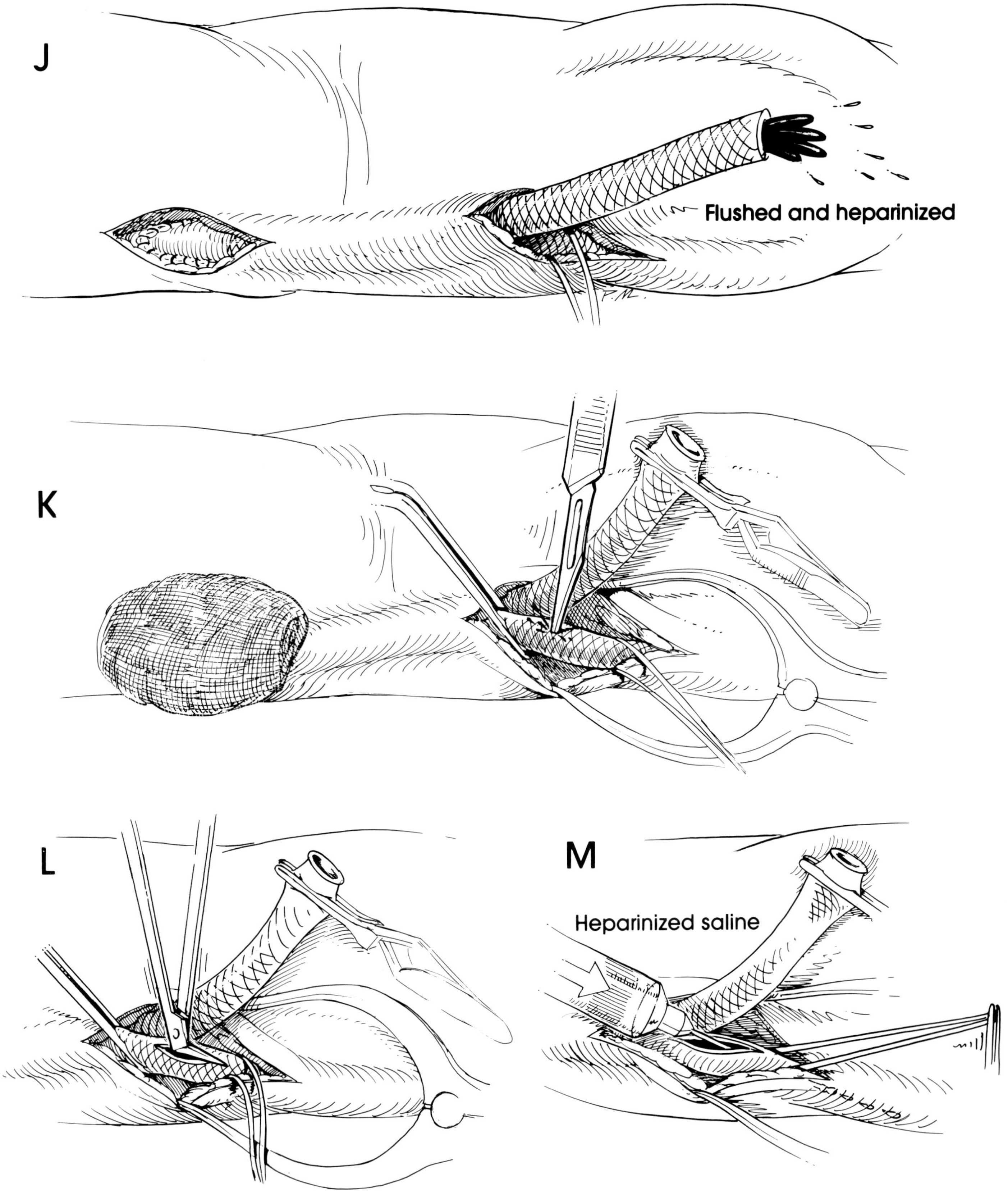
J
Flushed and heparinized
K
L
M
Heparinized saline

N After the interposition graft has been tapered appropriately, the end-to-side anastomosis is constructed with 6-0 vascular sutures in a running fashion.

O Clamps are removed, allowing the graft to fill.

P A palpable pulse and thrill confirm the relief of inflow tract obstruction. The incisions are closed with 3-0 absorbable suture for the subcutaneous layer and with staples to reapproximate the skin.

N

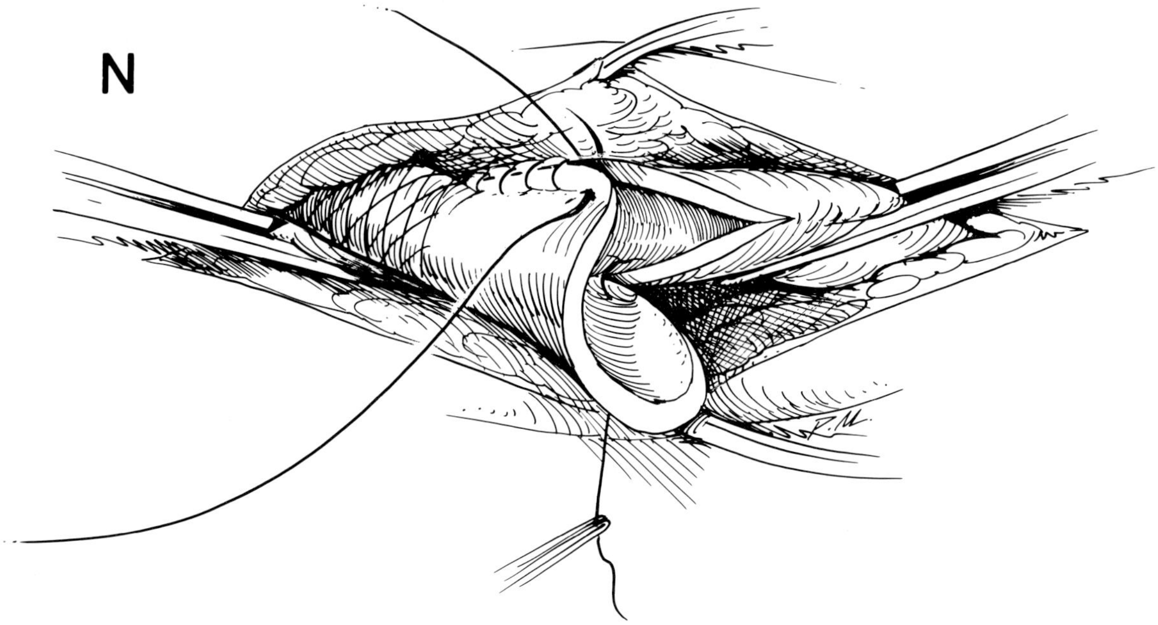

O

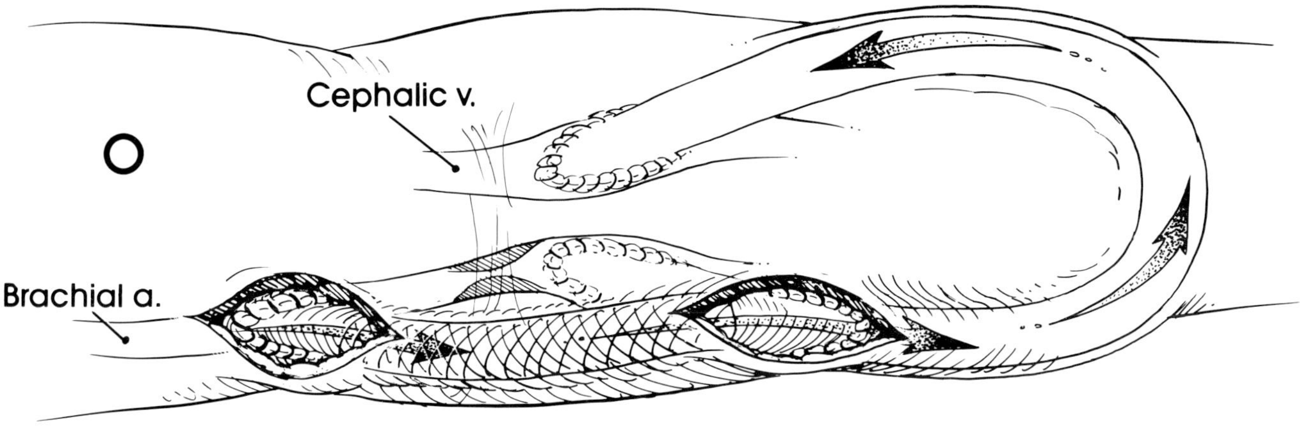

P

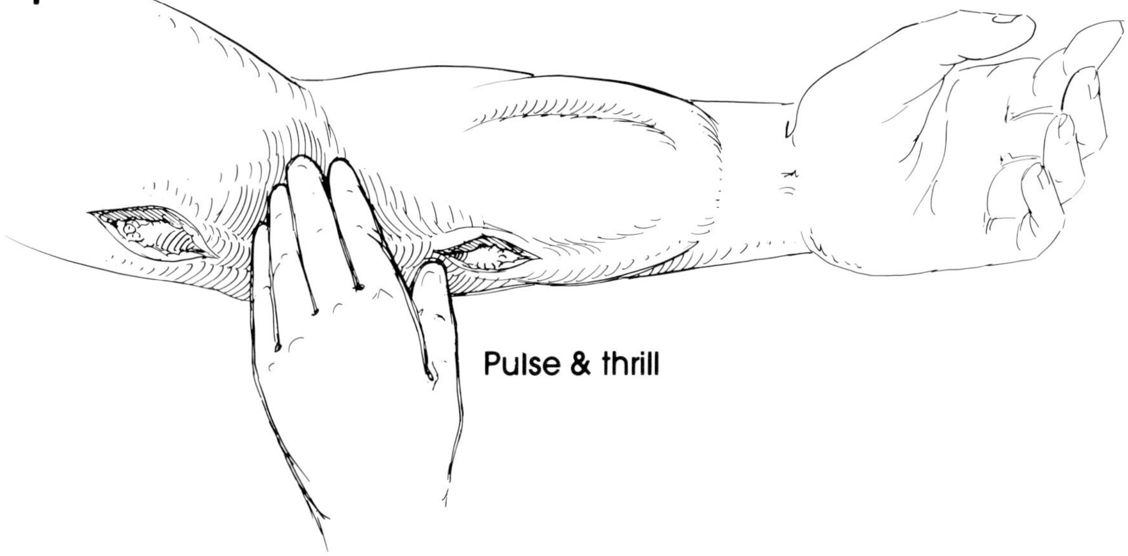

Recurrent arterial hyperplasia causing critical inflow tract obstruction may be treated in a similar manner. A series of bypass grafts may be used as needed to extend the functional life of the graft arteriovenous fistula.

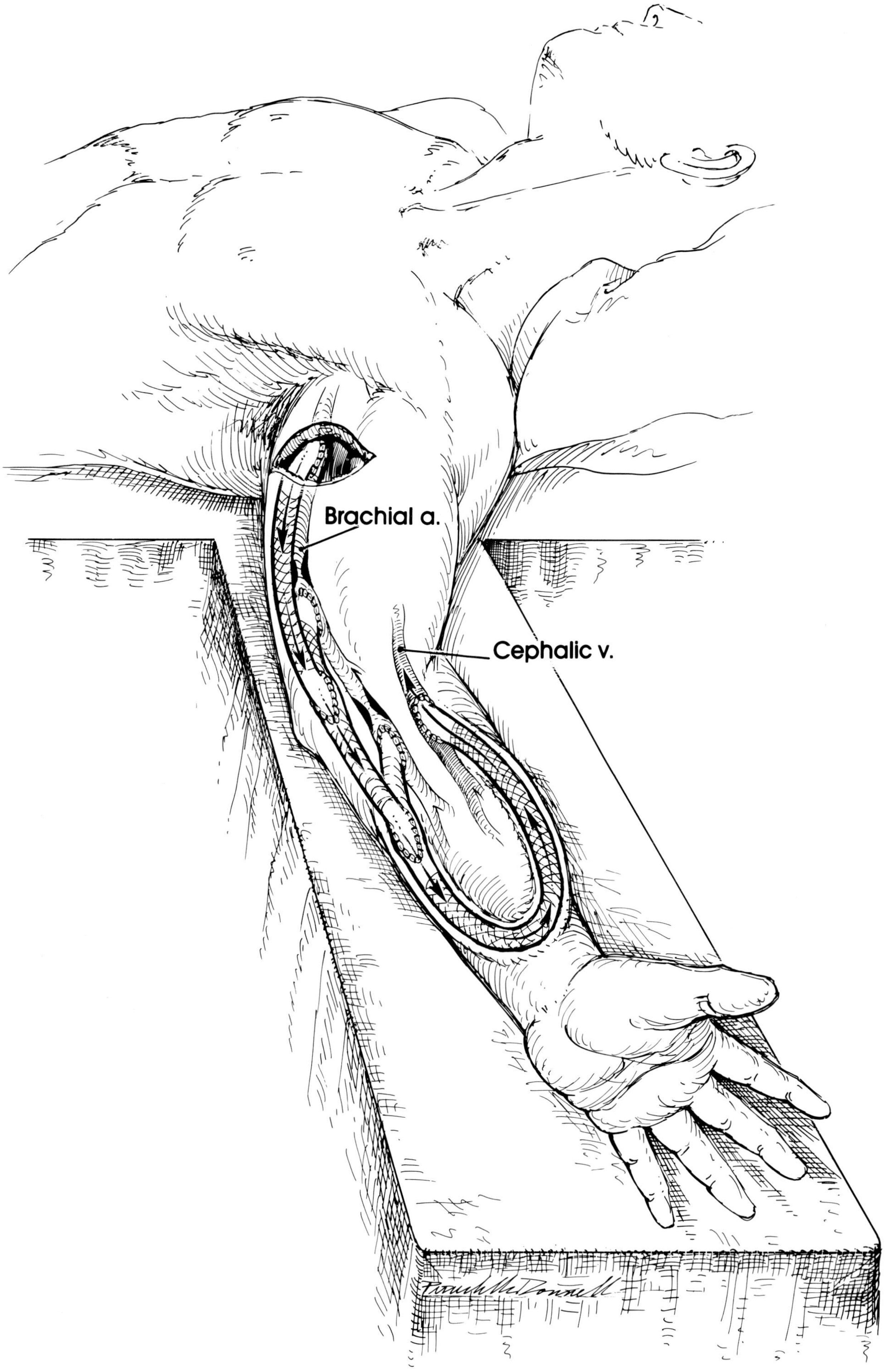
Brachial a.
Cephalic v.

Graft Dissection

A A graft arteriovenous fistula may be dissected during cannulation if the needle is advanced far enough to lacerate the back wall of the graft. This tear in the pseudointima develops into a false lumen corresponding to the cleavage plane between the graft wall and the dissected pseudointima. This flap impedes blood flow through the fistula, and graft thrombosis results.

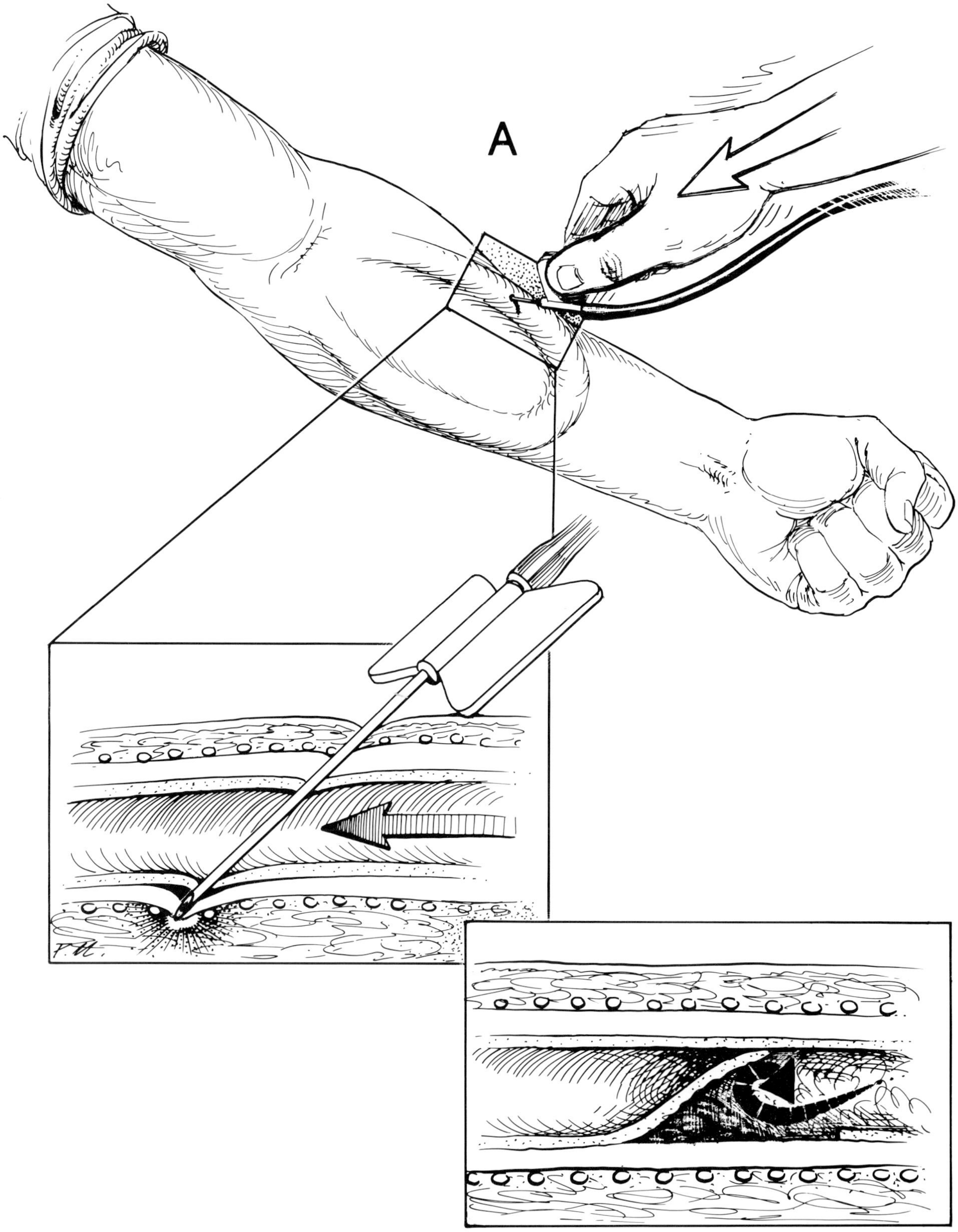
A

B At the time of thrombectomy, a first attempt to advance a 5 F balloon catheter through the venous limb of the graft is unsuccessful because of the cul-de-sac encountered. This makes it impossible to advance the catheter in the lumen.

C The balloon is inflated and the catheter withdrawn. Subsequent attempts to advance the catheter through the venous limb corroborate the obstruction.

D A thrombectomy of the arterial limb is performed. Vessels are heparinized, and the distal end of the arterial limb is clamped.

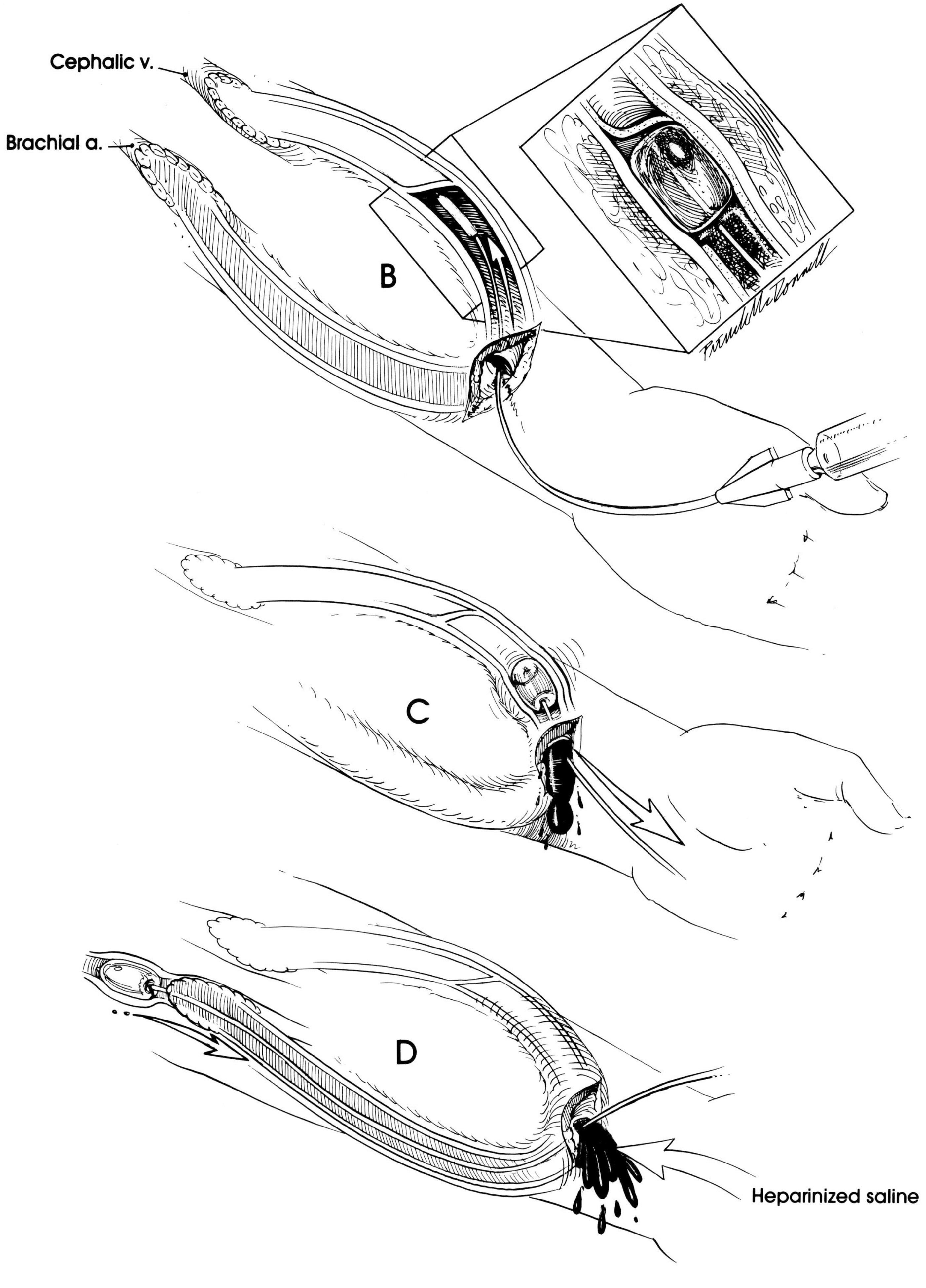
Cephalic v.
Brachial a.
B
C
D
Heparinized saline

E An angiogram of the venous limb confirms the presence of the dissected flap.

F A longitudinal incision is made overlying the area of graft dissection, as identified on the angiogram.

G–H The graft is mobilized, and the segment is opened with a no. 11 blade.

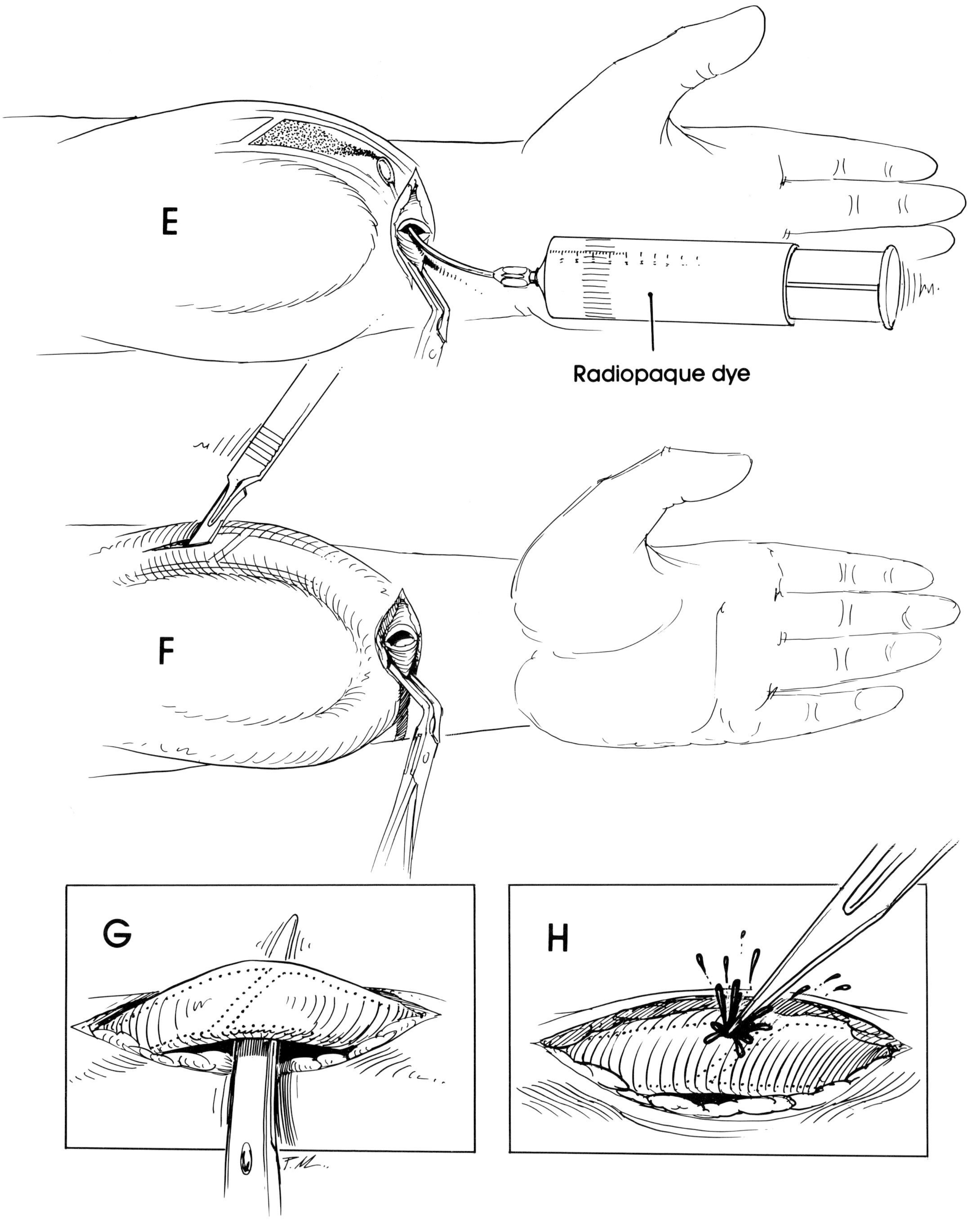
E
Radiopaque dye
F
G
H

I The internal surface of the graft is inspected and the dissection identified. The incision is extended to points proximal and distal to any pseudointimal involvement.

J Proximal and distal transection of the graft permits removal of the affected portion.

K An interposition graft is then incorporated into the remainder of the fistula. A proximal end-to-end anastomosis is constructed with 6-0 running vascular sutures, and the interposition graft is allowed to fill. It is then transected at the appropriate length, and the final end-to-end anastomosis is completed.

L A palpable pulse and thrill confirm adequate function. Incisions are closed with a layer of 3-0 absorbable suture for the subcutaneous layer and with staples for the skin.

I

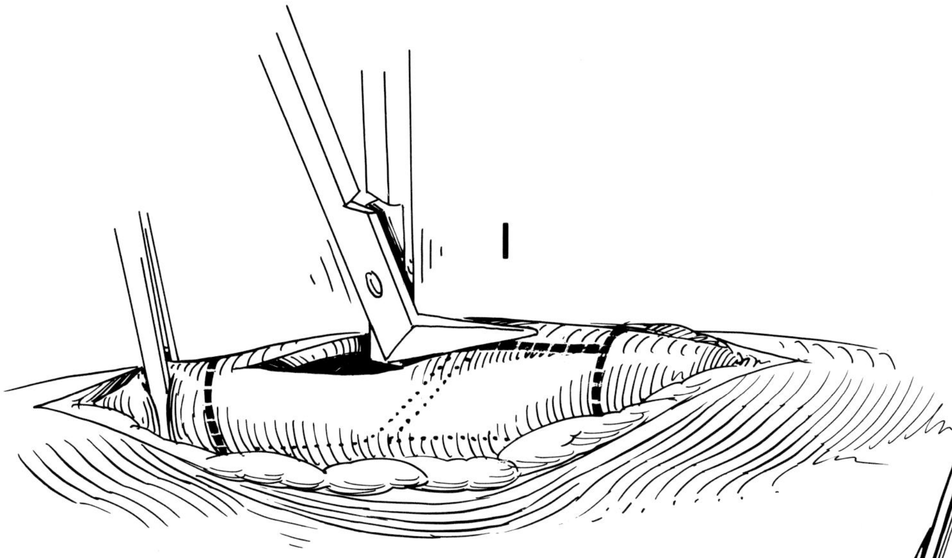

J

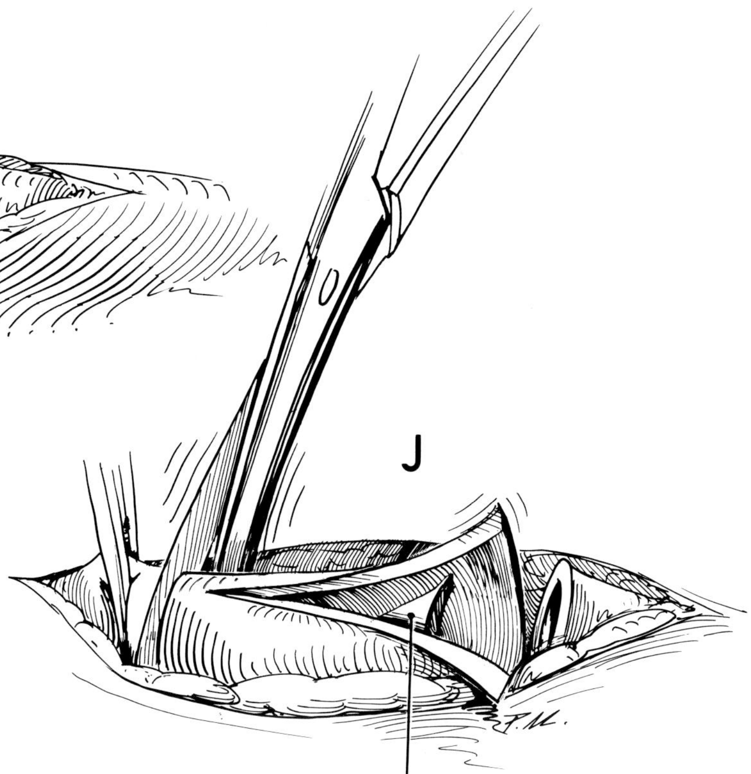

K

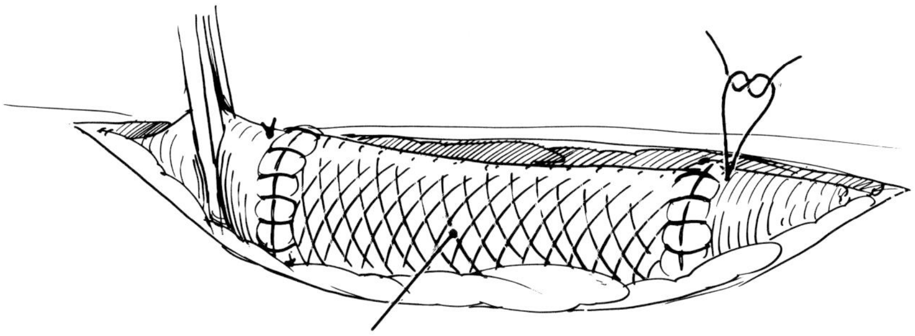

L

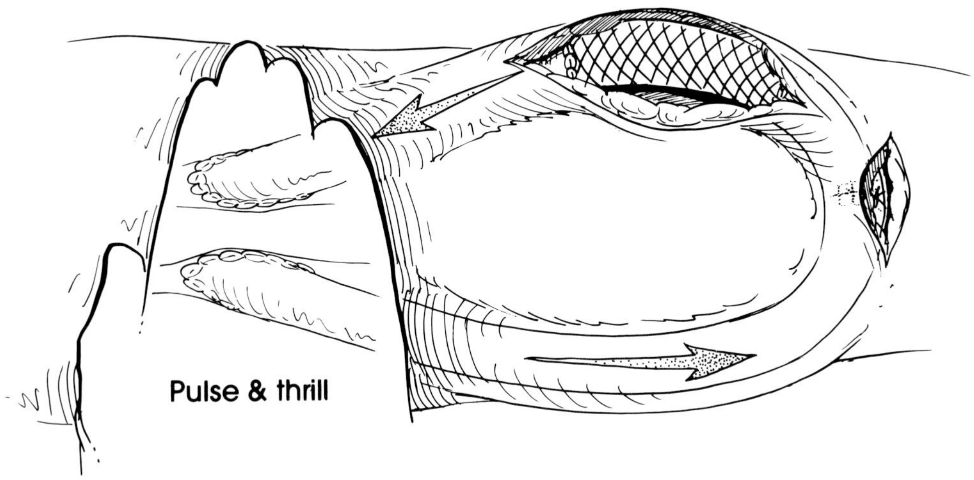

Graft Aneurysm

Staple Plication

A–B A longitudinal incision is made overlying the previously identified graft aneurysm.

C The incision is extended to expose graft segments of normal diameter on both sides of the aneurysm.

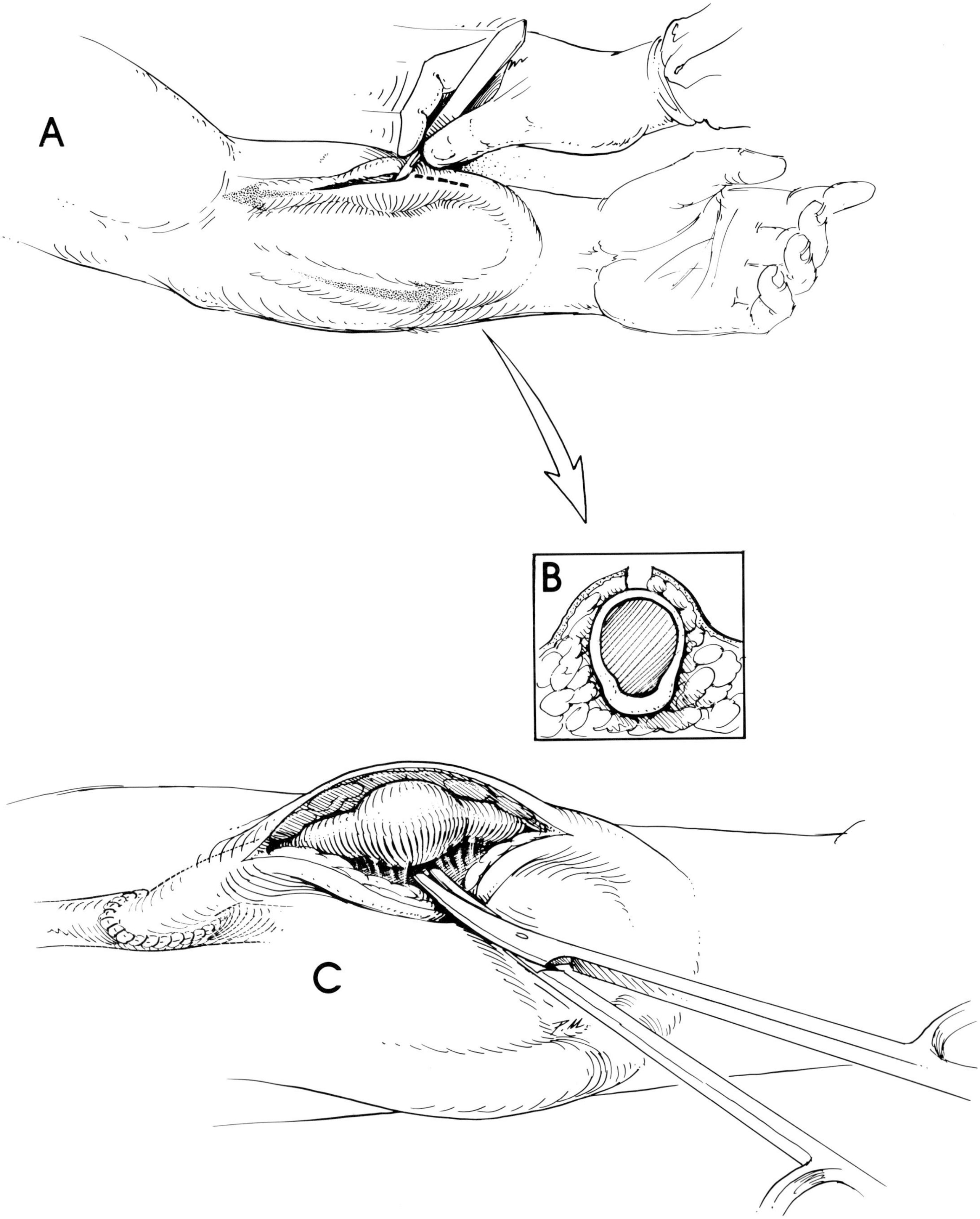
A
B
C

D The superior portion of the aneurysm is then grasped with two Allis clamps. A TA-55 stapler loaded with 3.5-mm staples is placed perpendicular to the clamps.

E The jaws of the stapler are closed on the aneurysmal sac, leaving a normal graft diameter. The staples are affixed, and the stapler is removed. The aneurysmal sac is then resected.

F A postoperative pulse and thrill confirm adequate flow through the fistula. Following inspection and hemostasis of the staple line, the subcutaneous tissue is closed with 3-0 absorbable sutures; 3-0 nylon sutures are used to reapproximate the skin.

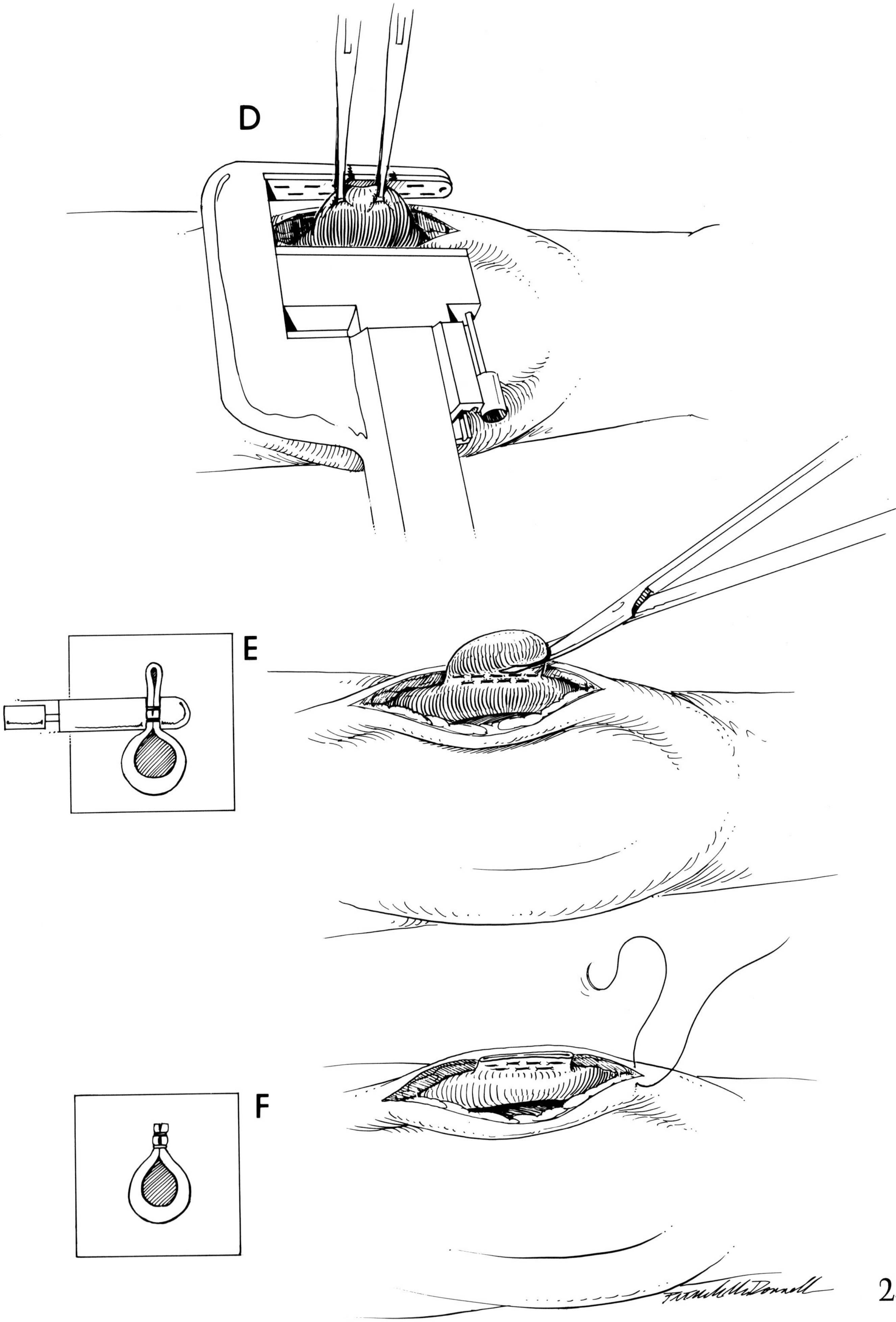
D
E
F

Graft Aneurysm

Resection

A A longitudinal incision is made overlying the aneurysmal portion of the graft.

B Dissection is carried out, and the aneurysm is identified and mobilized. Segments of the normal graft proximal and distal to the aneurysm are dissected free from the surrounding tissue to allow clamp placement and construction of the anastomoses after aneurysm resection.

C Proximal and distal vascular clamps are placed on the graft, and the aneurysm is resected. Short segments of normal graft are included in the aneurysmal resection to ensure strong tissue for construction of the anastomoses.

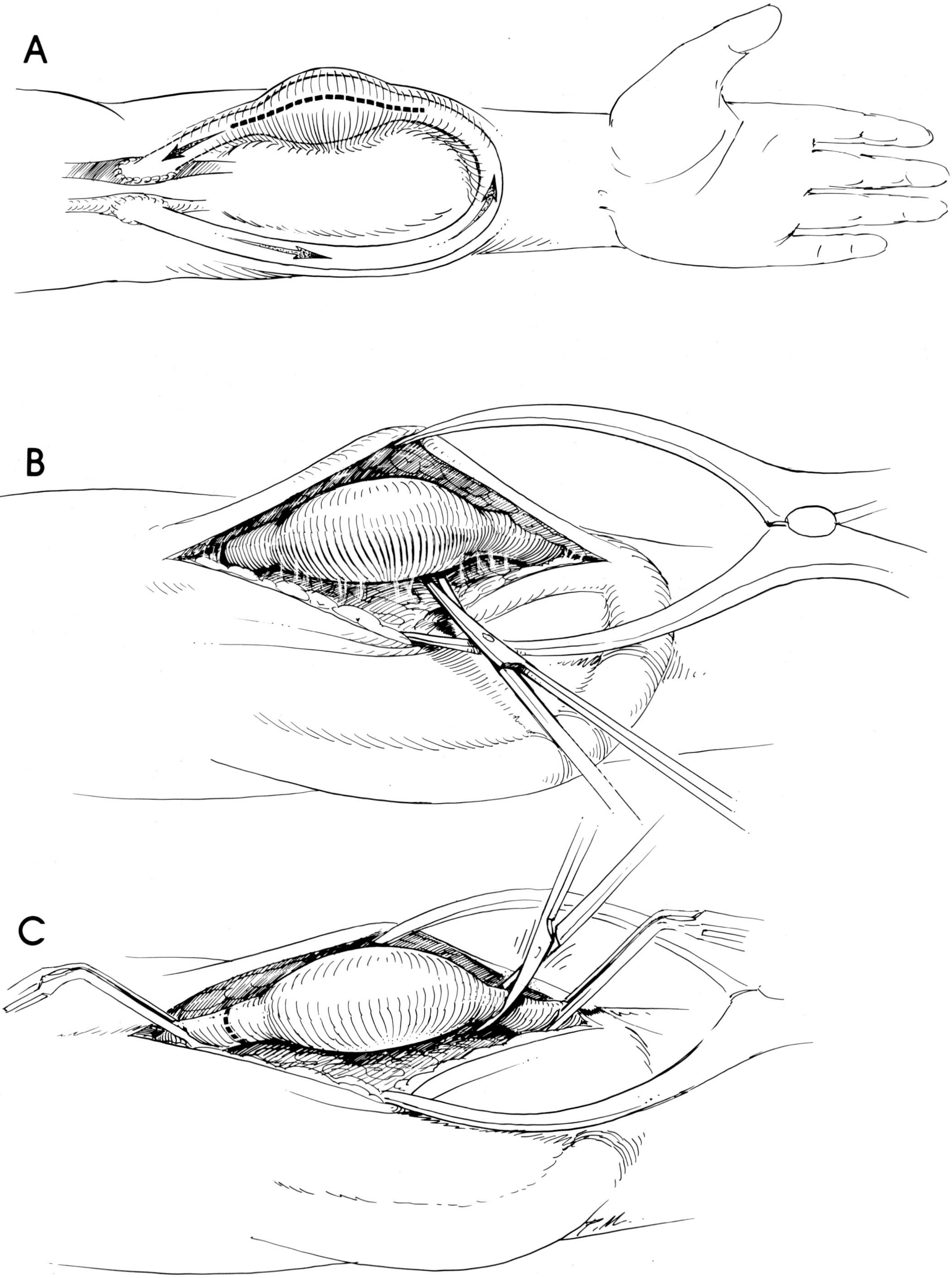
A
B
C

D Both portions of the fistula are filled with heparinized saline, and the clamps are replaced.

E The proximal end-to-end anastomosis between the fistula and the interposition graft is constructed with running 6-0 polypropylene sutures.

F After the anastomosis is completed, the interposition graft is flushed and allowed to fill.

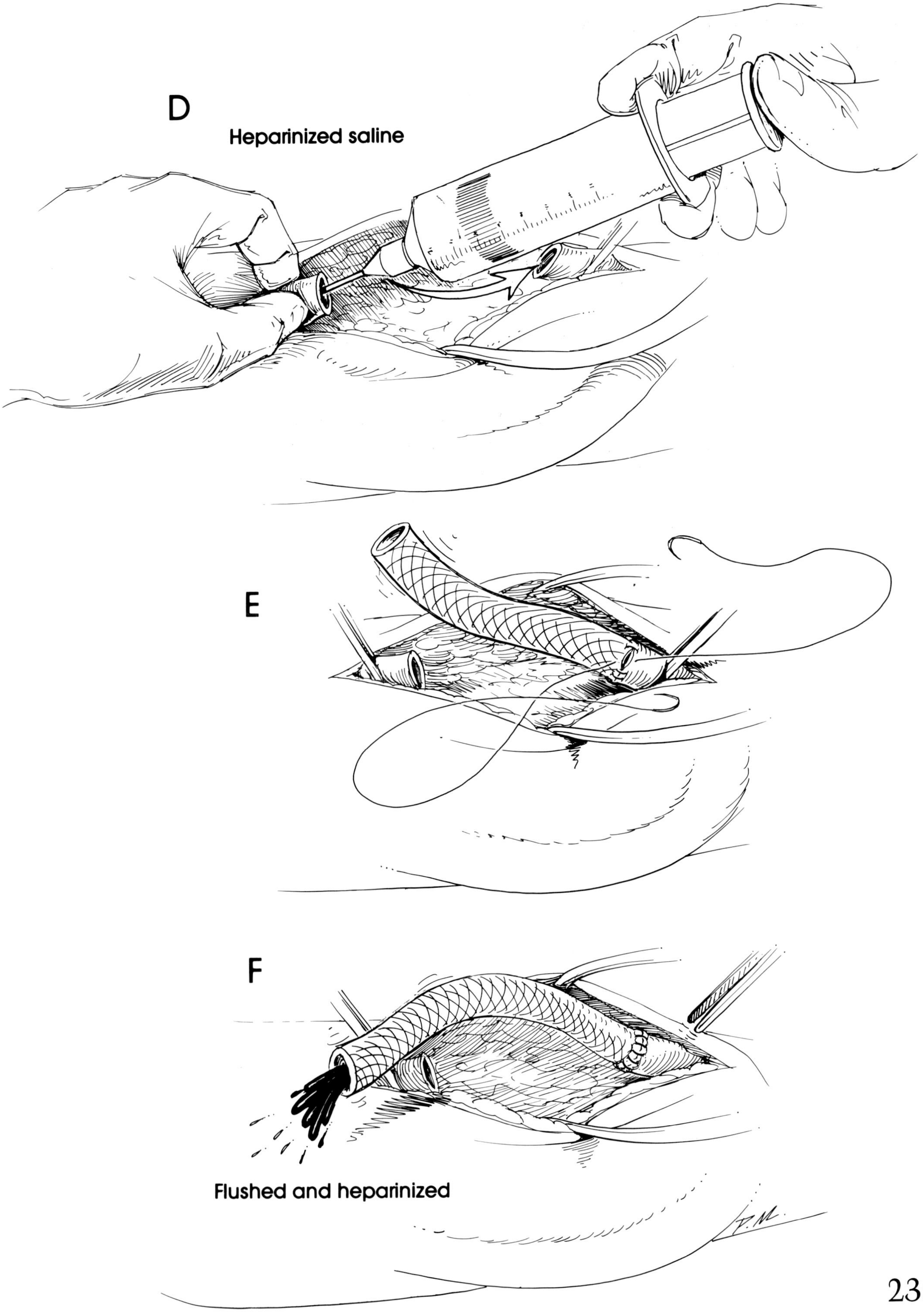
D
Heparinized saline
E
F
Flushed and heparinized

G The venous limb is clamped, and the distended interposition graft is measured and cut to the appropriate length.

H The final end-to-end anastomosis is completed, and the clamps are removed.

I A palpable pulse and thrill confirm adequate flow. Closure is performed with a single layer of subcutaneous sutures and with 3-0 nylon to reapproximate the skin.

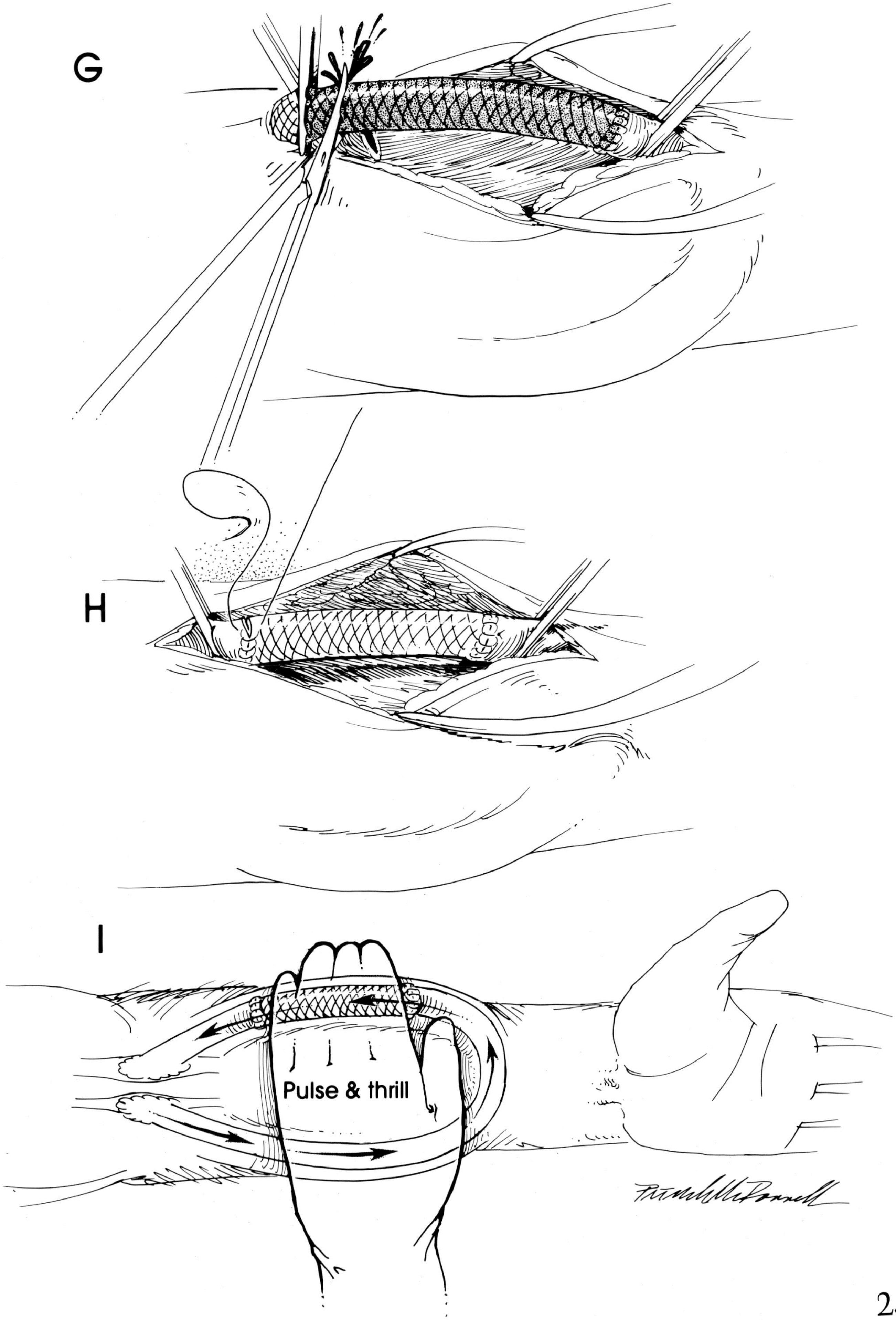
G
H
I
Pulse & thrill

Arterial Steal Syndrome

Sleeve Insertion

A Angiography demonstrates filling of the fistula at the expense of the arterial circulation distal to the graft anastomosis. Dye injected while the graft is occluded demonstrates normal filling of the palmar arch and digital branches.

B A 10-cm incision is made overlying the middle portion of the arterial limb.

C An 8-cm segment of the graft is mobilized.

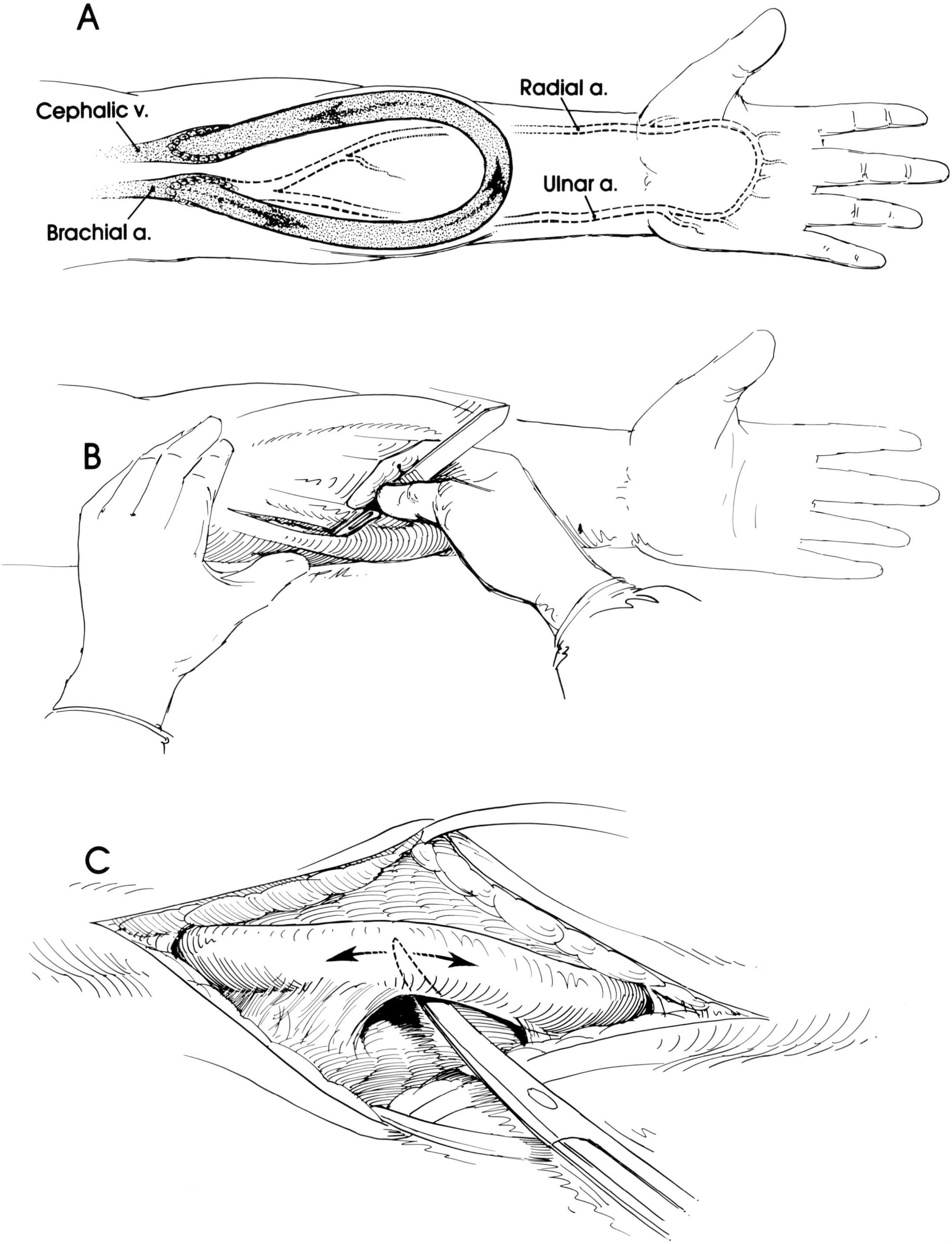
A
Cephalic v.
Brachial a.
Radial a.
Ulnar a.
B
C

D The graft is clamped proximally and distally and opened with a no. 11 blade.

E The graft incision is extended to expose a segment of the graft at least 6 cm long. Transverse extensions of the incision are made to gain access to the back wall of the open graft segment.

F An interposition graft 2 mm smaller in diameter than the fistula is used to create the graft insert. The proximal end-to-end anastomosis is constructed with running 6-0 sutures.

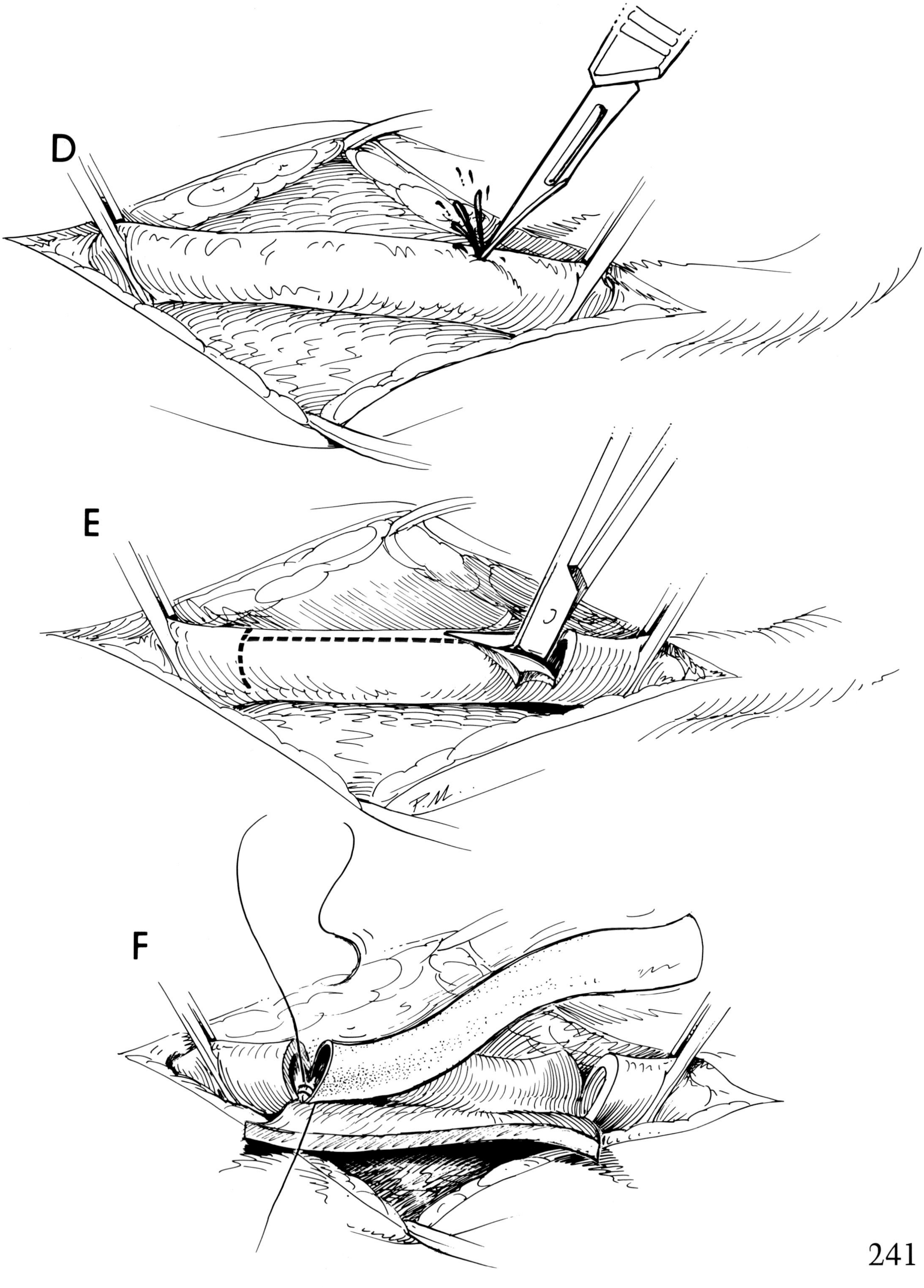
D
E
F

G The interposition graft is flushed and heparinized.

H The insert is transected in preparation for the distal anastomosis.

I A running 6-0 polypropylene suture is used to construct the anastomosis between the fistula and the smaller graft insert.

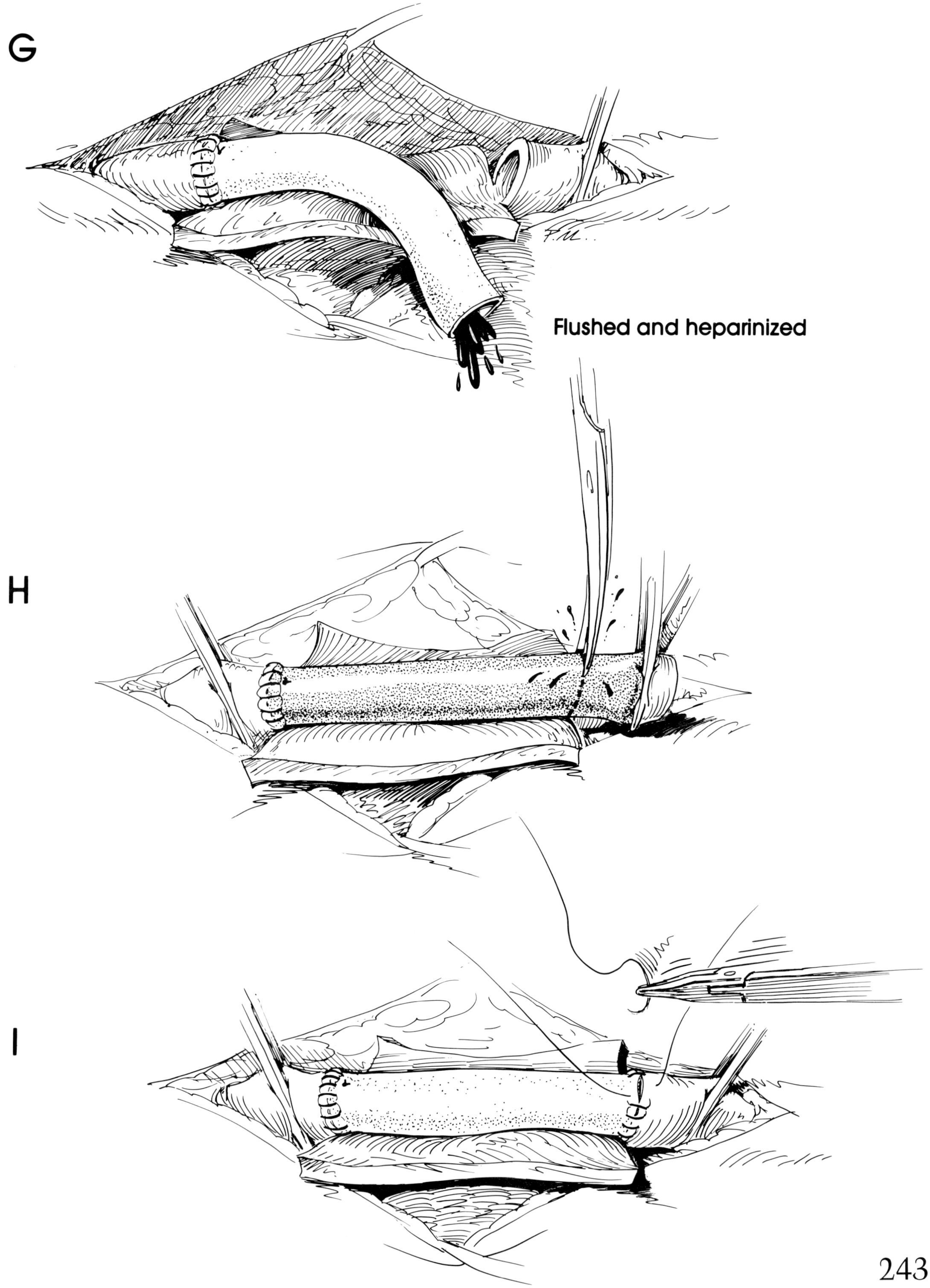
G
Flushed and heparinized
H
I

J After the anastomosis has been completed the clamps are removed, and flow through the fistula is assessed.

K The incisional flaps are reapproximated over the insert with running 6-0 vascular sutures.

L A palpable pulse and thrill confirm adequate flow through the graft. Repeated angiography should demonstrate restoration of the distal arterial circulation.

J

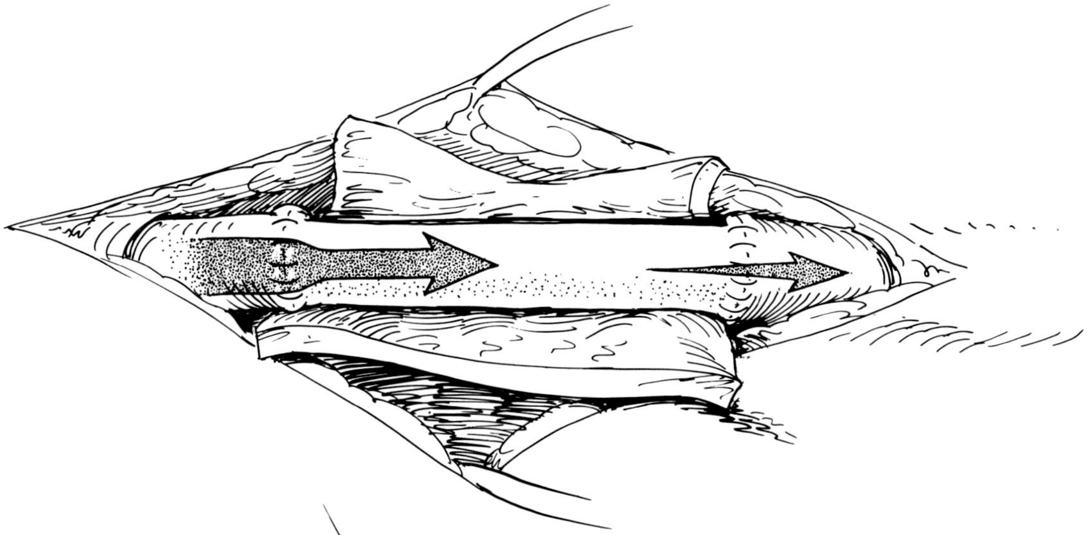

K

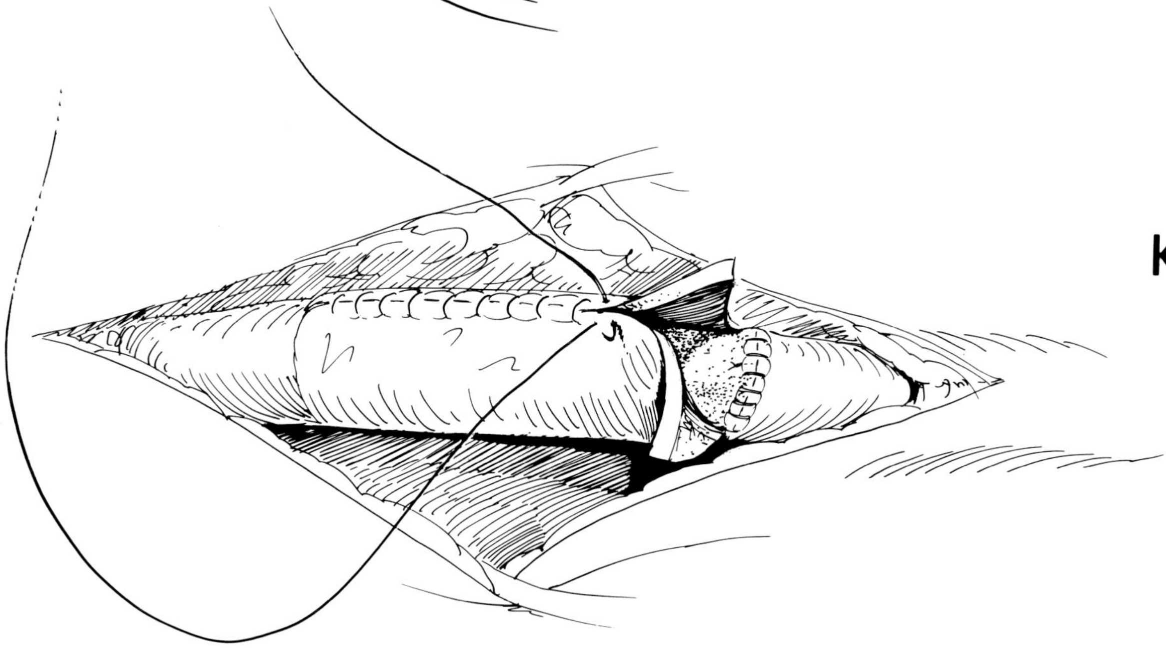

L

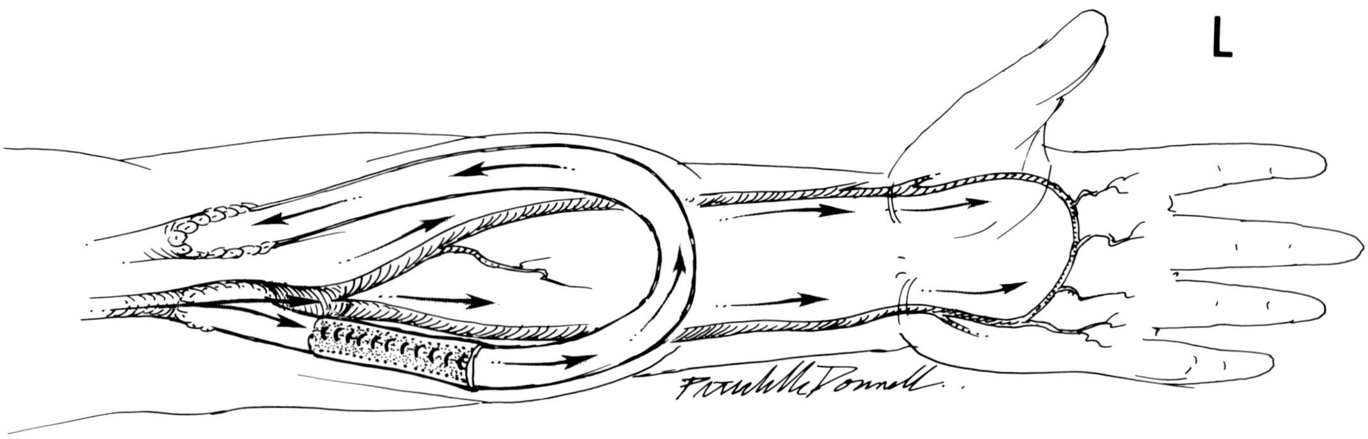

Arterial Steal Syndrome

Graft Closure

A A 4-cm transverse incision is made overlying the arterial limb of the graft and approximately 3 cm distal to the anastomosis.

B The graft is identified and mobilized sufficiently to allow insertion of the stapler.

C A TA-30 stapler with 3.5-mm staples is inserted through the incision and positioned around the graft.

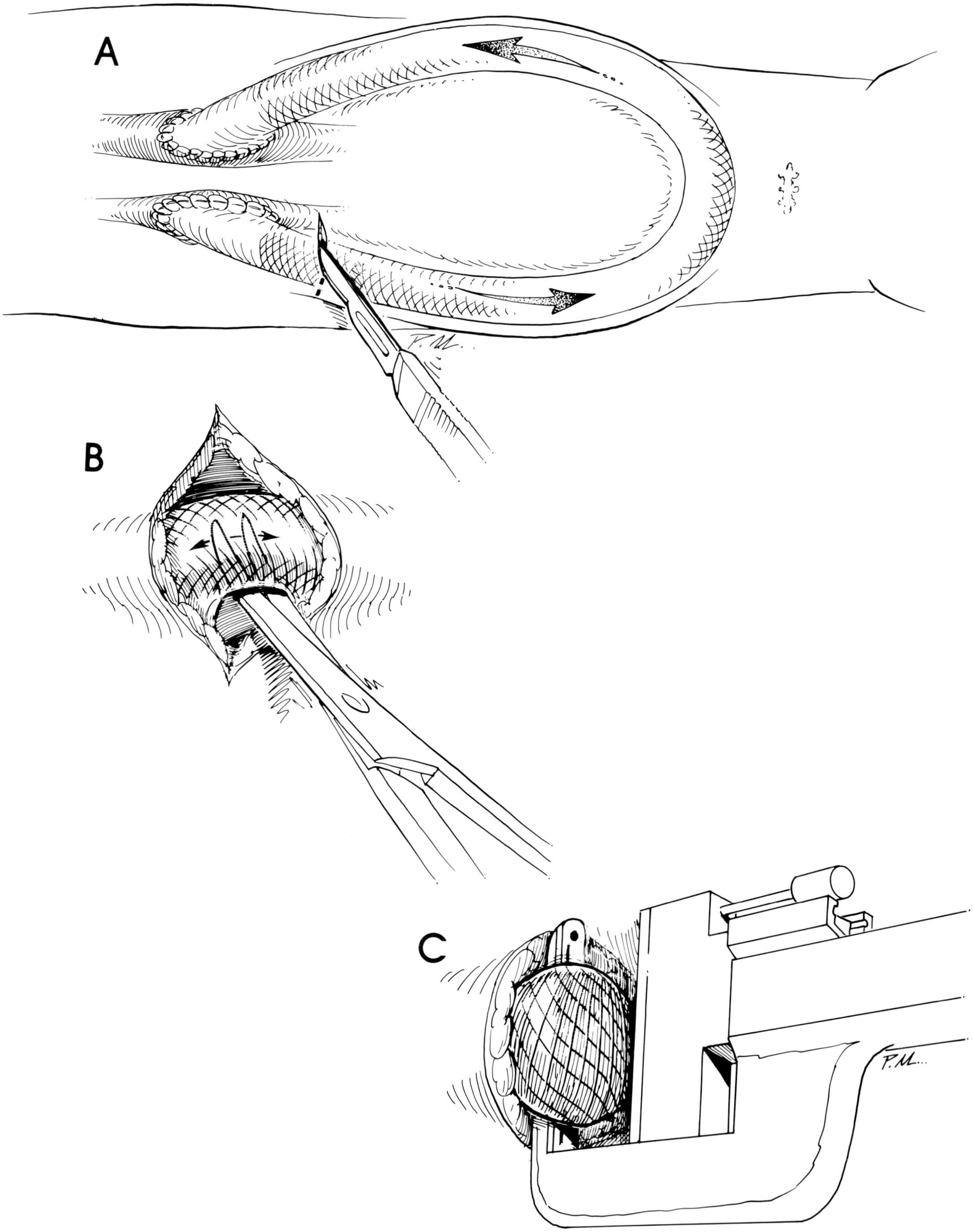
A
B
C

D–E The stapler is closed and fired. The double row of stainless steel staples is inspected.

F The graft is then decompressed in the patient's arm.

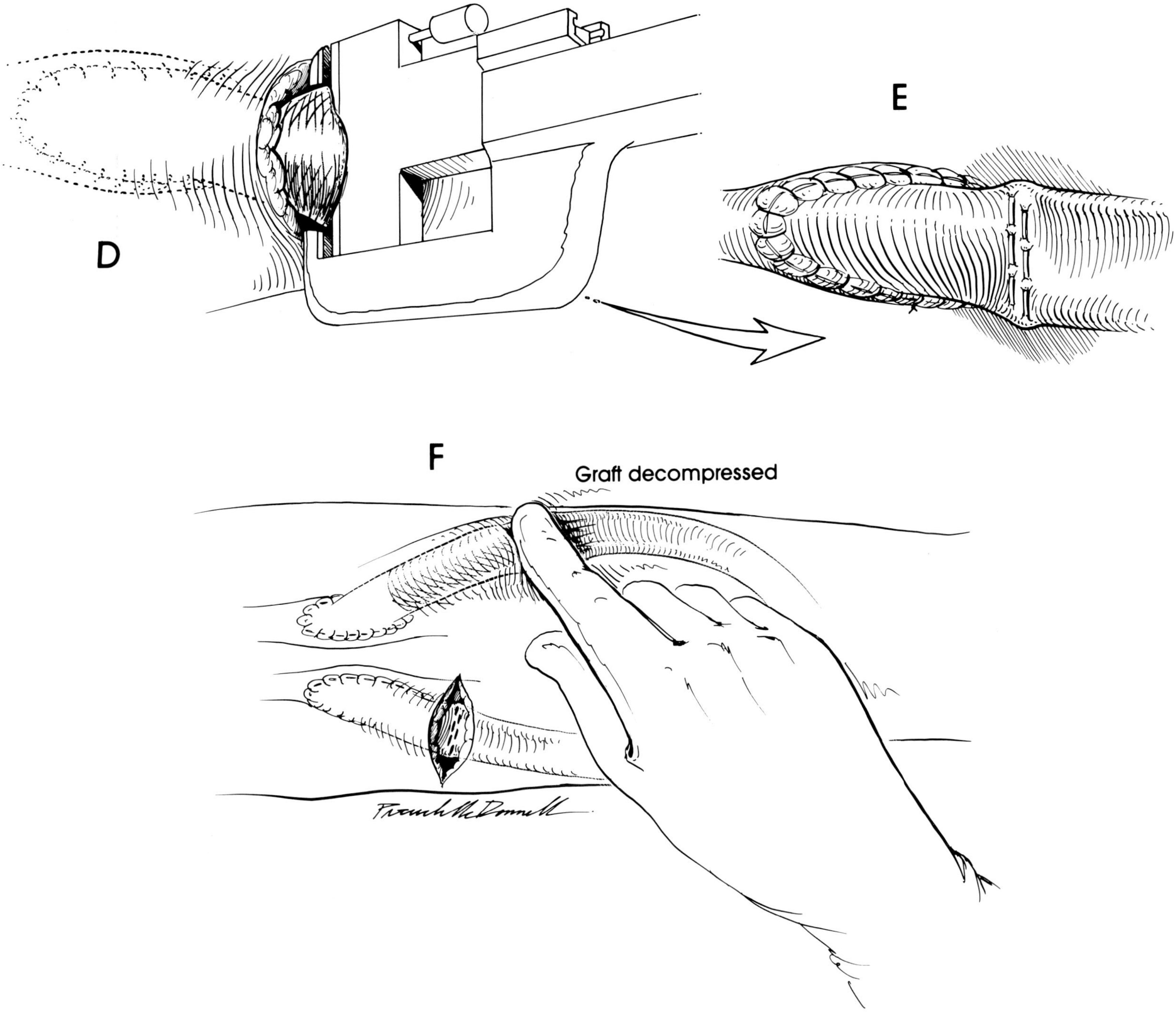
D
E
F
Graft decompressed

Infection

Graft Removal

A The skin is incised along the entire course of the graft fistula.

B Dissection is performed, and the graft is mobilized.

C The arterial limb is closed 2 cm from the anastomosis by means of a single application of the TA-30 stapler with 3.5-mm staples.

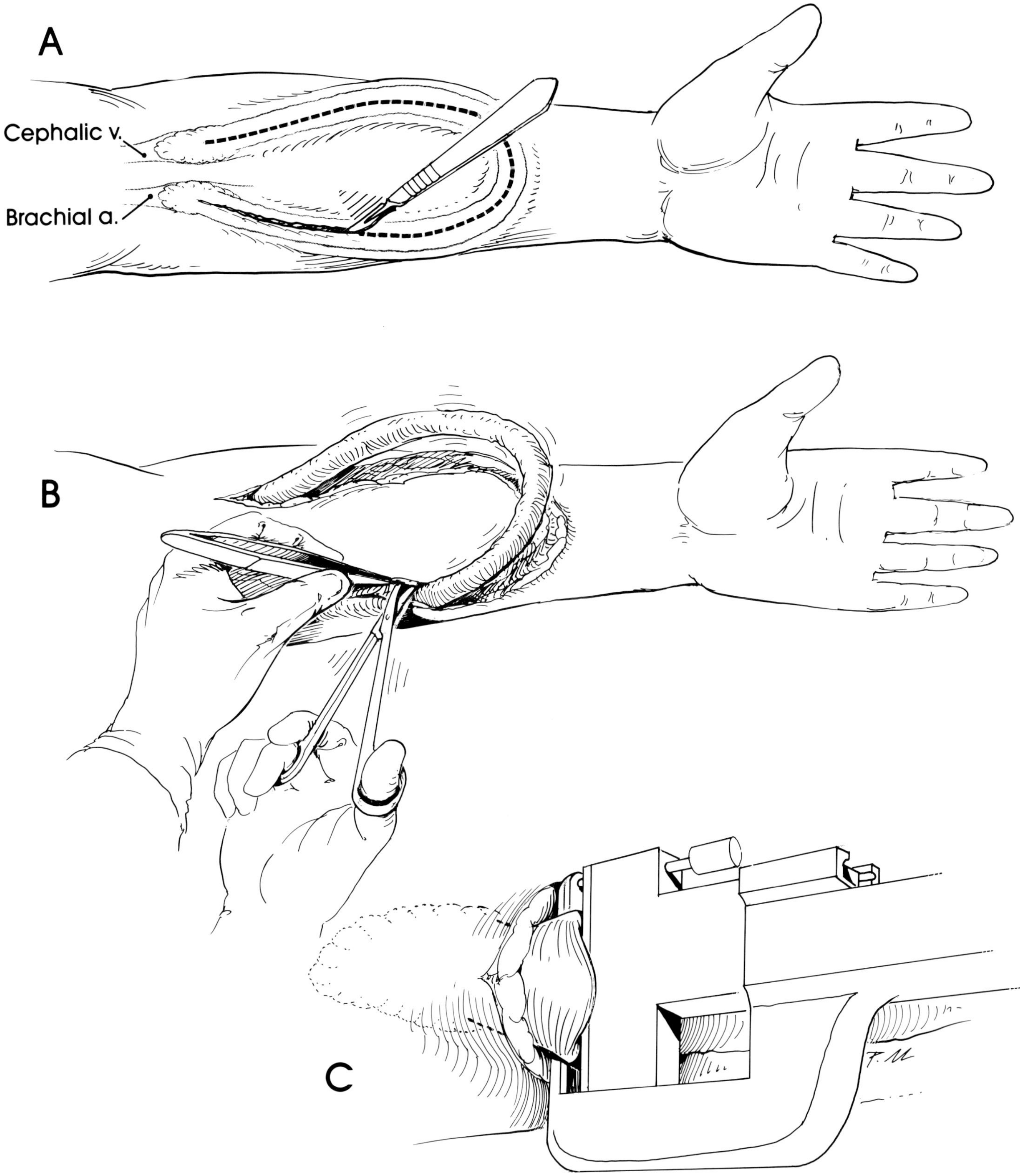
A
Cephalic v.
Brachial a.
B
C

D The graft is decompressed.

E The venous limb is closed in the same fashion as the arterial limb (pp. 246–249).

D

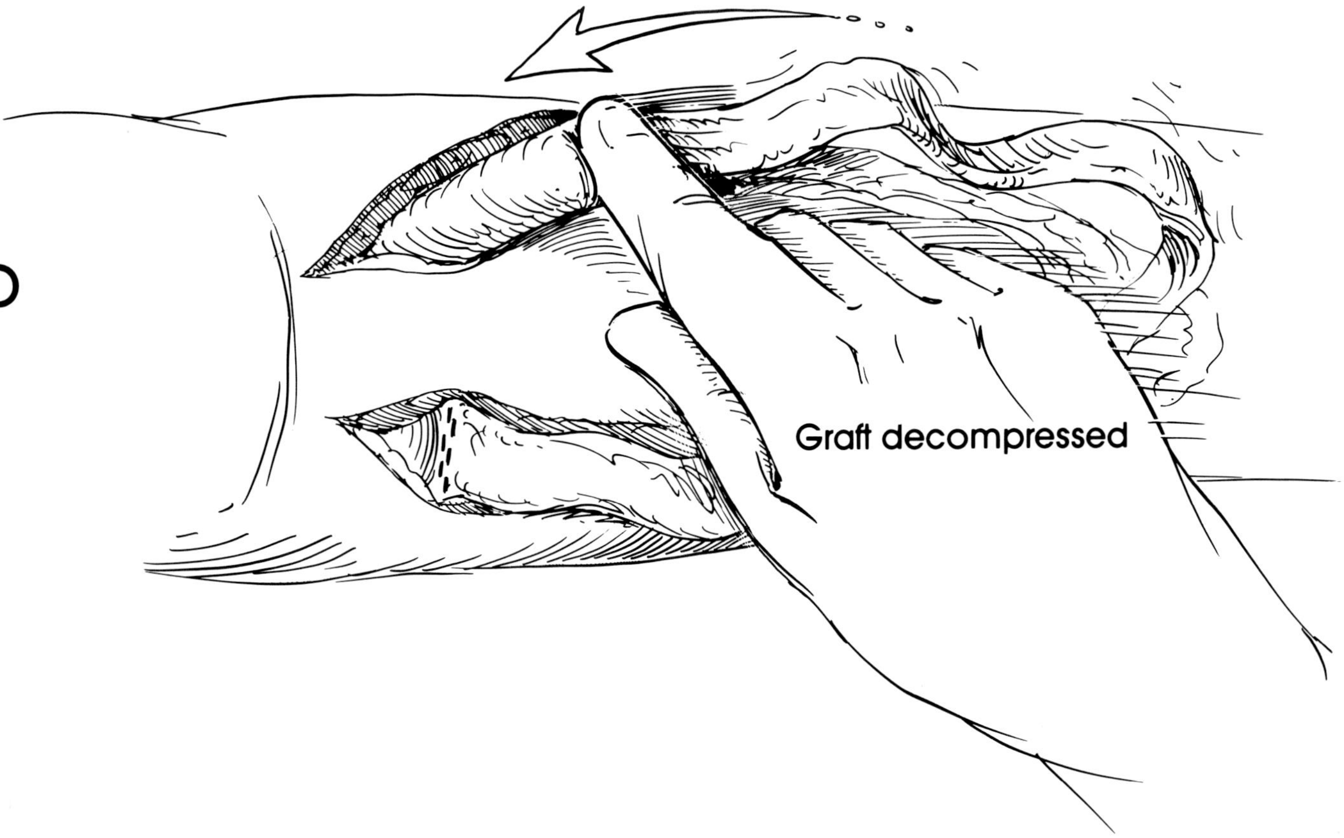

E

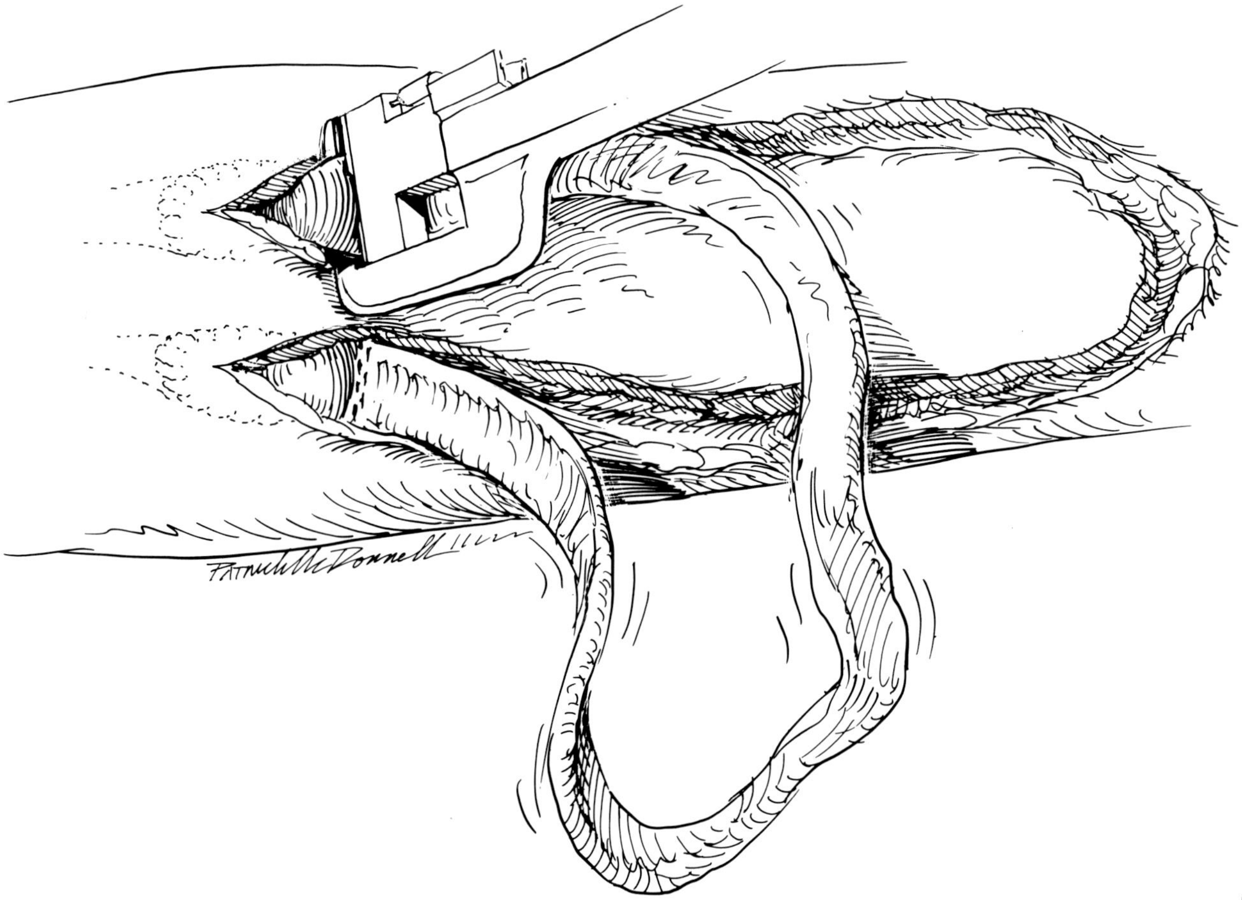

F The graft is transected distal to both staple lines.

G After copious irrigation with bactericidal solution, the skin is closed with running 3-0 nylon sutures.

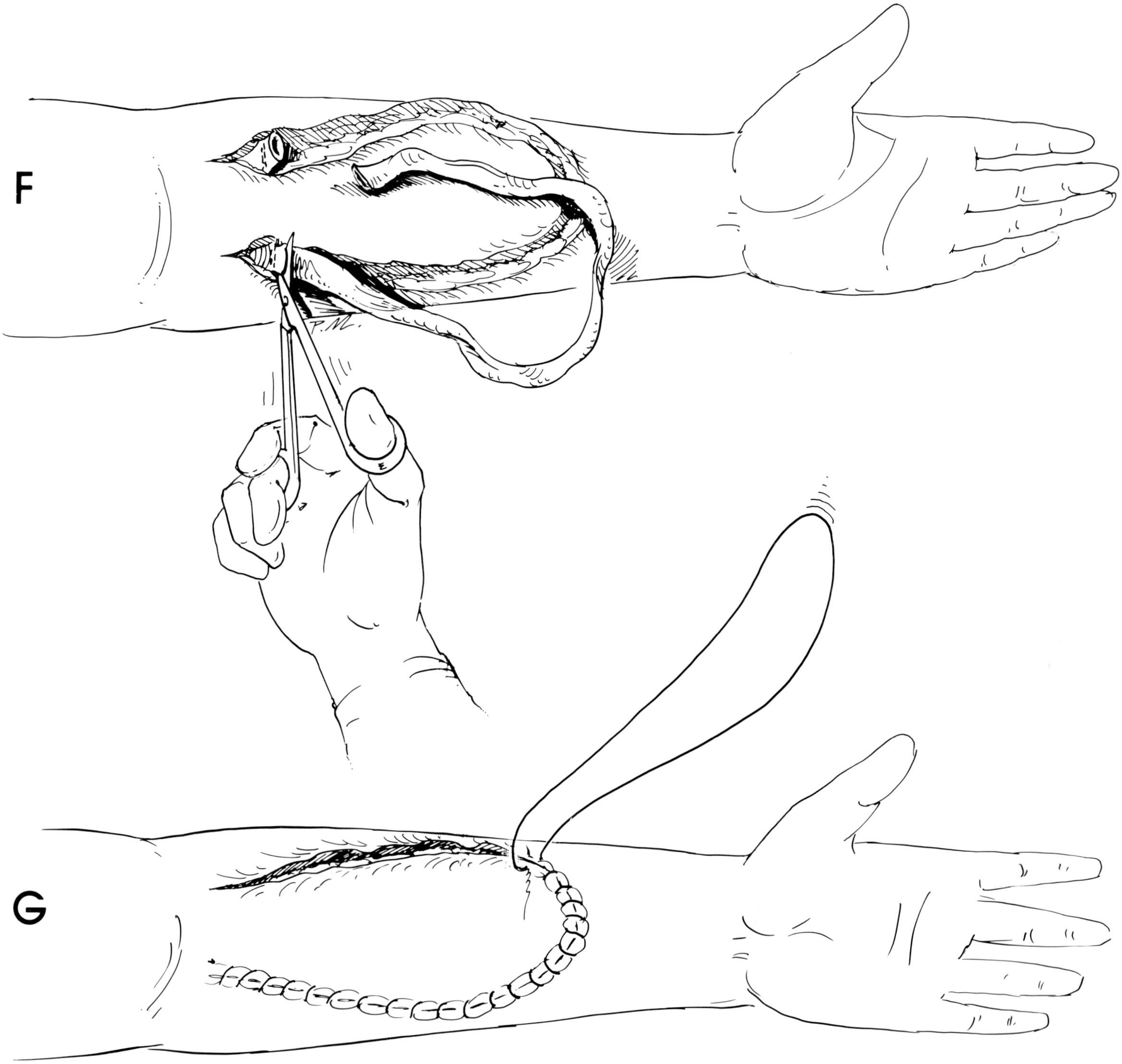
F
G

References

Arteriovenous Shunts

Ahearn D.J., Maher J.F.: Heart failure as a complication of hemodialysis arteriovenous fistula. *Ann. Intern. Med.* 77:201, 1972.

Allen L.E., Applegate G.: Arteriovenous shunts in the thigh for hemodialysis. *J. Urol.* 104:803, 1970.

Alwall N.: On the artificial kidney: Apparatus for dialysis of the blood in vivo. *Acta Med. Scand.* 128:317, 1947.

Foran R.F., Golding A.L., Treiman R.L., et al.: Quinton-Scribner cannulas for hemodialysis: Review of four years' experience. *Calif. Med.* 112:8, 1970.

Kisken W.A., Jones R.J., Bernhardt L.C.: Arteriovenous shunts for hemodialysis. *Arch. Surg.* 97:634, 1968.

Quinton W., Dillard D., Scribner B.H.: Cannulation of blood vessels for prolonged hemodialysis. *Trans. Am. Soc. Artif. Intern. Organs* 6:104, 1960.

Ramirez O., Swartz C., Onesti G., et al.: The winged in-line shunt. *Trans. Am. Soc. Artif. Intern. Organs* 12:220, 1966.

Thomas G.I.: Large vessel applique arteriovenous shunt for hemodialysis: A new concept. *Am. J. Surg.* 120:244, 1970.

Percutaneous Angioaccess Catheters

Acchiardo S.R., Cuestas C.A., White T.J. Jr.: Experience with percutaneous femoral vein catheterization. *Dial. Transplant.* 2:28, 1973.

Arana V.A., Hodson J.M., Menno A.D., et al.: Percutaneous femoral vein catheterization in patients receiving hemodialysis. *J. Urol.* 106:492, 1971.

Bernard R.W., Stahl W.M.: Subclavian vein catheterizations: A prospective study. Non-infectious complications. *Ann. Surg.* 173:184, 1971.

Bernard R.W., Stahl W.M., Chase R.M. Jr.: Subclavian vein catheterization: A prospective study. Infectious complications. *Ann. Surg.* 173:191, 1971.

Borja A.R.: Current status of infraclavicular subclavian vein catheterization. *Ann. Thorac. Surg.* 13:615, 1972.

DeCubber A., DeWolt C., Lameire N., et al.: Single needle hemodialysis with a double headpump via the subclavian vein. *Dial. Transplant.* 7:1261, 1978.

Herbst C.A.: Indications, management and complications of percutaneous subclavian catheters. *Arch. Surg.* 113:1421, 1978.

Nidus B., Matalon R., Katz C.: Hemodialysis using femoral vessel cannulation. *Nephron* 13:416, 1974.

Peters J.L., Armstrong R.: Air embolism occurring as a complication of central vein catheterization. *Ann. Surg.* 187:375, 1977.

Shaldon S., Chiandussi L., Higgs B.: Hemodialysis by percutaneous catheterization of the femoral artery and vein with regional heparinization. *Lancet* 2:857, 1961.

Shaldon S., Silva H., Pomeroy J., et al.: Percutaneous femoral venous catheterization and reusable dialysis in the treatment of acute renal failure. *Trans. Am. Soc. Artif. Intern. Organs* 10:133, 1964.

Smith B.E., Modell J.H., Gaub M.L., et al.: Complications of subclavian vein catheterization. *Arch. Surg.* 90:228, 1965.

Primary Arteriovenous Fistulas

Beven E.G., Hertzer N.R.: Construction of arteriovenous fistulas for hemodialysis. *Surg. Clin. North Am.* 55:1125, 1975.

Brescia M.J., Cimino J.E., Appel K., et al.: Chronic hemodialysis using venipuncture and a surgically created arteriovenous fistula. *N. Engl. J. Med.* 275:1089, 1966.

Byrne L., Stevens L., Weaver D., et al.: Advantages for arteriovenous fistulas in hemodialysis. *Arch. Surg.* 102:359, 1971.

Ferbino V., Tice D., Katz L.: A six-year clinical experience with arteriovenous bypasses and fistulas for hemodialysis. *Surgery* 76:1018, 1974.

Kurnival K., Beven E.G.: Arteriovenous shunts and fistulas for hemodialysis. *Surg. Clin. North Am.* 51:1227, 1971.

Complications of Primary Arteriovenous Fistulas

Bussell J.A., Abbott J.A., Lim R.C.: A radial steal syndrome with arteriovenous fistula for hemodialysis. *Ann. Intern. Med.* 75:387, 1971.

Delphin E.A.S.: Swelling of the hand after arteriovenous fistulas for hemodialysis. *Am. J. Surg.* 132:373, 1976.

Rubio P.A., Farrell E.M.: Arterialization syndrome of the hand caused by reversal of flow of malfunctioning arteriovenous fistulae. *Vasc. Surg.* 13:157, 1979.

Storey B.G., George C.R.P., Stewart J.H., et al.: Embolic and ischemic complications after anastomosis of radial artery to cephalic vein. *Surgery* 66:325, 1969.

Graft Arteriovenous Fistulas

Baker L.D., Johnson J.M., Goldfarb D.: Expanded polytetrafluoroethylene (PTFE) subcutaneous arteriovenous conduit: An improved vascular access for chronic hemodialysis. *Trans. Am. Soc. Artif. Intern. Organs* 22:382, 1976.

Burdick J.F., Scott W., Cosimi A.B.: Experience with Dacron graft arteriovenous fistulas for dialysis access. *Ann. Surg.* 187:262, 1978.

Chinitz J., Yokoyama T., Bower R., et al.: Self-sealing prosthesis for arteriovenous fistula in man. *Trans. Am. Soc. Artif. Intern. Organs* 18:452, 1972.

Dardik H., Ibrahim I.M., Dardik I.: Arteriovenous fistulas constructed with modified human umbilical cord vein graft. *Arch. Surg.* 111:60, 1976.

Dunn I., Frumkin E., Forte R., et al.: Dacron velour vascular prosthesis for hemodialysis. *Proc. Dial. Transplant. Forum* 2:85, 1972.

Garcia-Rinaldi R., Von Koch L.: The axillary artery to axillary vein bovine graft for circulatory access: Surgical considerations. *Am. J. Surg.* 135:265, 1978.

Girardet R.E., Hackett R.E., Goodwin N.J., et al.: Thirteen months' experience with the saphenous vein graft arteriovenous fistula for maintenance hemodialysis. *Trans. Am. Soc. Artif. Intern. Organs* 16:285, 1970.

Hertzer N.R., Beven E.: Venous access using the bovine carotid xenograft. *Arch. Surg.* 113:696, 1978.

Johnson J.M., Baker L.D., Williams T.: Expanded polytetrafluoroethylene: A subcutaneous vascular conduit for hemodialysis. *Dial. Transplant.* 5:52, 1976.

Kaplan M.S., Mirahmadi K.S., Winer R.L.: Comparison of PTFE and bovine grafts for blood access in dialysis patients. *Trans. Am. Soc. Artif. Intern. Organs.* 22:388, 1976.

Rubio P.A., Farrell E.M.: Human umbilical vein graft angioaccess in chronic hemodialysis: A preliminary report. *Dial. Transplant.* 8:211, 1979.

Rubio P.A., Farrell E.M.: Maintenance hemodialysis with modified human umbilical vein graft angioaccess. *Vasc. Surg.* 14:186, 1980.

Rubio P.A., Farrell E.M.: Modified human umbilical vein arteriovenous fistula for maintenance hemodialysis. *Arch. Surg.* 117:943, 1982.

Tellis V.A., Kohlberg W.I., Bhat D.J., et al.: Expanded polytetrafluoroethylene graft fistula for chronic hemodialysis. *Ann. Surg.* 189:101, 1970.

Complications of Graft Arteriovenous Fistulas

Arrants J.E., Locklair P.R. Jr.: Staple closure of an atriotomy incision. *Ann. Thorac. Surg.* 18:638, 1974.

References

Dart C.H. Jr., Scott S.M., Takaro T.: Six year experience using automatic stapling devices for lung resections. *Ann. Thorac. Surg.* 9:535, 1970.

Fogarty T.J., Cranley J.J., Krause R.J., et al.: A method for extraction of arterial emboli and thrombi. *Surg. Gynecol. Obstet.* 116:241, 1963.

Haimov M., Baez A., Neff M., et al.: Complications of arteriovenous fistulas for hemodialysis. *Arch. Surg.* 110:708, 1975.

Merickel J.H., Anderson R.C., Knutson R., et al.: Bovine carotid artery shunts in vascular access surgery. *Arch. Surg.* 109:245, 1974.

Owens M.L., Shinaberger J., Wilson S.E., et al.: Aneurysmal enlargement of e-PTFE AV fistulas. *Dial. Transplant.* 7:692, 1978.

Rubio P.A., Farrell E.M.: A technique for salvage of forearm looped bovine xenografts utilizing extension to the axillary vein. *Dial. Transplant.* 8:651, 1979.

Rubio P.A., Farrell E.M.: A technique for salvage of forearm graft arteriovenous fistulae utilizing a new reversal of flow method. *Vasc. Surg.* 13:336.